Communications
in Computer and Information Science 450

Kaija Saranto   Maaret Castrén
Tiina Kuusela   Sami Hyrynsalmi
Stina Ojala (Eds.)

Safe and Secure Cities

5th International Conference on Well-Being
in the Information Society, WIS 2014
Turku, Finland, August 18-20, 2014
Proceedings

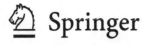 Springer

Volume Editors

Kaija Saranto
University of Eastern Finland
Kuopio, Finland
E-mail: kaija.saranto@uef.fi

Maaret Castrén
Karolinska Institutet
Stockholm, Sweden
E-mail: maaret.castren@ki.se

Tiina Kuusela
University of Turku, Finland
E-mail: takuus@utu.fi

Sami Hyrynsalmi
University of Turku, Finland
E-mail: sthyry@utu.fi

Stina Ojala
University of Turku, Finland
E-mail: stina.ojala@utu.fi

ISSN 1865-0929   e-ISSN 1865-0937
ISBN 978-3-319-10210-8   e-ISBN 978-3-319-10211-5
DOI 10.1007/978-3-319-10211-5
Springer Cham Heidelberg New York Dordrecht London

Library of Congress Control Number: 2014945643

Typesetting: Camera-ready by author, data conversion by Scientific Publishing Services, Chennai, India

Printed on acid-free paper

Springer is part of Springer Science+Business Media (www.springer.com)

Preface

The 5th International Conference on Well-Being in the Information Society (WIS) 2014, organized by the University of Turku, Turku School of Economics, and Baltic Region Healthy Cities Association, gathered researchers and developers under the topic of "Safe and Secure Cities" to Turku in August 2014. The core topic of WIS 2014 was livability and quality of (urban) living with safety and security strongly in the foreground. Among other issues, secure and equal use of information resources, safe and secure work environments and education institutions, cyberaggression and cybersecurity, as well as the impact of culture on urban safety and security were discussed.

The number of submitted papers and posters was 64, consisting of academic contributions on the topics of intersection of health, ICT, and urban ways of living, all manifested in the information society context of the conference program.

The review process was carried out by 49 international reviewers with each paper having at least two reviewers. We are grateful for their commitment to the process.

This book presents 24 papers in alphabetical order based on the first author's surname. The papers describe well-being and security in society from various perspectives giving the readers an excellent possibility to focus on areas not necessary known before. This is the great advantage of a multidisciplinary conference. One can really create innovative ideas for development in the future.

On behalf of the Organizing and the scientific Program Committees we hope you benefit from the knowledge gathered in this book.

June 2014

Kaija Saranto
Maaret Castrén

Organization

WIS 2014 Organizing Committee

Suomi, Reima
    Conference Chair   University of Turku
Li, Hongxiu
    Organizing Committee Chair University of Turku
Castrén, Maaret
    Program Co-chair   Karolinska Institutet
Saranto, Kaija
    Program Co-chair   University of Eastern Finland
Haanmäki, Birgit   University of Turku
Hyrynsalmi, Sami   University of Turku
Ilola, Agnieszka   Baltic Region Healthy Cities Association
Kuusela, Tiina   University of Turku
Kärkkäinen, Jukka   The National Institute for Health and Welfare
Machiewicz, Karolina   Baltic Region Healthy Cities Association
Ojala, Stina   University of Turku
Polvivaara, Kimmo   Turku University of Applied Sciences
Putkinen, Marjut   Turku University of Applied Sciences
Rautava, Päivi   Health Care District of South-West Finland
Reiman, Johanna   Baltic Region Healthy Cities Association
Sachdeva, Neeraj   University of Turku
Salanterä, Sanna   University of Turku
Suominen, Sakari   University of Turku
Widen, Gunilla   Åbo Akademi University

WIS 2014 Program Committee

Amdam, Roar   University of Volda, Norway
Bade, Dirk   Universität Hamburg, Germany
Bergum, Svein   Eastern Norway Research Institute, Norway
Borlund, Pia   Copenhagen University, Denmark
Cabral, Regis   FEBRO, Sweden
Carmichael, Laurence   University of the West of England, England
Cellary, Wojceich   University of Poznan, Poland
Dahlberg, Tomi   University of Turku, Finland
Deursen, Nicole   Edinburgh Napier University, UK
Hansen, Preben   Stockholm University, Sweden
Harnesk, Dan   University of Luleå, Sweden
Herbst, Andrea   University of Liechtenstein, Liechtenstein

Hori, Mayumi   Hakyoh University, Japan
Islam, A.K.M. Najmul   University of Turku, Finland
Jackson, Paul   Oxford Brookes University, UK
Järveläinen, Jonna   University of Turku, Finland
Kapocius, Kestutis   Kaunas University of Technology, Lithuania
Klein, Stefan   Universität Münster, Germany
Kokol, Peter   University of Maribor, Slovenia
Kurland, Lisa   Karolinska Institutet, Sweden
Lamersdorf, Winfried   Universität Hamburg, Germany
Lawrence, Roderick   University of Geneva, Switzerland
Li, Hongxiu   University of Turku, Finland
Liu, Yong   University of Oulu, Finland
Mandl, Thomas   Hildesheim University, Germany
Mettler, Tobias   University of St. Gallen, Switzerland
Moen, Anne   University of Oslo, Norway
Moring, Camilla   Copenhagen University, Denmark
Müller, Oliver   University of Liechtenstein, Liechtenstein
Norri-Sederholm, Teija   University of Eastern Finland, Finland
Paget, Dineke   EUPHA - European Public Health Association,
                                      Netherlands
Palsdottir, Agusta   University of Iceland, Iceland
Papacharalambous, Lefkada   TEI of Halkida, Greece
Päivärinta, Tero   University of Luleå, Sweden
Rapp, Birger   Blekinge Institute of Technology, Sweden
Rasmussen, Niels Kristian   Østfold County Council, Norway
Butleris, Rimantas   Kaunas University of Technology, Lithuania
Ryjov, Alexander   The Russian Presidential Academy of National
                                      Economy and Public Administration, Russia
Saranto, Kaija   University of Eastern Finland, Finland
Schellhammer, Stefan   Universität Münster, Germany
Sheerin, Fintan   University of Dublin, Ireland
Singh, Rajesh   Emporia State University, USA
Webster, Premila   University of Oxford, England
Wells, George   Rhodes University, Shout Africa
Wickramasinghe, Nilmini   RMIT University, Australia
Vom Brocke, Jan   Universität Liechtenstein, Liechtenstein
Womser-Hacker, Christa   Hildesheim University, Germany
Östergren, Per-Olof   University of Lund, Sweden
Österle, Hubert   Universität St. Gallen, Switzerland

Table of Contents

Finnish Health Journalists' Perceptions of Collaborating with Medical
Professionals 1
   *Ulla Ahlmén-Laiho, Sakari Suominen, Ulla Järvi, and
   Risto Tuominen*

Perceived Need to Cooperate in the Creation of Inter-organizational IT
Governance for Social Welfare and Health Care IT Services – A Case
Study 16
   Tomi Dahlberg

Aggression Management Training at Schools........................ 30
   Kirsi-Maria Haapasalo-Pesu and Tiina Ilola

FirstAED Emergency Dispatch, Global Positioning of First Responders
with Distinct Roles - A Solution to Reduce the Response Times and
Ensuring Early Defibrillation in the Rural Area Langeland 36
   *Finn Lund Henriksen, Per Schorling, Bruno Hansen,
   Henrik Schakow, and Mogens Lytken Larsen*

Tweeting about Diabetes and Diets – Content and Conversational
Connections 46
   Kim Holmberg, Kristina Eriksson-Backa, and Stefan Ek

Documentation of the Clinical Phase of the Cardiac Rehabilitation
Process in a Finnish University Hospital District 57
   *Lotta Kauhanen, Laura-Maria Murtola, Juho Heimonen,
   Tuija Leskinen, Kari Kalliokoski, Elina Raivo, Tapio Salakoski, and
   Sanna Salanterä*

Special Features of Counselling Work Carried Out through
Interactive TV... 68
   Sirppa Kinos, Sari Asteljoki, and Pia Suvivuo

Evaluation of Intravenous Medication Errors with Infusion Pumps 78
   Eija Kivekäs, Kaisa Haatainen, Hannu Kokki, and Kaija Saranto

Experiences on Telemedicine Solutions for Diabetes Care – Case eMedic
Project 88
   Elina Kontio, Ursula Hyrkkänen, and Teppo Saarenpää

Problem Limiting the Public Domain -Rawls's Veil of Ignorance
and Time 94
  Jani S.S. Koskinen, Kai K. Kimppa, and Ville M.A. Kainu

Utilising Social Media for Intervening and Predicting Future Health in
Societies 100
  Camilla Laaksonen, Harri Jalonen, and Jarkko Paavola

Practice-Oriented Safety Procedures in Work Environment with
Visually and Hearing Impaired Colleagues.......................... 109
  Riitta Lahtinen, Russ Palmer, and Stina Ojala

Revitalizing the Quantitative Understanding of the Digital Divide:
An Uptake on the Digital Divide Indicators 120
  Farooq Mubarak

Information Management Efforts in Improving Patient Safety in
Critical Care - A Review of the Literature 131
  Laura-Maria Murtola, Heljä Lundgrén-Laine, and Sanna Salanterä

Information Categories Used to Create Situational Awareness in
Emergency Medical Dispatch: A Scenario-Based Study................ 144
  Teija Norri-Sederholm, Juhani Seppälä, Jouni Kurola,
  Kaija Saranto, and Heikki Paakkonen

Serious Games and Active Healthy Ageing: A Pre-study 159
  Reetta Raitoharju, Mika Luimula, Aung Pyae,
  Paula Pitkäkangas, and Jouni Smed

A Proxy-Based Security Solution for Web-Based Online eHealth
Services.. 168
  Sampsa Rauti, Heidi Parisod, Minna Aromaa, Sanna Salanterä,
  Sami Hyrynsalmi, Janne Lahtiranta, Jouni Smed, and
  Ville Leppänen

Case Study: Using Assistive Technology to Cope with Unexpected
Blindness 177
  Neeraj Sachdeva

Data Mining in Promoting Aviation Safety Management 186
  Olli Sjöblom

Safe Community Designation as Quality Assurance in Local Security
Planning.. 194
  Brita Somerkoski and Pirjo Lillsunde

Patients Using Open-Source Disease Control Software Developed by
Other Patients... 203
  Jose Teixeira

Local Pilots, Virtual Tools - Experiments of Health Promotive and
Inclusive Services in Different Settings in the Western Uusimaa
Region 211
   Hanna Tuohimaa, Elina Rajalahti, Anne Makkonen, Liisa Ranta,
   Ulla Lemström, and Aila Peippo

The Influence of Tourists' Safety Perception during Vacation
Destination-Decision Process: An Integration of Elaboration Likelihood
Model and Theory of Planned Behavior 219
   Ping Wang

Patient Safety and Patient Privacy When Patient Reading Their
Medical Records 230
   Rose-Mharie Åhlfeldt and Isto Huvila

Author Index 241

Finnish Health Journalists' Perceptions
of Collaborating with Medical Professionals

Ulla Ahlmén-Laiho[1], Sakari Suominen[2,3,4], Ulla Järvi[5], and Risto Tuominen[6,7]

[1] Turku University Hospital, Finland
humahl@utu.fi
[2] Nordic School of Public Health, Gothenburg, Sweden
[3] Department of Public Health, Medical Faculty, University of Turku, Finland
[4] Folkhälsan Research Center, Helsinki, Finland
[5] Finnish Medical Journal, Helsinki
[6] Department of Public Health, Medical Faculty, University of Turku, Finland
[7] Primary Health Care Unit, Turku University Hospital, Finland

Abstract. Doctors are important collaborators with journalists specializing in health issues. A survey was conducted among Finnish health journalists about their views on doctor-journalist relationships, their opinions of source reliability and what sort of prejudices doctors and journalists might have of one another. In general the respondents had positive experiences of such collaboration. Most respondents identified more strongly with medical science than alternate therapies. Respondents considered scientific publications and research centers to be the most reliable information sources and considered online discussion forums and alternative therapy providers to be unreliable. Most common experiences of collaboration were positive or varying between individual doctors, although doctors' busy schedules sometimes make collaboration challenging. According to the respondents, not all doctors recognize the need for clarification of difficult topics for laypeople instead of favoring accurate scientific language. Potential prejudices that respondents felt doctors might have towards their profession was a sensationalist approach and inaccurate reporting of facts. Our findings could benefit both doctors and journalists in terms of fruitful collaboration.

Keywords: health journalism, medical journalism, media ethics, medical profession, source reliability.

1 Introduction

Science news, and medical news in particular, are very popular topics among media consumers [1]. It has been claimed that health reporting is dependent on the scientific community for information [2]. A suggested difference between health journalism and other types of media is that health information needs to be utilizable – that its value depends on whether people can use it for personal gain or not [3]. This requires the information conveyed to be clear and accurate, which entails that the language of

K. Saranto et al. (Eds.): WIS 2014, CCIS 450, pp. 1–15, 2014.

science needs to be translated into a form anyone can understand. Compared to general assignment journalists, journalists specializing in health topics may bring a higher level of prior knowledge to the table, which might affect their source and expert relationships [4]. Health journalists share a cultural community inside the greater media environment [5] and have formed their own associations in many countries [6], Finland included [7].

Dispersing important health information through the media has been an established health promotion strategy since the 1980s [8]. After use of the Internet at home has become widespread, health information is now more easily accessible to patients than ever before. Patients might bring the information they have discovered to their doctor's appointment [9] and media coverage on health topics has been proven to affect patients' opinions and behavior [10]. Doctors have recognized the need to participate in public discussion of health topics, thus making journalists an important affiliate in their profession. It could be said that scientists and health journalists are dependent on one another – the scientific community needs a way to relay new information to the public and journalists need expert collaborators and new topic ideas [2, 11].

The role that journalists themselves, their sources and the general public give to health journalism has strong implications for practices in the field [9]. For instance, The Union of Journalists In Finland and The Finnish Medical Association have issued a joint statement on medical journalism ethics [12] which attempts to benefit both parties in terms of common goals and ethical guidelines.

Negative news concerning health care seems to get more easily published than positive news [13]. Several studies and commentary articles have looked into how doctors are portrayed in the media and results have differed from negative [14, 15, 16] to balanced [17] atmosphere towards the profession. The question has been raised whether negative mass media coverage could even contribute to doctors' being unhappy in their profession [18]. Research has mostly focused on the end product of the collaboration process – the outcome and its effect - not the relationship between journalists and doctors.

Doctors do not complain to Finland's self-regulatory media body, The Council for Mass Media in Finland, more often than other groups of media collaborators, but some profession-specific issues may affect their interaction with the media, such as medical confidentiality [19]. What is not known is what kind of views health journalists hold of doctors – a particularly interesting question is, whether journalists feel that there are differences between doctors and other health experts when it comes to media collaboration. Making these differences visible could be useful in enhancing media-doctor collaboration.

Part of the journalistic process is selecting a suitable source or sources. It is not known when journalists want to employ doctors and when they would prefer other interviewees or experts. It has been suggested that some larger medias are increasingly employing doctors in order to strengthen the relaying of the health information they serve [20]. Journalists' views on source credibility might also play a role in the selection. Health journalism encompasses both the views of the scientific community and the field of alternate therapies. Doctors are likely to represent the former. There might be potential for conflict if doctors feel that they should have a vocal monopoly in health expertise but the purpose of journalism is not to be the outlet of just one interest group [21]. The medical community has been proven to impact the reporting of medical news [11].

A single previous Scandinavian study [8] focused on specific professional problems and concerns of health journalists, their views on drug and risk perceptions as compared with laymen and science experts and their views of potential further collaboration between health professionals and medical journalists. Although this study does focus on health journalists as their own subgroup it does not focus on collaboration with doctors and does not aim to describe the journalistic process between these parties.

2   Purpose of This Study

The purpose of this study was to find out whether Finnish health journalists perceive there to be differences between doctors and other expert collaborators in terms of the journalistic process. Another goal was to determine whether health journalists view themselves as representatives of medical science, alternative medicine or to a grey zone in between and whether this affects their opinions of doctors. A third topic covered was how these journalists evaluated different sources or health information in terms of source credibility. A fourth point of interest closely linked to the aforementioned issues is what sort of function health journalists view their field to have in society.

3   Data and Methods

The Finnish Association for Health Journalists was selected as a potential group of journalists who have considerable experience of working with doctors. There are likely other journalists who share a similar amount of experience, but due to the subject matter in which health journalists focus on they might utilize medical professionals more in their work than the average "generalist" reporter. In order to formulate a set of suitable questions used in the survey, four experienced health journalists were in depth interviewed about the study topics.

The association has 284 members in total. All members were sent information about the study by e-mail. Members who had never been or were no longer employed in the field, and those who had informed the research group that they did not consider themselves health journalists, were excluded from the actual respondent group.

Using an automated, web-based survey tool (Webropol), we presented an anonymous questionnaire to those members who we identified as potential respondents. All were sent a personal link by e-mail to the electronic questionnaire. Two reminder messages were sent to those who did not fill the survey within the allotted time of two weeks. If they still did not return a completed questionnaire, an SMS message requesting either participation or stating the reason for not filling out the survey, was then sent to their mobile phones. Afterwards, those who still had not responded in any way, were contacted by phone to inquire why they did not wish to participate and whether they at all could be considered representing a potential respondent after all. Those who still were willing to participate were then given an additional chance to fill the questionnaire. If non-responding members could not be reached via e-mail of phone, an online search was made to find out whether they could be considered to be working as health journalists. Some members were further excluded from the pool of potential respondents through this information.

Out of the potential participants (249 members), 118 filled the questionnaire, resulting in a response rate of 47%. Table 1 contains the non-respondent analysis results.

Table 1. Reasons for non-participation in the survey

Reason for non-participation	N:o of persons (total = 131)	Percentage
Too busy or forgot	27	21%
Dislike of such surveys or not interested	10	8%
Technical difficulties with the survey	19	15%
Did not feel competent enough to fill the survey despite being a health journalist	7	5%
Unknown or person could not be contacted	67	51%

Final survey results were analyzed with the internal statistical tools offered by the polling service (Webropol). Numerical data was analyzed utilizing basic statistical analysis and open questions were analyzed using standard word-mining algorithms offered by the Webropol toolkit.

4   Results

4.1   Demographic Profile

Women formed a clear majority among our respondents (86%). Health journalists aged between 30 and 39 years represented 25% of our respondents. Only one respondent was younger than this. Of all respondents, 32% were between 40 and 49 years of age. 42% were aged more than this. The median age was 55 years. Altogether, 61% of respondents had been working within journalism for 10 to 30 years. Only 6% had been active in the field for less than five years. Overall, 21% had more then thirty years' experience in the field.

Magazines were the most common media represented by the respondents (64% did magazine work). The second most common media were newspapers (23%) and assorted non-mass media forms of health journalism such as books, customer magazines, publications released by non-governmental organizations (NGO) and advertorials for medical companies (19%). Television and radio were a small minority, a little less then six percent of respondents worked for television and less than two percent covered health topics for radio broadcasts.

Of the respondents, 42% worked as freelancers. A great majority of all respondents spent at least 50% of their working hours among health topics and 23% stated that all of their journalistic work was about health.

Four respondents held a university degree in natural sciences (including two academic dentists). Five respondents had either a degree in healthcare or substantial work experience in health care. One respondent had a degree in psychology. The by far most common training was an university degree of varying level in humanities, social sciences, linguistics or journalism (76% of respondents). Only 14% of respondents held either a degree from a lower level educational institution or no formal training beyond high school at all.

4.2   The Definition of Health Journalism and Its Role in Society

Respondents were asked to define the term "health journalism". Altogether, 39% defined it merely as media reporting on topics of health, illnesses and wellbeing. Of all respondents, 19% felt that health journalism is a much broader field and includes health politics, ethics and healthcare economics among those topics listed by respondents whose perspective was somewhat narrower. Common characteristics of health journalism listed by respondents are listed in Table 2.

Table 2. The most common listed defining characteristics of health journalism

Characteristic	N:o of mentions
A narrow definition of health journalism being merely reporting about health, illnesses and well-being with no broader perspective or no set function or paradigm	46
A broad social perspective beyond individuals and their health and illnesses	22
Translating scientific content to laymen, popularization of science	19
Reliability/being fact-based/neutrality	16
Utilizable by its consumers in improving their own life or health	12
A scientific/medical paradigm	8

Respondents were asked to evaluate Finnish health journalism in terms of its general tone and how critical journalists tend to be towards source material in their writing on a Likert scale ranging from 1 to 9 (1 standing for very critical/negative and nine being very uncritical/positive). The data gave an average of 5.6 for the general tone and 5.6 for critical thinking (both ranges between 2 and 9).

When enquired whether health journalism can influence readers' and viewers' health choices 95% of respondents felt that this was indeed possible. Those who disagreed felt either that they could merely strengthen already existing opinions or the effect of a media piece was short-lived. One respondent stated that readers are looking for feelings, not facts.

Respondents were asked to set themselves on a Likert scale ranging from 1 to 9 concerning whether they felt they represented medical science or the alternate sector in their work. (1 stood for solely medical science and 9 for singularly alternative medicine). The average was 2.7. Only 5.9% of respondents placed themselves at 6 or higher. Respondents were then asked to evaluate what the balance was in Finnish health journalism in general. The same scale was used. The average given was 3.8. Only 8.5% felt that the scales were tipped towards alternative medicine.

The respondents were then asked to list characteristics of a high-quality piece of health journalism. Most common properties are listed in Table 3. One respondent felt that a good piece of health journalism should always include a doctor's view. Many respondents stated that characteristics of any good journalism apply to health journalism as well. Three respondents stated that a good piece of health reporting takes into account the self-corrective nature of science and thus doesn't represent anything as entire and permanent truth.

Table 3. Most common characteristics of quality health journalism given by respondents

Characteristic	N:o of mentions
Reliable/fact-based/facts have been checked/experts have been used as collaborators	52
Easy to understand/language suitable for the selected readership/clarifies things	31
Interesting/enticing/emotionally touching	19
Has a impact on readers' lives/encourages readers to seek further information/is useful for readers	19
Neutral in tone	14
Represents scientific consensus	13
Fresh/contains new information/is topical	10

4.3   Source Reliability

Respondents were requested to evaluate different information sources on a Likert scale ranging from 1 to 9; 1 standing for extremely unreliable, and 9 standing for extremely reliable (Table 4).

The greatest reliability was enjoyed by 1) Finnish scientific publications (although 3% considered these to be very unreliable), universities and other research centers, The Finnish National Institute for Health and Welfare, the ministry of Health and Social Welfare and associations for different medical specialties. The most unreliable sources (sources that scored below 5) were: online discussion forums, representatives of alternative therapies and individual patients. Of all participants, 20% scored alternative therapy representatives with at least 6. Opinions varied concerning individual patients – 30% of respondents gave them at least a 6. In terms of unreliability, there seemed to be a strong consensus that online forums are not reliable: only 3% of respondents considered them reliable to any extent.

Table 4. Source reliability according to the respondents. 1 = very unreliable, 9 = very reliable. Numbers represent percentages.

	1 - 2	3 - 4	5	6 - 7	8 - 9	Average
Finnish scientific publications	3%	2 %	0 %	13 %	83 %	**7,92**
Foreign scientific publications	2 %	2 %	3 %	34 %	60 %	**7,45**
TV, radio	0 %	24 %	26%	41 %	8 %	**5,57**
Newspaper health reporting	0 %	20 %	21%	47 %	13 %	**5,78**
Magazines focusing on health topics	1 %	16 %	9 %	58 %	16 %	**6,11**
News agencies	1 %	14 %	21%	46 %	19 %	**6,07**
Universities and other research facilities	3 %	0 %	1 %	17 %	78 %	**7,92**
Administration of a public healthcare unit	1 %	6 %	5 %	40 %	47 %	**7,1**
Individual researchers or research groups	2 %	3 %	3 %	45 %	49 %	**7,21**
Finnish Ministry of Health and Social Services	1 %	4 %	4 %	40 %	52 %	**7,28**
The National Institute for Health and Welfare	1 %	4 %	1 %	25 %	70 %	**7,69**
Patient organizations	1 %	11 %	8 %	52 %	28 %	**6,5**
Pharmaceutical companies	7 %	18 %	27%	43 %	6 %	**5,25**
General medical associations	1 %	8 %	7 %	46 %	39 %	**6,86**
Medical specialty associations	1 %	7 %	3 %	35 %	54 %	**7,13**
Alternate therapy providers	38 %	28 %	13%	17 %	3 %	**3,58**
Individual doctors working in the private sector	4 %	15 %	14%	52 %	14 %	**5,95**
Individual doctors working in the public sector	2 %	11 %	8 %	63 %	17 %	**6,32**
Individual patients	15 %	30 %	24%	25 %	5 %	**4,6**
Online discussion forums	68 %	26 %	4 %	1 %	2 %	**2,23**

Participants were requested to list properties of both particularly reliable and particularly unreliable sources. Text mining resulted in the most common characteristic stated being: 1) experience in subject matter, 2) expertise, 3) being based on scientific research. Other common terms were independence and impartiality. 54% of respondents listed scientific research, verifiability of information and/or peer review of source material as a characteristic.

Most common properties given by respondents are listed in Table 5. Text mining gave very similar results: attempt to further individual gain, commercial or financial ties to subject matter, single-mindedness and lack of expertise were the most common results.

Table 5. Most common characteristics of unreliable sources stated by respondents

Characteristic	N:o of mentions
Personal gain / commercial interests / attempt to further the interests of a certain group	47
Single-mindedness / fanaticism / highly emotional / black and white thinking	31
Lack of expertise / opinions not based on any data, lack of scientific rationale	30
Opinions based on a single case or personal experience	18
Source representing alternative medicine	8
Seeks media attention / seeks ego-boosting	7

Some respondents stated that although single patients' personal experiences were not valid data for generalizations concerning their illness, but could still be very useful as sources if the aim was to highlight what it was like to live with such an ailment. According to the respondents, personal gain could also mean the ulterior motives of a patient association or medical association when they attempted to further the interests of their members through the media.

4.4   Collaborating with Doctors

Altogether 75% of respondents stated that they have doctor contacts they have utilized as experts or interviewees more than once. Common criteria stated for the selection of such experts are listed in Table 6.

Table 6. Most common reasons for utilizing the same doctor in journalistic several times

Reason	N:o of respondents
Expertise	33
Good prior experiences of collaboration, reliability	30
Ability to popularize and clarify difficult scientific material	9
Understanding of journalistic work, favorable attitude towards the media	8
Availability	5
Proximity (works in same organization, is a leader in local health administration etc)	5

Respondents were requested to evaluate how well doctors know the Finnish Guidelines for Journalists [23], which outline acceptable conduct in Finnish media. A score of 1 represented an opinion that doctors knew these guidelines very well and a score of 9 indicated that they were perceived to have very poor knowledge of these issues. The respondents gave an average score of 4.1 but scores varied a great deal. Of all respondents, 14% gave a score of 1 or 2 and 18% a score of at least 6.

When requested to freely describe journalistic collaboration with doctors, most common comments are listed in Table 7.

Table 7. The responding health journalists' most common descriptions of journalistic collaboration with doctors

Description	N:o of mentions
Positive experiences or working with doctors, and/or doctors having positive attitudes towards media	74
Strong variance in whether collaboration is easy and fruitful or not; depends on the individual doctor	24
Doctors can be busy and difficult to contact	23
Doctors act superior to journalists and/or try to take over the journalistic process / don't trusts journalists' skills or motives	20
Doctors are meticulous about facts being correct or carefully exercise their right to check the media product before publication	12
Doctors often express things in ways that are difficult to understand / don't see the need to translate things to laypeople	11
Doctors are cautious about what they say / are nervous about expressing their opinions, especially if they feel it might reflect on their own image among their colleagues	8

Text mining gave the results that the most common descriptions were: 1) collaboration is good and positive, 2) doctors are busy and 3) quality of collaboration varies greatly between individual doctors. Two respondents stated that there were no differences between doctors and other kinds of collaborators. Singular interesting statements included: doctors expected the journalist to have basic knowledge on the subject in question and that some doctors aggressively requested money in exchange for collaboration.

Participants were asked whether doctors decline collaboration requests more often than other potential collaborators and interviewees. Altogether, 66% replied that doctors did not decline more often than others. 17% were unsure and 17% said yes. When enquired about potential reasons, the most common answers were: 1) doctors are too busy, 2) the doctor in questions doesn't think he's the best expert in the subject and 3) distrust towards media.

Respondents were also enquired whether they felt doctor-media collaboration had changed in some ways through the years and if yes, how they would describe these changes. In all, 46% felt that there had been changes, 33% were uncertain and 21% felt there had been no substantial change. Most common statements concerning the name of these changes were: 1) attitudes and collaboration have become more positive and open; doctors appreciate journalists more, 2) attitudes have become more precautious and negative due to sensationalist press and lowering quality of journalism and 3) doctors are increasingly busy which makes them less likely to want to collaborate.

4.5 Potential Prejudices between Journalists and Doctors

In all, 55% of the respondents perceived that doctors and journalists had prejudices towards one another. Altogether, 30% were unsure and 15% felt that no such prejudices exist. When asked to describe what kind of such views they imagined doctors might harbor towards journalists, the most common answers are as listed in Table 8.

Table 8. Most common prejudices given by respondents that doctors might have of journalists reported by the respondents

Potential prejudice	N:o of mentions
Journalists twist things or don't report things accurately	19
Journalists are after sensationalist pieces or have questionable motives	17
Journalists don't have enough training or background information to understand the medical topics they are reporting on	7

Respondents were also requested to list prejudices that their own colleagues might have of doctors. The most common answers are listed in Table 9.

Table 9. The most common prejudices that health journalists might have of doctors as reported by the respondents

Potential prejudice	N:o of mentions
Doctors don't know how to express themselves in a way that non-medical professionals can understand	11
Doctors don't appreciate journalists' skills and/or act superior or omnipotent	5
Doctors try to take over/dominate the journalistic process	5
Doctors have a personal agenda when collaborating with the media or are corrupt	4

5   Discussion

According to the results of the study, the respondents can be considered to represent individuals who have a lot of experience on health journalism and who devote the majority of their working time to health topics. Most respondents had at least 10 years of journalistic work experience which is favourable in terms of survey results. They can thus be considered health journalism experts. What should be taken into account, however, is that not all who write about health and medicine are members of the association but it feels safe to assume that journalists who strongly identify themselves working with health topics might feel compelled to belong to such an organization. We excluded those members of the Health Journalist association who were not journalists and who had not been employed in the field for some time. However, we were unable to contact a substantial number of members and there might be some among them who should have been excluded.

When studying a relationship between two parties, information needs to be gathered from both sides. Similar data needs to be collected from doctors and these results should be reflected in a comparative perspective in order to recognize differences in the views of journalists and doctors that might make collaboration either particularly troublesome or particularly fruitful between doctors and journalists. This survey is one-sided in that it only gives voice to the journalists.

The piloting method of our study (interviews with experienced health journalists) was comparable to the aforementioned previous Swedish health journalism study [8] which utilized a group discussion among a similar focus group to gain insight into the issues before formulating a questionnaire.

Even though our response rate was not as high as would have been desirable, it was somewhat comparable to the response rate in a previous Swedish study of health journalists where the rate was 55% (with 110 potential respondents who comprised of all members of the Swedish Association for Medical Journalists) [8]. An effort was made to find out why members had not participated in the survey. This was largely due to the journalists in question being very busy during the time of the survey. There did not seem to be an attitude bias dividing potential participants according to response status although we could not obtain a reason for non-responsiveness from a considerable number of respondents. In the previous Swedish study reasons for unresponsiveness remained equally unknown in most cases, but some individually approached non-respondents stated that they out of principle never answered questionnaires (one of our non-respondents gave this answers as well) or felt that they were not active enough in the field [8].

The percentage of women was much higher than is the average among Finnish journalists, which is 57.2%. In the Swedish study, women comprised 66% of respondents [8] so these figures might suggest a female majority among health journalists in Scandinavia. The respondents' age distribution was quite similar to that of Finnish journalists in general [24].

The amount of freelancers among respondents was much higher than is the average among all Finnish journalists which is 15% [22]. Magazines and newspapers were strongly presented among the medias employing the respondents, as well as newer or miscellaneous medias such as online portals. Our results echo those of the Swedish medical journalist study [8] in terms of health journalists' background – although a great majority have a university-level education most have no formal scientific training, which together with the technical nature of medical information strengthens the dependency of health journalists on science professionals. University-level training might bridge the educational gap to some degree.

In a prior study, only one third of interviewed television health journalists said that they devoted all their work time to health reporting – most were obliged to cover other topics as well [2]. This might affect the extent of their knowledge base on health topics since they had less time to devote to the field. The majority of respondents in our study spent more than half of their working time among health topics, which likely lessens this problem. If doctors, like some respondents suggested, might assume or downright demand that the journalist interviewing them is familiar with the subject matter, allowing journalists to specialize in health topics might be a good way to enhance doctor-media collaboration. In a Swedish study, many health journalists felt that a lack of medical background knowledge was their primary professional shortcoming [8]. We do not know, however, how common the observation that doctors might demand this, is a prominent characteristic of doctor-media relationships. In our study, only a few respondents stated that doctors might be prejudiced towards journalists because of their lack in scientific training.

A considerable majority of the respondents identified with a medical science paradigm. This result is similar what was obtained in the Swedish health journalists study: 61% of Swedish respondents agreed with the statement that "biomedical research is a cornerstone of society" and 74% agreed with a negative statement about alternative medicine [8]. When asked about defining characteristics of quality health stories, our respondents listed reliability and a scientific basis as the important properties. The previous Swedish study did not ask such a question, but replies to their question concerning the most important qualities of a medical journalist could be considered comparable [8]. The Swedish medical journalists listed a respect for facts, good sources and a sense of responsibility as such premier properties and many considered a lack of medical knowledge as their greatest self-perceived deficit [8]. Whether this is due to an internal ideal of medical journalism or reflective of demands made by collaborators, is not known.

When asked to rank their role attributes according to importance, Swedish medical journalists considered "giving facts about medical advances to be the most important, followed by "critical" and "stimulating" [8]. Our Finnish results are compatible: responsibility, fact-checking and a scientific paradigm were strongly present in respondents' perceptions about quality health journalism. Many respondents don't limit their view of health journalism to merely reporting about health and illness phenomena. Instead they give health journalism a wide function in discussing social issues, health politics, healthcare, individual patient experiences and advances in science. There seems to be an emphasis on reliable information that can be utilized by its audience to improve their health and their lives. This goal is very compatible to the ethos of medical professionals and can serve well in doctors' need for the media in order to convey important health information. According to our data, Finnish health journalists strongly feel that journalism can affect readers' opinions and behaviour. Our respondents characterized good quality health journalism as having an impact on readers' lives and that good health journalism thus needs to be utilizable by readers in some way. Our survey results also reveal that health journalists rely on science as the most reliable resource material.

Due to these ideals it is clear that health journalists need experts – one study indicated that reporters need to consult medical experts regardless of how experienced the reporter is in the field [2]. Cultivation of these journalist-expert relationships is thus probably very important for the success of the journalistic process when covering health topics. Several respondents wrote of this translational role between their readers and the scientific world, i.e. health journalists are tasked with translating scientific messages into a form that laypeople readers and viewers can understand and utilize in their personal lives. Doctors have often been accused for not being able to convey their message to laypeople and a skilled journalist could well be a desired companion in utilizing media for spreading important health information to patients. Some respondents reflected on this by saying that some doctors tend to cling to scientific expressions, not understanding that their potential readers could be alienated by such an approach. Several respondents also listed "not being able to popularize/clarify scientific facts into a form that laymen can understand" as a potential prejudice that journalists might have of doctors.

Previous studies have claimed that perceptions of information sources' motives might affect journalists' acceptance of information [3]. When asked about potential prejudices that doctors might have of journalists, sensationalism and inaccurate reporting of facts were the most common ones among those listed by the respondents. It has also been suggested that journalists could be categorized into "audience advocates" who are more favourable to PR-type source material, and "skeptics" who closely scrutinize all types of information [3]. Some of the open question answers in this study indicated that many Finnish health journalists employ this "skeptic" type of attitude and feel that medical science and medical journalism should share a scientific paradigm.

Respondents' views on source reliability were not surprising when taking into account their emphasis on medical science. Alternative therapy providers were deemed to be the second most unreliable after online discussion forums, whereas scientific journals and larger research units were viewed as the most reliable. Health magazines were thought to be more reliable than newspapers' health reporting which could perhaps be because magazine reporters often have much more time to verify facts and build bigger articles compared to more hectic life and limited text space of daily newspapers. Medical associations were thought to be more reliable than pharmaceutical companies, but some respondents commented that they felt that general medical associations could be biased because they wanted to protect the benefits of being a doctor. The comparatively low perceived reliability of individual patients is interesting, considering that patient stories are a commonly used source material in health reporting and a popular way in bringing a human-interest –type approach to a story which makes it more relatable to laymen readers [25]. They bring emotional content and a narrative to health reporting [26].

Some researchers have pointed out that much of the criticism of media being inaccurate in their reporting of facts might actually be due to disagreement and uncertainty within scientific communities and not due to the actions of journalists per se [8]. Fear of sensationalism was a common potential prejudice doctors might have, as listed by our respondents.

Overall, our respondents seemed to think rather favourably of collaborating with doctors. This echoes the results of our previous study [19], which illustrated that doctors are not frequent complainants about journalists' conduct to the Finnish self-regulatory body of journalism ethics. Potential prejudices listed by our respondents offer tools for both parties to improve understanding considering challenges of doctor-media collaboration and making potential prejudices visible could particularly help journalists prepare for this collaboration. Several respondents listed a fear of sensationalist publicity as a potential prejudice doctors might have. This is linked to the fact that when asked if and how doctor-media collaboration has changed through the years, those who felt that there had been changes usually stated that doctor's attitudes towards the media had changed for the positive. The most common descriptions that respondents gave of journalistic collaboration with doctors were positive and fruitful. This study verified that Finnish health journalists share common ideals of health journalism as a tool for improving the lives of their readers and that medical science should form a basis for such journalism.

Aknowledgements. The authors wish to thank the Finnish Society for Health Journalists for assistance.

References

1. The Association for Science Information in Finland, http://www.tieteentiedotus.fi/files/ Tiedebarometri_2013_net.pdf (read April 19, 2014)
2. Tanner, A.H.: Agenda Building, Source Selection, and Health News at Local Television Stations: A Nationwide Survey of Local Television Health Reporters. Science Communication 25, 350 (2004), doi:10.1177/1075547004265127
3. Len-Ríos, M., Hinnant, A., Park, S.-A., Cameron, G.T., Frisby, C., Lee, Y.: Health News Agenda Building: Journalists' Perceptions of the Role of Public Relations. Journalism & Mass Communication Quarterly 86, 315 (2009)
4. Gans, H.J.: Deciding what's news: A study of CBS Evening News, NBC Nightly News, Newsweek and Time. Pantheon Books, New York (1979)
5. Nelkin, D.: Selling science: How the press covers science and technology. Freeman, New York (1995)
6. The Finnish Association of Health Journalists, http://terveystoimittajat.fi (read April 18, 2014)
7. Healthwriters.com, http://www.healthwriters.com (read April 18, 2014)
8. Finer, D., Tomson, G., Björkman, N.M.: Ally, advocate, analyst, agenda-setter? Positions and perceptions of Swedish medical journalists. Patient Educ. Couns. 3(1), 71–81 (1997)
9. Larsson, A., Oxman, A.D., Carling, C., Herrin, J.: Medical messages in the media— barriers and solutions to improving medical journalism. Health Expect 6(4), 323–331 (2003), doi:10.1046/j.1369-7625.2003.00228.x, PMID 15040794
10. Haas, J.S., Kaplan, C.P., Gerstenberger, E.P., Karlikowske, K.: Changes in the Use of Postmenopausal Hormone Therapy after the Publication of Clinical Trial Results. Ann. Intern. Med. 140, 184–188 (2004)
11. Corbett, J.B., Mori, M.: Medicine, media, and celebrities: News coverage of breast cancer, 1960-1995. Journalism and Mass Communication Quarterly 76(2), 229–249 (1999)
12. The Finnish Medical Association, http://www.laakariliitto.fi/ edunvalvonta-tyoelama/suositukset/tiedotussuositus/ (read April 18, 2014)
13. Bartlett, C., Sterne, J., Egger, M.: What is newsworthy? Longitudinal study of the reporting of medical research in two British newspapers. Br. Med. J. 325, 81–84 (2002)
14. Ali, N.Y., Lo, T.Y.S., Auvache, V.L., White, P.D.: Bad press for doctors: 21 year survey of three national newspaper. Br. Med. J. 323(7316), 782–783 (2001)
15. Goodman, N.: The steady drip of biased reporting. Br. Med. J. 320, 1414 (2000)
16. Keep, P.: Why are doctors being hounded by the media? Hosp. Doctor 17, 42 (2000)

17. Lupton, D., McLean, J.: Representing doctors: discourses and images in the Australian press. Soc. Sci. Med. 46, 947–958 (1998)
18. Smith, R.: Editorial: Why are doctors so unhappy? Br. Med. J. 322, 1073 (2001)
19. Ahlmén-Laiho, U., Suominen, S., Järvi, U., Tuominen, R.: Complaints Made to the Council for Mass Media in Finland Concerning the Personal and Professional Lives of Doctors. In: Eriksson-Backa, K., Luoma, A., Krook, E. (eds.) WIS 2012. CCIS, vol. 313, pp. 91–103. Springer, Heidelberg (2012)
20. Schwitzer, G.: The magical medical media tour. Journal of the American Medical Association 267(14), 1969–1972 (1992)
21. Väliverronen, E.: Lääketiede mediassa. Duodecim 121, 1394–1399 (2005)
22. The Finnish Association of Journalists, http://www.toimittajaksi.fi/freelancerit/ (read April 18, 2014)
23. The Council for Mass Media in Finland, http://www.jsn.fi (read April 19, 2014)
24. The Finnish Association of Journalists, http://www.journalistiliitto.fi/liitto/liiton_jasenet/jasentilastoja/ (read May 2, 2014)
25. Hujanen, E.: Lukijakunnan rajamailla. Sanomalehden muuttuvat merkitykset arjessa. Dissertation, Univerisyt of Jyväskylä studies in humanities. University of Jyväskylä (2007)
26. Järvi, U.: Media terveyden lähteillä : miten sairaus ja terveys rakentuvat 2000-luvun mediassa. Dissertation, University of Jyväskylä studies in humanities. University of Jyväskylä (2011)

Perceived Need to Cooperate in the Creation of Inter-organizational IT Governance for Social Welfare and Health Care IT Services – A Case Study

Tomi Dahlberg

Turku School of Economics At University of Turku, Finland
tkmdah@utu.fi

Abstract. How to establish IT governance for social welfare and health care IT is an issue faced by organizations within this sector. Needs to establish inter-organizational IT governance arrangements have increased. They facilitate data sharing, pooling of development efforts and IT purchases, etc. This research investigates the creation of inter-organizational IT governance involving over 100 organizations. They provide specialized medical care, basic health care and/or social welfare services. Attention is placed especially on the role of perceived need to cooperate in the creation of IT governance. Empirical data range from notes, emails and project documents to survey data. Results achieved suggest that the perceived need to cooperate is necessary to the creation of inter-organizational IT governance arrangements. This finding augments the knowledge base of both IT governance research and best practice standards.

Keywords: Social welfare and health care IT, IT Governance, Resource Based View on Strategy (RBV), Case Research.

1 Introduction

Governance of IT [25], IT Governance [14] and Corporate Governance of IT [10], [17] concepts emerged some thirty years ago. IT governance is a practical IT management concern and an academic research topic. Although IT governance has become a widely used concept it has many definitions. This article follows the definitions of IT Governance Institute [14] and the ISO/IEC 38500:2008 Corporate Governance of IT standard [10, 11, 12].

Several reasons contributed to the emergence of IT governance. As the deployment of IT and digital data increased, the need to ensure that IT provides value increased. This issue was debated as the IT investment and productivity paradox [5]. Clearer and more transparent accountabilities for IT management were also called for [19], [21]. The purpose of IT governance became to establish structures, processes and cooperation mechanisms [19] including decision-making rights for key IT decisions [25], and by doing so secure clear accountabilities and IT value delivery. Another purpose is to guide relevant stakeholders to use IT responsibly [14], [10]. Increased deployment of IT makes organizations more vulnerable to IT-related risks. Therefore IT governance extends IT accountabilities also to IT risk management [14], [19].

K. Saranto et al. (Eds.): WIS 2014, CCIS 450, pp. 16–29, 2014.

IT governance has influenced IT management practice and research in many ways. Link to regulatory reporting is probably the most visible outcome. The reporting of IT accountabilities including IT-related risks has become a common regulatory disclosure requirement. Regulations include OECD corporate governance recommendations, Basel II and III accords for financial institutions, Sarbanes-Oxley Act (SOX) for securities issued in the US but also the requirement to report medical and other incidents with serious adverse impacts on patient health. Two other IT governance influences are even more important for this research. It is generally acknowledged that accountabilities for IT decisions and their implementation need to be clear and well communicated. Accountabilities can no longer be allocated to IT professionals only [10], [14], [19], [21]. Secondly, IT governance distinguishes IT governance and IT management [10], [21]. For example, the ISO/IEC 38500:2008 standard specifies that the responsibility of an IT governance function/body is to evaluate for what purposes IT is used, then direct IT management to pursue the objectives of evaluation and finally monitor IT management so that the objectives are achieved. This is called the Evaluate-Direct-Monitor (EDM) process. Correspondingly, the responsibility of an IT management function/body is to plan and implement needed IT-related development activities and service operations.

IT governance research has revealed that clear accountabilities improves IT but also organizational performance, such as revenues, return on assets and return on IT investments [21], [6]. Research findings also indicate that key IT decisions could have different IT governance arrangements. For example, the accountabilities of IT architecture and business application decisions usually differ. Similarly organizations with the target to grow have different allocation of accountabilities than organizations with focus on productivity [20,21]. When compared to the long tradition of centralized versus decentralized IT decision-making [25], this approach advocates more varied IT governance arrangements. The idea is to design IT governance so that the arrangements fits to the nature and needs of each governed issue [20, 21].

Research on how to design and implement IT governance has been conducted mainly in single organizations. This research explores how to create inter-organizational IT governance in a complex multi-organizational environment. The environment is complex since organizations participating to the arrangement are legally independent, have operated previously in isolation, are of different size and are public entities where politicians participate to decision-making. Furthermore, past efforts had failed.

This study contributes to research also by considering the role of perceived need to cooperate in the creation of IT governance. This issue is explored both on individual and organizational levels. The research idea is, that if participants perceive that cooperation is beneficial to them as individuals and also to their organizations, that will influence positively the creation of an inter-organizational IT governance arrangement [1, 2]. In summary, the generalized research question of this study is: How does the creation of inter-organizational IT governance differ from the creation of intra-organizational IT governance, and especially what is the role of perceived need to cooperate?

The empirical part of this research is a case study. During May 2013 - February 2014, an IT governance arrangement was created for the Oulu University Hospital's Social Welfare and Health Care Special Catchment Area (OYS-ERVA). OYS-ERVA is one of the five Special Catchment Areas in Finland. Geographically it covers almost half of the country. OYS-ERVA consists of 68 cities, towns or municipalities, 5 hospital districts, 9 hospitals including one of Finland's five University Central Hospitals, 33 health care centers and 5 social welfare development districts. No comparable IT governance arrangement had existed previously in OYS-ERVA or in any other Special Catchment Area with a history of prior failures. The created IT governance arrangement consolidated the IT services of specialized medical care, basic health care and social welfare services for the first time. Previously each sector and each organization within them had arranged, developed and operated IT services independently. Although there were strong pressures to increase inter-organizational IT cooperation, the creation of the arrangement was voluntary.

Matrixed approach to IT governance, COBIT, other "best practice" IT governance methods and ISO/IEC 38500 IT standards as well as social psychological theories and resource based view on strategy are discussed in section 2 as the theoretical background. Section three covers research approach, other methodology issues and the case. The results of the research are presented and discussed in the final two sections.

2   Theoretical Background

Several models and approaches to craft IT governance have been proposed [6], [19, 20, 21]. Some approaches emphasize IT governance structures and others processes [7]. The matrixed approach to IT governance [21, 22] is probably the best-known structural approach. Although academics have proposed process models [e.g. 7], probably the most-widely used models are embedded in best practice methods [13, 14, 15] and in ISO/IEC 38500 standards [10, 11]. Best practice methods apply generic process models and usually label the modified model as development method. Best practice methods typically consist of domains and IT processes. Domains and processes define the scope of IT management and governance. For example, COBIT version 5 has five domains, which break down to 36 processes.

Van Grembergen et al [19] claim that in addition to structures and processes cooperation mechanisms are needed to create IT governance. Even with best possible structures, such as allocation of decision making-rights for IT, and best possible processes, such as well executed evaluate – direct – monitor cycle, individuals with different competencies and responsibilities need to work together. The purpose of cooperation mechanisms is to ensure that individuals share the same objectives, and are able to resolve disputes and organize work efficiently. My interpretation is that these mechanisms are needed to address the need to cooperate.

What other theories explain why individuals and organizations want to cooperate? This research builds on cognitive social psychology [1, 2] and the resource based view on strategy [8]. As explained earlier the proposition is that perceived need to cooperate with envisioned benefits of cooperation is necessary for cooperation to happen. Perceived need to cooperate was deemed to be highly important for the creation of voluntary inter-organizational IT governance. In the investigated case IT governance is voluntary since the Constitution of Finland stipulates that cities, towns and municipalities are independent autonomous legal entities. Decisions made in any inter-organizational IT governance body have to be confirmed be city, town or municipality councils. On the other hand, several powerful actors advocated strongly for increased IT cooperation between organizations providing specialized medical care, basic health care and social welfare. These actors included the Government of Finland, Ministry of Social Welfare and Health Care and the Association of Finnish Local and Regional Authorities (Kuntaliitto). OYS-ERVA became the pilot area in the creation of inter-organizational IT cooperation and governance for social welfare and health care IT services.

2.1   Matrixed Approach to IT Governance

The matrixed approach to designing IT governance [21,22] proposes that there is five IT decision areas for which the decision-making rights need to be agreed. Weill and Ross list 22 issues under these areas. They identified first six [21] and later five [22] governance archetypes. When IT decision areas and governance archetypes are mapped together, the result is the IT governance matrix. Weill and Ross compared governance performance between enterprises with four criteria ranging from cost-efficient use of IT to effective use of IT for business flexibility [22].

One of the key findings of the matrixed approach to IT governance is that all IT decisions are not made in the same way. Applicable governance archetype varies from one IT decision area to the next. As a whole, IT governance matrix should reflect to the business priorities of the governed entity. The governance archetype concept combines business – IT and senior executive - business unit executive - IT executive dimensions. Matrixed approach to IT governance has helped to identify IT arrangements outside of the centralization versus decentralization axis [25].

Three features of the matrixed approach to IT governance were applied in the case. IT processes were classified into the five IT decisions areas (the Final Report of the case [26]). Secondly, governance archetypes were operationalized as actual governance bodies. Existing IT governance bodies included city, town, municipality, hospital district, etc. councils and boards, departmental and IT committees. Two new IT governance bodies were established; OYS-ERVA level IT development unit and OYS-ERVA level IT strategy and governance council. Thirdly, the principle that IT decisions could have different IT governance arrangements was applied.

2.2   COBIT and Other Best Practice Methods

Matrixed approach to IT governance distinguishes IT governance and IT management. However, as that approach focuses on decisional structures it does not describe how IT governance and management processes are linked. COBIT version 5 [13] not only separates IT governance and IT management but also describes in detail how these two processes are linked. COBIT calls them as the process for governance of enterprise IT and the process for management of enterprise IT. This feature of COBIT reflects the participation of ISACA (organization responsible for the development of COBIT) to the standardization of ISO/IEC 38500 IT governance standards.

Three characteristics of COBIT and other best practice methods were applied in the case. COBIT and also the ISO/IEC 38500 standards emphasize that IT management processes need to be both governed and managed and that governance and management have interactions. Secondly, best practice methods have comprehensive lists of IT tasks and processes that need governance. IT management processes listed in COBIT 5 [13], IT service management processes listed in ITIL version three [3] and architectural work products listed in TOGAF version 9.1 [15], were compiled. Overlaps were removed and the list was used to determine key IT services within OYS-ERVA. The final list contained 24 IT services/processes. Services were grouped into five IT decision areas by applying the matrixed approach to IT governance. Thirdly, best practice methods apply the RACI (responsible, accountable, consulted, informed) role model to allocate IT governance and management accountabilities. Accountable and responsible roles were defined for each of the 24 key IT services/processes by allocating them to the actual IT governance bodies mentioned in section 2.1. The result was a detailed IT governance matrix where the IT governance arrangement was optimized for each 24 IT service/process within the five IT decision areas.

2.3   ISO/IEC 38500 Standards Family

The ISO/IEC 38500:2008 Corporate Governance of Information Technology standard [10] defines the EDM (evaluate–direct–monitor) process of IT governance and how it steers the IT management processes. The standard also specifies six principles of good IT governance practice. The ISO/IEC DTS 38501:2014 is the implementation guide for IT governance. The ISO/IEC TR 38502 depicts the background ideas of the EDM IT governance framework and other models in the ISO/IEC 38500:2008 standard.

Two characteristics of the ISO/IEC 38500 standards family were applied in the case. The principles of how IT governance process steers IT management process were used in the design of IT governance and management processes for each of the 24 IT service/process. Secondly, the six principles of good IT governance practice were applied to craft the five design principles of the created IT governance arrangement.

2.4   Perceived Need to Cooperate and Envisioned Benefits of Cooperation

In this research two sets of theories were selected from alternative theories, which describe why individuals and organizations cooperate. Selected theories were deemed to cover both the individual and the organizational levels of the perceived need to cooperate. They were also considered to support the definition of envisioned concrete benefits of cooperation in the creation of the IT governance arrangement.

Cognitive social psychological theories, such as the theory of reasoned action (TRA) [1] and the theory of planned behavior (TPB) [2], explain that attitudes, beliefs and values with their antecedents (e.g. past experiences and education) impact behavioral decisions in social contexts. Individuals cooperate - that is, they choose to behave in this way - if they perceive that cooperation is beneficial to them for personal and/or social reasons. Social reasons, such as the perceived attitudes of an individual's colleagues and strong lobbying for cooperation from authorities, may result in cooperation behavior, as the individual perceives that such behavior is expected. In the current case, welfare and health care professionals had to decide whether or not to participate to the creation of IT governance for OYS-ERVA.

Resource based view on business strategy (RBV) [8], also known as relational view, was applied to include organizational level behavior. RBV proposes that inter-organizational cooperation happens if cooperation provides win-win value to the participating organizations by aggregating, sharing and exchanging their valuable unique resources, and if this value cannot be achieved otherwise. Social psychology theories and RBV were used to enhance IT governance knowledge basis rather than operationalize the constructs of those theories (e.g. [27]).

3   Methodology Issues and the Case

The researcher acted as the consultant recruited by Kuntaliitto during the creation of the IT governance arrangement for OYS-ERVA. The Assignment lasted 9 months from June 2013 to February 2014. The assignment was run in parallel and as a part of the "Support Project of Planning and Documenting National Enterprise Architecture" for social welfare and health care services (VAKAVA). That project designed the national target architecture for social welfare and health care IT services. VAKAVA project took its mandate from the Law of Organizing IT steering in the Public Sector (Tietohallintolaki), which became effective in 2011. This law stipulates that enterprise architecture has to be used to steer IT in public sector organizations unless they are exempted from the Law.

OYS-ERVA became the pilot for the creation of inter-organizational IT governance arrangement. The group that designed IT governance included the chief medical officer of one health district, CIOs of three health districts, the CIO of a major city, two enterprise architects of health districts, three specialist from social welfare development centers, health districts and National Institute for Health and Welfare, one IT expert from another Special Catchment Area, two senior advisors from STM and two senior advisors from Kuntaliitto. Majority of project material was delivered to these 16 persons. During the assignment the experiences of other Special Catchment Areas and social welfare development centers were presented and the outlines of the revised social welfare and health care legislation was reviewed. Selected interim and final materials of the case were made public and presented both within OYS-ERVA and nationally.

Due to the role of the researcher this research follows the reflective observation approach in a single case context. Guidelines outlined for case studies [24], [9] and for the building of research constructs [16], [18] are followed. Several types of material created during the assignment are used as empirical research material. Workshop materials represent a large proportion of data volume. Workshop materials range from RACI charts to handwritten discussion notes, from agendas to thick pre-reading documents, and from draft revisions to the Law on Arranging Social Welfare and Health Care Services to the draft and final memorandums of the assignment with motions for decisions. Empirical data includes also project memos, emails, presentation slides, and documented answers to questions and feedback. A final report with recommendations and motions for decisions was written.

In November-December 2013 a web-based self-administrated survey was conducted to evaluate the benefits of IT cooperation and the guiding principles of the created IT governance arrangement. Survey design followed guidelines provided by [16], [18], [24]. The survey had five background questions about respondents and their organizations. In data analysis they were used as independent (explaining) variables. The second category of variables consisted of 20 evaluative questions about IT and its role in social welfare and health care, about the status of IT deployment within the respondent's organization, and about the accountabilities in the development of welfare and health care IT services. In data analysis responses were used both as dependent (explained) and as independent (explaining) variables. The third category of questions evaluated the benefits of IT cooperation (10 questions) and the principles of the created IT governance arrangement (7 questions). In data analysis responses were treated as dependent (explained) variables.

The 37 evaluative questions were formulated into statements. Respondents were asked to evaluate each statements on a 7-point Likert scale from totally disagree (=1) to totally agree (=7). Comments in writing were also collected.

Invitation to participate to the survey was emailed to 260 Finnish social welfare and health care experts throughout the country. After one reminder 68 responses were received (26% response rate). Slightly over half (37) of the 68 responses were from OYS-ERVA. Seven respondents had participated into the creation of the IT governance arrangement. Slightly over half of the respondents worked in hospital districts, 37 % in cities, towns or municipalities and 10 % in other organizations. Of the respondents 43 % were social welfare or health care managers or executives and 12 % specialists. Social welfare or health care IT managers and executives accounted for 23 % and IT specialists for 22 %.

Due to the limited number of responses structured equation models and other multivariate statistical methods could not be used. Statistical significance of differences in the means of dependent variables was analyzed with the two-tailed Student t-test by grouping responses on the basis of background and evaluative variables (the latter into agree and disagree groups). A more profound statistical analysis is, however, left to future study since this research focuses on the role of cooperation and its ability to enrich IT governance knowledge.

As a whole, the work in the assignment was organized around workshops. Table 1 below shows the workshops, their topics, and the theoretical background applied in each workshop and between two workshops. In addition to the workshops shown in the table three teleconference workshops were organized.

Table 1. Workshops organized to design the IT governance Arrangement with the theoretical basis of each workshop

#	Description of the workshop / assingment given to participants in between two workshops	Matrixed approach to IT governance	Best practice methods (RACI, lists of IT processes)	ISO/IEC 38500 standards family (EDM model, principles)	Benefits of cooperation for individuals - social psychological theories	Benefits of cooperation for organizations - Resource Based View on Strategy
1	Intoduce IT governance concepts, craft first lists of IT services and decision making entities, craft 1. version of RACI matrix	Primary	Primary	Primary	None	None
	Participant were given the task to list current IT services and IT decision making entities within their respective organizations	In the background	In the background	In the background	None	None
2	Define reasons for IT cooperation with concrete measurable benefits, discuss alternative IT governance arrangements	In the background	In the background	In the background	Primary	Primary
	Evaluate the list of reasons for cooperation and cooperation benefits as well as evaluate alternative IT governance arrangements	None	None	None	Primary	Primary
3	Agree to cooperate, draft for the principles of the IT governance arrangement, present proposal for the arrangement	Apply	Apply	Apply	Primary	Primary
	Consider what kind of presentation material is needed to communicate the results of the work	None	None	None	None	None
4	Evaluate and improve the proposed arrangement and presentation materials, discuss the governance of EA	Apply	Apply	Apply	Apply	Apply
5	Guidance to the final report, recommendations and other materials, review of survey questions	Apply	Apply	Apply	Apply	Apply
	Provide feedback and revision requests to the final report to incorporate comments from presentations in the organizations of the participants	None	None	None	None	None
6	Present survey results, accept the final report with revisions, end the work	Apply	Apply	Apply	Apply	Apply

4   Results

4.1   Contributions of the IT Governance Arrangement

From practical perspective the most important result is the creation and acceptance of IT governance arrangement for OYS-ERVA. The recommendations and the motions for decisions of the final report were accepted in February 2014. The implementation of the IT governance arrangement started immediately. The created IT governance arrangement included the establishment of two new OYS-ERVA level IT governance bodies. The accepted IT governance arrangement divided the accountabilities of 24 IT services/processes into three categories; OYS-ERVA level governed and locally managed (12 services), locally governed and managed (5 services) and into services/processes the governance of which is decided later case by case (7 services).

As a whole, the proposed IT governance arrangement was labeled "the model of shared management". The final report and full survey results are publicly available from the web page of Kuntaliitto (www.kuntaliitto.fi, both documents are in Finnish, [26]).

Here scientific contributions are more important. This case proposes strongly that in addition to IT governance knowledge also other factors need to considered in the context of inter-organizational IT governance. Perceived need to cooperate with concrete and measurable benefits from cooperation is a strong candidate. In this case, where previous efforts to build inter-organizational IT governance had failed, this factor proved decisive.

This research links resource based view on strategy and social psychological theories to IT governance. The pooling and sharing of local resources, competencies and experiences in the development and operation of IT services combined was envisioned to lead to benefits that would not be achieved otherwise. It is noteworthy that the created IT governance arrangement leaves most IT resources and assets to their current organizations but makes them better available by resource pooling and by OYS-ERVA level steering of IT services sourcing, enterprise architecting and implementation of national IT services.

Thirdly, this research supports findings [21] according to which the centralization versus decentralization of IT decisions should be replaced with more sophisticated models. In this case that was done by involving senior executives, business professionals and IT professionals and by making them agree accountabilities for each key IT service/process. This case also shows that it is possible to agree accountabilities on IT service/process level rather than IT decision area level. The distinction of IT governance and management processes opened up new arrangement opportunities. In this case, the governance of some IT services/processes was OYS-ERVA level and their management was local whereas both could also be local.

4.2   Perceived Need to Cooperate in the Creation of IT Governance

As stated above the perceived need to cooperate with concrete benefits was decisive for the creation of the IT governance arrangement. The work on the assignment started by applying solely IT governance knowledge, best practices and standards (first workshop). That approach proved insufficient in terms of participants' commitment. One of the CIOs coined the problem "Although I understand the governance matrix with RACI roles, it is useless in my organization. Doctors do not understand from the matrix the benefits of IT cooperation. They ask me, why should we use time to consider cooperation when there are so many burning IT issues in our organization."

It became necessary to reschedule work and use next two workshops to answer questions: Do we really need to increase IT cooperation from its current status? What can we learn from our past failed efforts? What concrete benefits does IT cooperation offer? Answers to these questions proved valuable when the proposal to establish two new OYS-ERVA level IT governance bodies was presented. After a long silent moment one of the participants stated, "if we are logical with our statements that we need more IT cooperation, then something like this has to be established." That was the decisive moment for the creation of the IT governance arrangement.

Survey results provided strong support to the envisioned benefits of cooperation as Figure 1 illustrates. Furthermore, the means (t-test) of responses did not differ statistically significantly between groups formed on the basis of background variables no between agree/disagree groups formed on the basis of the 20 evaluative variables. This means that respondents answered similarly despite of differences in profession, type of organization, organizational position, IT-expertise and geographical area. Respondents answered also largely similarly despite differences in their attitudes to the use of IT, implementation of IT in their organization.

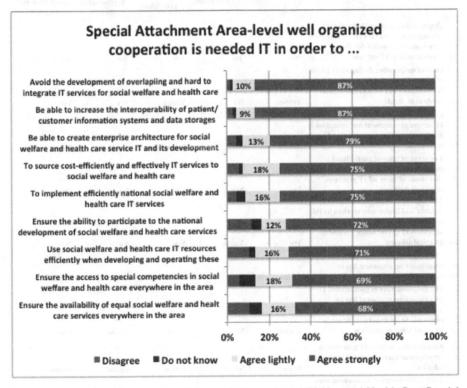

Fig. 1. Evaluations on the benefits of IT cooperation in Social Welfare and Health Care Special Attachment Areas (n=68)

4.3   Principles of the Created Inter-organizational IT Governance Arrangement

The theoretical background discussed in chapter 2 was condensed into five principles that guided the creation of the IT governance arrangement. As a whole, they operationalized for the case IT governance knowledge on how to create an inter-organizational IT governance arrangement, and integrated perceived need to cooperate into that knowledge. For the survey they were broken down to seven statements. The statements reflect also the environment of the case. Each principle and its breakdown to survey questions with relation to theoretical background are shown in Table 2. The number in the first column refers to a principle number and S# refers to a survey statement.

Table 2. Principles of the IT governance arrangement

PRINCIPLE		THEORETICAL BASIS USED AND/OR APPLIED				
#, S#	Description of the workshop / assingment given to participants in between two workshops	Matrixed approach to IT governance	Best practice methods (RACI, lists of IT processes)	ISO/IEC 38500 standards family (EDM model, principles)	Benefits of cooperation for individuals - social psychological theories	Benefits of cooperation for organizations - Resource Based View on Strategy
1, S1	Organization responsible for the arrangement of social welfare and healt care is also responsible for the arrangement of IT services	No	Yes	Yes	Yes	Yes
1, S2	Lack of cooperation during early phase of IT service development and operation is an obstacle to IT cooperation (and needs to be fixed)	Yes/no	No	Yes/no	Yes	Yes
1, S3	Lack of cooperation during operation of IT service development and operation is an obstacle to IT cooperation (and needs to be fixed)	Yes/no	No	Yes/no	Yes	Yes
2 na	The scope of inter-organizational governance of social welfare and health care needs to cover all IT processes, tasks and decisions	Yes	Yes	Yes	No	None
3, S4	Although IT is deployed in all social wellfare and health care services its role is different in each service Atachmen area level IT goveernance is a useful practical solution	Yes	Yes/no	Yes	No	None
4, na	The proposed inter-organizational IT governance arrangement has to implemtable in steps	Yes/no	No	Yes/no	Yes/no	Yes/no
5, na	The proposed inter-organizational IT governance arrangement has to organization independent, that is, adaptable to the ongoing changes in laws and other regulations	Yes/no	No	Yes/no	Yes/no	Yes/no
& 5, S5	Attachment area level IT governance development team is a useful practical solution	Yes/no	No	Yes/no	Yes/no	Yes/no
& 5, S6	The establishment of Attachment area level IT governance council is a useful practical solution	Yes/no	No	Yes/no	Yes/no	Yes/no
& 5, S7	Start small from selected IT services and process on the basis of experience is a useful practical solution	Yes/no	No	Yes/no	Yes/no	Yes/no

Survey results support the validity of the IT governance principles of the case. Figure 2 illustrates the means and medians to each statement of the survey.

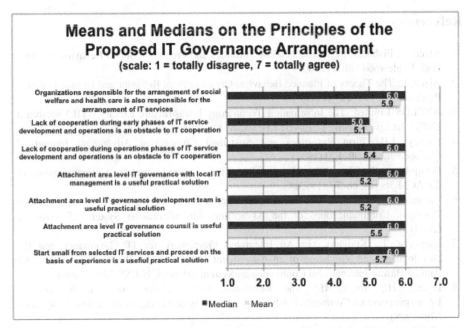

Fig. 2. Evaluations of statements on the principles of the created inter-organizational IT governance arrangement (n=68)

5   Discussion

This research has shown that IT governance knowledge alone was insufficient to create an inter-organizational IT governance arrangement. Results achieved suggest that perceived need to cooperate with concrete benefits could be critical to the creation of inter-organizational IT governance. By doing so this research linked resource based view on strategy and cognitive social psychology theories to IT governance knowledge. These findings answer the research question raised in section 1. However more studies are necessary as this research is a single case study.

Practitioners are adviced to consider willingness to cooperate on individual and organizational levels when they craft inter-organizational IT governance. They should ensure that visible benefits are identified on both levels. Similar to some other studies this research suggests that key IT decisions, services and processes can have different IT governance and management arrangement rather than force everything to one "single truth". It is even possible to arrange IT governance and IT management accountabilities in many ways.

In addition to the single case setting this research has also other limitations. The case covers one Special Attachment Area in one country. Different results could be obtained in other environments. The researcher acted as a consultant. Although there are no reasons to interpret the empirical material from some predetermined perspective that might still have happened. Changing legislation together with the strong objective of the Finnish Government to integrate social welfare and health care may have created strong incentives for cooperation, which could explain the findings of this research.

References

1. Ajzen, I., Fishbein, M.: Understanding Attitudes and Predicting Social Behavior. Prentice Hall, Englewood Cliffs (1980)
2. Ajzen, I.: The Theory of Planned Behavior. Organizational Behavior and Human Decision Processes 50, 179–211 (1991)
3. AXELOS Limited: The Information Technology Infrastructure Library (ITIL) version 3 (2007), http://www.itil-officialsite.com
4. Barney, J.B.: Firm Resources and Sustained Competitive Advantage. Journal of Management 17, 99–120 (1991)
5. Brynjolfsson, E.: The productivity paradox of information technology. Communications of the ACM 36(12), 66–77 (1993)
6. Brown, A.E., Grant, G.G.: Framing the Frameworks: A Review of IT Governance Research. Communications of the Association for Information Systems 15, 696–712 (2005)
7. Dahlberg, T., Kivijärvi, H.: An Integrated Framework for IT Governance and the Development and Validation of an Assessment Instrument. In: Proceedings of the 39th Annual Hawaii International Conference on System Sciences, HICSS 2006 (2006)
8. Dyer, J.H., Singh, H.: The Relational View: Cooperative and Sources of Interorganizational Competitive Advantage. Academy of Management Review 23(4), 660–679 (1998)
9. Eisenhardt, K.M.: Building Theories from Case Study Research. Academy of Management Review 14(4), 532–550 (1989)
10. International Organization for standardization and the International Electrotechnical Commission: ISO/IEC 35800:2008 Corporate Governance of Information Technology standard, http://www.iso.org
11. International Organization for standardization and the International Electrotechnical Commission: ISO/IEC 38501:2014 Corporate Governance of Information Technology – Implementation Guide, http://www.iso.org
12. International Organization for standardization and the International Electrotechnical Commission: ISO/IEC 38502: Corporate Governance of Information Technology – Framework and Reference Model, http://www.iso.org
13. ISACA: COBIT 5: A Business Framework for the Governance and Management of Enterprise IT, http://www.isaca.org
14. IT Governance Institute: Board Briefing on IT Governance, 2nd edn. (2003), http://www.itgi.org
15. The Open Group: TOGAF® Version 9.1 - The Book, http://www.opengroup.org
16. Sireci, S.G.: The Construct of Content Validity. Social Indicator Research 45, 83–117 (1998)
17. Standards Australia: AS8015-2005 Corporate Governance of Information and Communication technology standard
18. Tenopyr, M.L.: Content-construct Confusion. Personnel Psychology 30, 47–54 (1977)
19. Van Grembergen, W., De Haes, S., Guldentops, E.: Structures, Processes and Relational Mechanisms for IT Governance. In: Strategies for Information Technology Governance, pp. 152–168. Idea Group Global, Hershey (2004)
20. Van Grembergen, W., De Haes, S.: Implementing Information Technology Governance: Models, Practices and Cases. Idea Group Global, Hershey (2008)
21. Weill, P., Ross, J.: IT Governance: How Top Performers Manage IT Decision Rights for Superior Results. Harvard Business School Press, Boston (2004)

22. Weill, P., Ross, J.: A Matrixed Approach to Designing It Governance. Sloan Management Review 46(2), 25–35 (2005)
23. Williamson, O.: The Economic Institutions of Capitalism. Free Press, New York (1985)
24. Yin, R.K.: Case Study Research, Design and Methods, 4th edn. SAGE publications, Thousand Oaks (2009)
25. Zmud, R.W.: Design Alternatives for Organizing Information Systems Activities. MIS Quarterly 8(2), 79–93 (1984)
26. The Final Report of the case and survey results are available,
    http://www.kunnat.net/fi/asiantuntijapalvelut/soster/
    tietojarj-sahkoiset-palv/vakava-projekti/Documents/
    00SOTE%20tietohallintoa%20koskevan%20kyselyn%20tulokset_
    26012014_OSA1.pdf
27. How to design theory of planned behavior research instruments. Francis, J.J., Eccles, M., Johnston, M., Walker, A., Grimshaw, J., Foy, R., Kaner, E.F.S., Smith, L., Bonetti, D.: Constructing Questionnaires Based on the Theory of Planned Behaviour – A Manual for Health Services Researchers, University of Newcastle (2004) and Ajzen, I.: Constructing a TpB Questionnaire: Conceptual and Methodological Considerations (2002) , http://www.people.umass.edu/aizen/pdf/tpb.measurement.pdf

Aggression Management Training at Schools

Kirsi-Maria Haapasalo-Pesu[1] and Tiina Ilola[2]

[1] Satakunta Hospital District, Harjavalta, Finland
kirsi-maria.haapasalo-pesu@satshp.fi
[2] Satakunta Hospital District, Pori, Finland
tiina.ilola@satshp.fi

Abstract. Behavioral problems, such as, aggressiveness and disregard for the rules are common in adolescence. Inappropriate behavior may disturb learning and disrupt the atmosphere in the school. Within the Satakunta Hospital District, a project was implemented to introduce the Aggression Replacement Training (ART) method in schools. In the schools involved in the project, staff members were instructed in this method and ART courses were arranged for students. The ART groups provided the participating students with training in anger control, social skills and moral reasoning. According to the feedback, the behavior of the participants improved and the students learnt how to control themselves better. The schools gained a calmer work environment. The results of this project indicate that it may be useful to further expand the use of the ART method at schools.

Keywords: adolescent, aggression, school, prevention.

1 Introduction

Behavioral problems are common in adolescence. Approximately 10–13% of adolescent boys and 4–6% of girls suffer from behavioral problems and conduct disorders. A conduct disorder refers to a persistent and extensive behavioral pattern with indifference to the rights and well-being of others, and disregard for the laws, norms and rules of the community, which has a significant negative impact on the functioning capacity of the young person [1]. At school, disorderly behaviors include the neglecting of one's studies, instigation of disturbances, and disobedience of rules and regulations. In many cases, the student behaves in an impulsive and aggressive manner and uses inappropriate language. If no rehabilitation support measures are taken, the conduct disorder may result in underachievement at school [2]. A conduct disorder is a major risk factor for marginalization. Of juvenile offenders, 70-90% have some type of conduct disorder. It appears that conduct disorders with an onset in childhood or adolescence are associated with an antisocial personality disorder in adulthood [3,4]. Thus, it is a serious phenomenon. Being able to effectively tackle the problem at an early stage would be of great importance for both the individual and the community.

Aggressive behavior can be due to many different causes, for example, lacking impulse control. Sometimes adolescents can construe situations wrong: such misconstruction is common among young people suffering from ADHD or Asperger

K. Saranto et al. (Eds.): WIS 2014, CCIS 450, pp. 30–35, 2014.

syndrome. Shouting, hitting and kicking can also be a behavioral model that is learnt at home. Propensity to violence may be genetic and social learning can strengthen the tendency to aggressiveness [5].

Depressive youth can be hot-tempered and anxious. There are also young people who, for one reason or other, behave deliberately aggressive.

Often students' problems are reflections of the problems of the adults at home: substance abuse, domestic violence, mental health problems and difficult life situations [5]. Numerous studies demonstrate that aggression can also be associated with peer difficulties [6]. The overall school climate also has an impact on adolescents' behavior. Research has shown that students feel less safe in schools with higher levels of aggression [7].

It is common at schools that teachers feel irresolute when facing youth with behavioral disorders. Misbehaving students are not focused on learning, and they also disturb the rest of the class. The fact that teachers lack proper tools to deal with these youngsters also affects the teachers' work wellness and ability to cope.

In Finland, student counseling and school health care systems are in place within the schools. Students have access to the services of a nurse, psychologist and student counselor. Short-term interactive interventions can be initiated in order to deal with mild mental disorders [2]. The most successful mental health promotion programs include those that are designed to advance positive knowledge and skills, provided that they are targeted at the school community at large [8]. The possibilities for treating behavioral problems and conduct disorders within the school health care system have, in practice, proven insufficient, and conduct disorders are a common cause for students to be referred to specialized care, such as an adolescent psychiatry clinic.

2   Aim

As part of a national health care development project (KASTE) in 2008-2013, the Unit of Adolescent Psychiatry within the Satakunta Hospital District implemented a project to introduce the Aggression Replacement Training (ART) method in schools. There is promising evidence of a connection between the use of ART and a reduction in crime [9].

3   Methods and Materials

The project was resourced with one nurse who arranged training in the ART method for the staff members in the participating schools. When the method was being launched at a school, she served as a partner to the trained staff member in guiding the ART groups, and also, otherwise, contributed to the group arrangements.

The ART method was developed in the United States in the 1980s. Based on research, it appeared that dialogical counseling was not of much help for the purpose of changing an individual's aggressive behaviour [10]. Psychologist Arnold Goldstein developed the ART method. Understanding that an adolescent's aggressive behavior results from a number of factors, Goldstein developed a multimodal method that targeted precisely those skill deficiencies that are known to underlie aggressive behaviors. Multimodality means that aggression is approached through reasoning, action and emotions. ART is a group-based skills training method that utilizes the power of working together, and relies on the principles and practices of advanced learning theories [10].

The main components of training cover anger control, social skills and moral reasoning.

The idea is to make pro-social behavior more rewarding than aggressive behaviour. The role of the adult group leader is to guide and encourage the group.

Through the anger control training in the ART group, the adolescents are encouraged to respond to provocation in a socially acceptable manner, instead of behaving aggressively. They are taught that they can manage their anger by breaking up their fury or rage in stages that form the process of anger management. The stages are conquered one by one. Through this process, the adolescents learn to identify their physical excitement, the anger-triggering events and their own individual interpretations, and to calm down so that they can respond by using their social skills [11].

Modeling is used as the method to help adolescents advance their social skills. They are given an opportunity to practice social skills through role playing, and they are encouraged and praised throughout the exercise. The method includes a total of 50 different social skills, such as listening to other people, saying thanks, introducing oneself and complimenting other people.

In terms of moral reasoning, the group training aims to influence values and promote behaviors such as the keeping of promises, sticking to the truth, helping others, respecting life and obeying the law.

During the course of the project, if a student behaved badly at school, one of the staff members raised the issue for discussion with the adolescent and his or her parent or guardian. They were informed about the ART group work at the school, and the adolescent was given an opportunity to take part in a group.

The ART groups were closed groups, and they convened a total of ten times, for one hour at a time. At the start of each session, the participants were served a light snack, for example, juice and cookies. The group size was 4-6 adolescents, and each group was guided by two adults. The method comprised of a training program in which a new social skill was trained every week. It was possible to give homework so that the adolescents could try their new skills also outside the group.

At the end of the program, the adolescents were asked to give written feedback (a structured form) on the atmosphere of the group, its usefulness, what they found difficult and what was nice in the group. Feedback was requested from the group leaders as well.

Within the project, all of the 20 municipalities within the Satakunta Hospital District were invited to take part in the training.

4   Results

A total of nine municipalities took part in the project. The number of individual schools was 20.

The ART training enabled employees in various fields of administration to work together when guiding the groups. People from municipalities or local parishes could work jointly with the staff members in the schools. Teachers, psychologists, student counselors and school nurses from various schools took part in the training.

Written feedback was received from eight schools.

According to the group leaders, those adolescents who benefited most from the groups were personally motivated to take part in the groups and also backed by solid support from their parents. The adolescents enjoyed taking part in the ART groups. According to the feedback, the behavior of the participants improved, there was less quarrelling and fighting during the breaks, the students learnt to control themselves better than before and they were able to settle quarrels by themselves.

Of the responding adolescents, 70-83% felt that they had benefited from the ART group. They stated that they were able to control their anger better than before, and they had learnt to apologize, listen and show gratitude. They appreciated peer support and adult encouragement. Some adolescents felt that role playing was difficult. Some hesitated at first to express their opinions, because they were afraid of criticism. Over one half of the respondents reported that they had, in their leisure time, thought about the topics discussed in the group. The adolescents felt it was especially important that they received positive feedback in their everyday lives from friends, parents and other personally important individuals. They also learnt self-evaluation, that is, to subjectively assess how they had managed in conflict situations and if they could have handled the situation better.

I was taught ways to avoid fights. At home, there were not as many fights anymore.
–Girl, 15
I understood that good behavior matters.
–Girl, 14
It was great that a grown-up was listening to me and gave me clear instructions so I could solve my problems.
–Boy, 15
Anger control was not easy at first, but then I realized what I was like myself and that I can control myself.
–Boy, 15
The prizes were encouraging. I've told my friends only good things about ART. Acting in front of the others made me nervous at first, but then I got used to it.
–Boy, 14
Social skills [training] was good; in moral [reasoning], the stories were interesting, and you could say your own opinion.
–Boy, 14
Positive feedback and encouragement from the adults felt good.
–Boy, 15

5   Discussion

The causes of aggressiveness are various, and the severity of problems varies. The ART method is helpful when the behavior of an adolescent is too retiring or aggressive. The limitation of the method is that it does not provide sufficient care for actual mental health problems such as affective or psychotic disorders.

Still it makes sense to organize ART groups in the schools and it is useful to train the staff of the schools to use this method. It is possible to detect early the behavior problems of the pupils in the school, and it is important to give the support to the young people as early as possible. It is natural to render basic services for young people close to their everyday life. Early intervention can give pragmatic problem solving skills and may prevent bigger problems and thereby reduce the need and utilization of adolescent psychiatric services [12]. The arranging of ART groups was a signal to students that the adults in their school are interested in their well-being and they found that they are not alone with their problems. The change of the behavior is not so easy. It needs much training and persistent work: the more repetitions, the more possible the change is. Adolescents need encouragement from adults in the school and at home, but also the support of their peers.

The ART groups were mainly experienced as positive and pleasant. The groups have continued working after the project ended. Those who served as group leaders have asked for additional training related to the method, and they have reported that they have drawn advantage from the ART ideology in other contexts outside the groups as well. The training provided them with new practical tools. The word about the good feedback has spread, and municipalities that were not involved in the project have become interested in the ART training. It appears that taking part in the ART groups has helped adolescents to better cope with the daily routines of the school. The schools have a calmer work environment. On the basis of the results of this project, it might be useful to expand the use of the method.

In the future, it is important that the long-term effects of the ART groups are followed up and that the results from the groups are investigated scientifically.

References

1. Lindberg, N.: Nuoruusikä ja psykopatia [Adolescence and psychopathy]. Duodecim 126, 1568–1574 (2010) (in Finnish)
2. Kaltiala-Heino, R., Ranta, K., Fröjd, S.: Nuorten mielenterveys koulumaailmassa [Adolescent mental health promotion in school context]. Duodecim 126, 2033–2039 (2010) (in Finnish)
3. Frick, P.J., Kimonis, E.R., Dandreaux, D.M., Farrell, J.M.: The 4 year stability of psychopathics traits in non-referred youth. Behav. Sci. Law 21, 713–736 (2003)
4. Loney, B.R., Taylor, J., Butler, M.A., Lacono, W.G.: Adolescent psychopathy features: 6-year temporal stability and the prediction of externalizing symptoms during the transition to adulthood. Aggress. Behav. 33, 242–252 (2007)

5. Fröjd, S., Mansikka, L., Ahonen, M., Kaltiala-Heino, R.: Oppilaan aggressiiviseen käyttäytymiseen puuttuminen. [Intervening with a student's aggressive behavior] Pirkanmaan Sairaanhoitopiirin Julkaisuja 6, 7–9 (2008) (in Finnish)
6. Card, N.A., Stucky, B.D., Sawalani, G.M., Little, T.D.: Direct and indirect aggression during childhood and adolescence: A meta-analytic review of gender differences, intercorrelations, and relations to maladjustment. Child Develop. 79, 1185–1229 (2008)
7. Goldstein, S.E., Young, A., Boyd, C.: Relational aggression at school: Associations with school safety and social climate. J. Youth Adolesc. 37, 641–654 (2008)
8. Santor, D.A., Bagnell, A.L.: Maximizing the uptake and sustainability of schoolbased mental health programs: commercializing knowledge. Child Adolesc. Psychiatric Clinics of North America 21(1), 81–91, ix, doi:10.1016/j.chc.2011.09.004
9. Reddy, L.A., Linda, A., Goldstein, A.P., Arnold, P.: Aggression Replacement intervention for aggressive adolescents. Res. Treat. for Child. Youth 18, 47–62 (2001)
10. Lipsey, M.: What do we learn from 400 research studies on the effectiveness of treatment with juvenile delinquents? In: McGure, J. (ed.) What Works: Reduicing Reoffending - Guidelines from Research and Practice, pp. 63–78. Wiley, Chichester (1995)
11. Röning, T., Kivelä, K., Jokinen, J., Kilvelä, R., Savolainen, J.: ART - Aggression Replacement Training – ryhmäharjoitusmenetelmä aggressiivisesti käyttäytyville nuorille [ART – Aggression replacement Training – A group training method for aggressively behaving adolescents]. In: Moring, J., Martins, A., Partanen, A., Nordling, E., Bergman, V. (eds.) Kansallinen mielenterveys- ja päihdesuunnitelma 2009-2015. Kehittyviä käytäntöjä 2011 [National plan for mental health and substance abuse work 2009-2015: Developing practices 2011]. National Institute for Health and Welfare (THL). Report, vol. 46, pp. 178–186 (2011) (in Finnish)
12. Puolakka, K., Kiikkala, I., Haapasalo-Pesu, K.-M., Paavilainen, E.: Mental health promotion in the upper level of comprehensive school from the viewpoint of school personnel and mental health workers. Scand. J. Caring Sci. 25, 37–44 (2011)

FirstAED Emergency Dispatch, Global Positioning of First Responders with Distinct Roles - A Solution to Reduce the Response Times and Ensuring Early Defibrillation in the Rural Area Langeland

Finn Lund Henriksen[1], Per Schorling[2], Bruno Hansen[2], Henrik Schakow[1], and Mogens Lytken Larsen[1]

[1] The AED Center, Dept of Cardiology, Odense University Hospital, Odense, Denmark
finn.l.henriksen@rsyd.dk
[2] The Langeland AED Association, Langeland, Denmark

Abstract. FirstAED is a supplement to the existing emergency response systems. The aim is to shorten the first responder response times at emergency calls to below 5 minutes. FirstAED defines a way to dispatch the nearby three first responders and organize their roles in the hope of reducing response times, ensuring citizens safety and equal possibility to early defibrillation.

First aid is provided by first responders who use their smartphone (iPhone 4S/5). FirstAED Global Positioning System GPS-track the nine nearby first responders and enables the emergency dispatcher to send an organized team of three first responders with distinct roles to the scene.

During the first 21 months the FirstAED system was used 588 times. Three first responders arrived in 89 % of the cases, and they arrived before the ambulance in 95 % of the cases. FirstAED entailed a significant reduction in median response time to 4 minutes 9 seconds.

Keywords: Cardiopulmonal resuscitation, response time, first responder, dispatching, Public Access Defibrillation (PAD), Global Positioning System (GPS).

1   Introduction

Sudden out-of-hospital cardiac arrest (OHCA) is the leading cause of death in developed countries. In Denmark, approximately 3.500 people suffer an out-of-hospital cardiac arrest every year. The overall survival rate for out-of-hospital cardiac arrest is low, approximately 10 % [1]. International guidelines recommend cardiopulmonal resuscitation (CPR) within 5-6 minutes [2] and early defibrillation with an automated external defibrillator (AED) with the purpose to increase the survival rate [3]. Shortening the ambulance/paramedic response times to less than five minutes in the rural areas of Denmark including the island of Langeland, is however extremely expensive and unrealistic. Therefore dispatch of volunteer trained first responders is a good, cheap, alternative solution.

K. Saranto et al. (Eds.): WIS 2014, CCIS 450, pp. 36–45, 2014.

Dispatching of volunteer first responders are established in the Netherlands [4] and in the RUMBA study in Stockholm, Sweden [5]. In both studies many volunteer laypersons can be alerted at the same time by the system. The Dutch system uses CPR-AED-Alert text messages to the local (living and/or working in the area) first responders to pick up the AED or to go to the victims of suspected out-of-hospital cardiac arrest and provide early cardiopulmonal resuscitation and defibrillation.

The Dutch model of emergency pre-hospital cardiac care began around five years ago, when it was clear that standard ambulance response times around 15 minutes were too long to provide an effective cardiopulmonal resuscitation service. Some rural Dutch regions have reduced the time from first emergency call to defibrillation to 7-8 minutes and increased the overall survival rate to 23 % [4].

In the RUMBA study, when an alarm call of a suspected out-of-hospital cardiac arrest is received by the EMS dispatch operator a Mobile Positioning System (MPS) is activated. The MPS uses the mobile phone network to geographically locate all lay volunteers connected to a tailored mobile phone service called Mobile Life Saver (MLS). The MPS then locates all lay volunteers within a pre-defined radius from the suspected out-of-hospital cardiac arrest and alerts them with a computer generated voice call and a sms containing data about where the suspected out-of-hospital cardiac arrest is located. A map is also sent in order to make route finding easy.

The island of Langeland is a part of the rural Denmark. Langeland is just around 60 kilometres (km) long and around 10 km at its widest. The island is characterized by long ambulance response times and long distances to the local Svendborg Hospital approximately 20 – 50 km.

The island has a population of 13.000 inhabitants, but in the summertime the population grows, when approximately 260.000 tourists visit the holiday island.

The island has only one ambulance and one paramedic vehicle. That can cause very long response times in the case that the ambulance is reserved for another duty. The average ambulance response time is 12 minutes, but more than 33 % of the ambulances arrives after more than 15 minutes. There are additionally plans for closing the Emergency Unit at the local Svendborg Hospital and building a new common Emergency Unit at the Odense University Hospital, located approximately 85 kilometres from the distal parts of the island.

The messages about the long ambulance response times and closing down the local Emergency Unit were very essential for the inhabitants 6 years ago, when the idea about founding the Langeland AED association was born. The inhabitants understood that they could not expect the Public Emergency Services to save their lives in a case of an acute emergency or cardiac arrest. They needed to take part in the first aid, the cardiopulmonal resuscitation and to establish Public Access Defibrillation (PAD).

The Langeland AED association was established in March 2008 and the members collected money, raised funds for buying AEDs, AED cabinets and resuscitation kits. They also established small local AED associations and provided first aid training to the volunteer first responders. Today there are 32 local AED associations in the Langeland AED association. The population purchased 96 AEDs which are available around the clock and placed less than two kilometres apart. Some of the AED's are placed in a temperature regulated, GPS controlled AED cabinets, which are localized and activated (emergency light and siren) by the new FirstAED alert system. The total fundraising amounted to approximately 340.000 €.

Adverts in the local newspaper, posters in the town and streamers on the cars were the media used to encourage the citizens to become first responders. Two hundred and fifteen volunteer first responders in the age 18-72 years were recruited in 2011 and they all received a 12 hours basic first aid training course (Airway, Breath, Circulation, Disability protocol) including cardiopulmonal resuscitation and how to use an AED. Every year all the first responders receive a 3 hours back up training course including a new theme like bacic pediatric life support, basic trauma life support (assess injuries, stabilization of cervical spine, seal wounds etc.).

In the beginning of the project, various models for calling the first responders where tried. At first, a model with information cards/posters with the AED owner contact details in combination with local telephone calls was tried, but very soon, this model proved not to be effective. Next an emergency telephone call to the first responder registered in the Danish AED registry (www.hjertestarter.dk) was tried, again without major improvement in response times. At last a model with emergency text messages sent to the local first responders was tested. But it became obvious that none of the models where effective enough in a rural area like the island of Langeland to shorten the response time for first responders to less than 5 minutes.

Often the first volunteer first responder was too far away to help, and the next volunteer first responder on the list had to be called loosing valuable seconds or even minutes in the resuscitation process. Generally the first responder arrived to the emergency scene after 8-10 minutes. They were often alone helping the patient, providing comfort to the relatives and sometimes giving cardiopulmonary resuscitation or basic trauma support, which could be a very dramatic and stressful experience – especially since the outcome was often dubious.

The Langeland AED association experienced that they needed to develop a more optimal dispatching system to the volunteers on the island. The smartphone application FirstAED was developed. The FirstAED solution GPS track the first responders smartphones. FirstAED is an auxiliary to the public services and it enables the emergency dispatcher to send an organized team of first responders with distinct roles to the scene.

All the 200 first responders were asked to buy their own rescuer smartphone (iPhone 4S/5). Some of the first responders were too old to use smartphones or to poor to buy the smartphone for the price 530 €, but a lot of new younger people were attracted by the smartphone solution.

2   Aim

2.1   Reduction in First Responder Response Time and AED on Site Time

The smartphone application FirstAED was developed with the target to reduce the first responder response time at emergency calls to below 5 minutes and to secure arrival of an AED within 6 minutes in a rural part of Denmark.

2.2   Organization of First Responders in a Rescue Team Structure

The project defines a new way to dispatch the nearby first responders and organize their roles in a rescue team structure in the hope of reducing response times, establishing early Public Access Defibrillation (PAD) and improving survival rates.

2.3 Assessment of the Cowork between First Responders and Paramedics/ Ambulance Staff

The project assess the extent to which volunteer first responders can help the paramedics and the ambulance staff in the rescue missions.

3   Methods

3.1   Setting

This study evaluate (preevaluate) all initial calls to EMS Ambulance Funen from April 1, 2012 to December 31, 2013 in which an emergency situation or out-of-hospital cardiac arrest was suspected and first responders had been alerted by the FirstAED Alert on the island of Langeland.

The project was designed in collaboration between the department of Cardiology at the Odense University Hospital, the Region of Southern Denmark and the Langeland AED association.

3.2   Emergency Medical System and FirstAED

Emergency Medical System (EMS) Ambulance Rudkoebing serves the island of Langeland in Denmark. Like all EMS's in Denmark, a national emergency telephone number, 112, is connected to the regional dispatch centre of the EMS. The dispatch centre is manned by experienced nurses who instruct different ambulance services with ambulance posts spread over the Region of Southern Denmark. When the nurse at the dispatch centre suspect an emergency situation or a cardiac arrest in the initial call (Danish Category A duty), one ambulance is dispatched. Immediately after dispatching the ambulance, the health care assistant manager at the dispatch centre activate the FirstAED GPS Alert system to dispatch three GPS tracked first responders. When the health care assistant manager activates the FirstAED GPS Alert system, the system GPS track all available first responders and the EMS FirstAED iPad shows the position of all the first responders and AEDs (Fig 1).

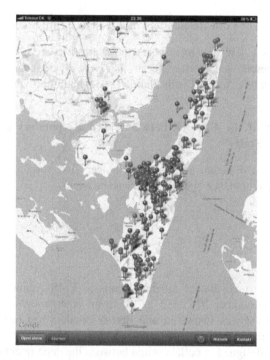

Fig. 1. Photo from EMS iPad showing the position of anonymised first responders (purple pushpins) and the 96 AEDs (green pushpins) a random day at the island of Langeland

The nurses uses following dispatching categories: Disease, Accident, Cardiac Arrest, Traffic Accident, Others (hanging, birth, diver with decompression sickness).

3.3   FirstAED-GPS-Alert Process

The FirstAED technology deployed on Langeland uses the Global Positioning System (GPS). GPS is a space-based satellite navigation system that provides location and time information anywhere on the Earth.

FirstAED is activated by the nurses at the central dispatch centre either on an iPad or by automatic signal from the Computer Aided Dispatch System. FirstAED Alert starts an automated communication sequence, GPS-track and send a push-message to the nine nearby first responders who can choose to accept or reject the alarm (Fig. 2).

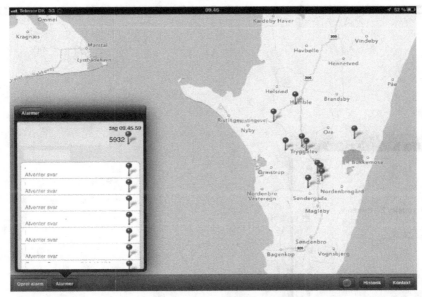

Fig. 2. Dispatch category Cardiac Arrest – 20 seconds after activation of the system. Photo from the EMS iPad showing the location of the geographically nearest nine first responders (purple pushpins) which were alerted via their iPhone. The place of the cardiac arrest is marked with the red pushpin.

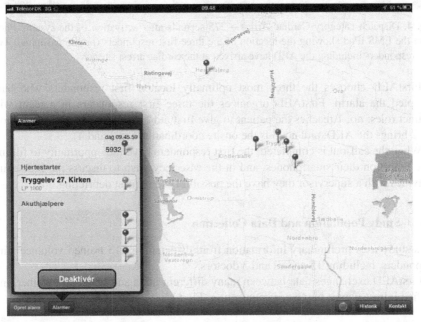

Fig. 3. Dispatch category Cardiac Arrest – 35 seconds after activation of the system. Photo from the EMS iPad showing the location of the three first responders (purple pushpins) who received distinct resuscitation tasks on their iPhone. The place of the cardiac arrest is marked with red pushpin and the place of the nearest AED is marked with the green pushpin.

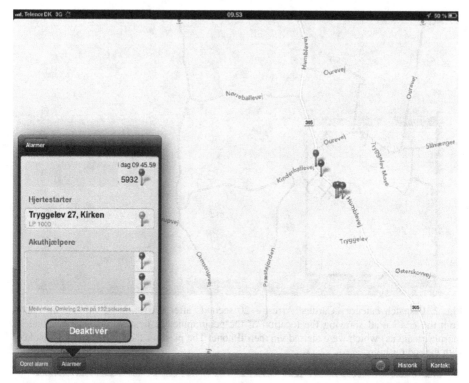

Fig. 4. Dispatch category Cardiac Arrest – 275 seconds after activation of the system. Photo from the EMS iPad showing the location of the three first responders (purple pushpins). Two first responders including the AED have arrived at the cardiac arrest site.

FirstAED chooses the three most optimally located first responders who have accepted the alarm. FirstAED organizes the three first responders in a team with distinct roles: no. 1 reaches the patient to give first aid/cardiopulmonary resuscitation; no. 2 brings the AED; and no. 3 is the onsite coordinator (Fig 3 and 4).

When the call-out is completed, the first responders have the opportunity to fill in a case report on their smartphones, and in the case they wish to discuss the life-saving activities with a supervisor they have the possibility to request debriefing.

3.4   Study Population and Data Collection

This study uses preliminary information from dispatching 215 trained volunteer first responders, including 15 nurses and 3 doctors.

FirstAED exchanges data between many different units and ties it all together, in a unified infrastructure-based communication (Fig 5).

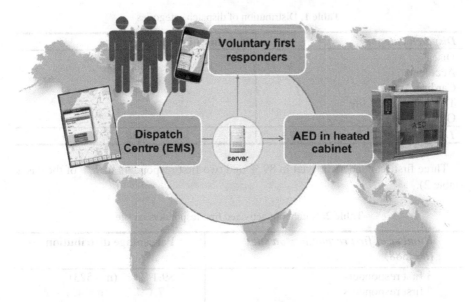

Fig. 5. FirstAED modern IT technology connects the healthcare assistant manager at the EMS dispatch centre, first responders and AEDs located in GPS controlled AED cabinets

The FirstAED IT-system collect dispatching data about the dispatching category, the emergency place location, the nine first responders involved in the alarm, the three first responders in the rescue team and their tasks, the GPS tracked first responder arrival time and the first responder case report.

Another part of the study compare the dispatching data with the Regional and University Hospital database, Cosmic. This part of the study will in the future look upon patient diagnoses, professional versus first responder response times, and evaluate 30 days and 12 months survival rates.

3.5 Statistical Analysis

Summary statistics (percentages, median value and range). All statistical analyses were performed with the use of the Excel statistical package.

4 Results

April 2012 the FirstAED system was implemented. During the first 21 months the FirstAED alarm system was used 588 times (table 1).

Table 1. Distribution of dispatch categories

Dispatch category	Number of dispatches
Disease	484
Accident	45
Cardiac Arrest	26
Traffic accident/ fire	21
Others	12
Total april 2012- december 2013	**588**

Three first responders arrived in 89 % and two first responders in 7 % of the cases (table 2).

Table 2. Number of activated first responders on site

Number of first responders on site (n = 588)	Percentage distribution	
3 first responders	89,1 %	(n = 523)
2 first responders	7,1 %	(n = 42)
1 first responder	3,1 %	(n = 18)
0 first responder	0,7 %	(n = 5)

The first first responder arrived before the paramedic/ambulance staff in 90 % or at the same time as the paramedic/ambulance staff in 8 % of the cases.

FirstAED entailed a significant reduction in first responder median response time from more than 8-10 minutes before to 4 minutes 9 seconds after (table 3). The first responder was on site in less than 5 minutes in more than 60 % of the cases.

Table 3. First first responder response time (median response time + range)

Response time – First first responder	Time
Median	249 sek.
Range	[1 – 1200 sek.]

The AED was on site within a median time of 5 minutes and 58 seconds (table 4).

Table 4. AED on site (median response time + range)

Response time – AED on site	Time
Median	358 sek.
Range	[1 – 1813 sek.]

During the first 21 months, the first responders were involved in 8 cardiac arrests (3 patients survived, 1 more than 30 days), 3 hangings (1 patient survived more than 30 days), 6 patients with serious respiratory insufficiency (5 patients survived more than 30 days), 25 patients with acute myocardial infarction (all survived more than 30 days), 1 patient with subarachnoid haemorrhage (complete restituted), 5 children with febrile seizures, two divers with decompression sickness (complete restituted) and positioning of more than 10 traffic accidents.

5   Conclusions

The new FirstAED solution has reduced the time to first responder and AED on site remarkably. It is ensured that in 98 % of the cases help from more than one person is quickly on-site. Peer support and feedback is provided to the first reponders.

The FirstAED technology implement strategic location of the AEDs, development of a team with responsibility for monitoring and maintaining the devices, training and retraining programmes for the volunteer first responders. FirstAED GPS-tracking reduces the first responder response times, and the quality of the effort improves as all the first responders who accept the FirstAED alarm have distinct roles. FirstAED localize and activate all the GPS activated AED cabinets, which makes it easy to collect the AED from the AED cabinet in foggy weather and dark nights. FirstAED is a logistic solution to reduce response times to below 5 minutes for first responder programmes. FirstAED defines a way to dispatch the nearby first responders and organize their roles in the hope of reducing response times, ensuring citizens safety and equal possibility to early defibrillation.

References

1. Wissenberg, M., Lippert, F.K., Folke, F., et al.: Association of National Initiatives to Improve Cardiac Arrest Management With Rates of Bystander Intervention and Patient Survival After Out-of-Hospital Cardiac Arrest. JAMA 310(13), 1377–1384 (2013)
2. Deakin, C.D., Nolan, J.P., Soar, J., et al.: European Resuscitation Council Guidelines for Resuscitation 2010. Section 4. Adult advanced life support. Resuscitation 81, 1305–1352 (2010)
3. Koster, R.W., Baubin, M.A., Bossaert, L.L., et al.: European Resuscitation Council Guidelines for Resuscitation 2010. Section 2. Adult basic life support and use of automated external defibrillators. Resuscitation 81, 1277–1292 (2010)
4. Dutch emergency care a global model - Response time down to eight minutes when locals gets involved. ESC Congress News 2013 - Amsterdam (2013)
5. Ringh, M., Fredman, D., Nordberg, P., et al.: Mobil phone technology identifies and recruits trained citizens to perform CPR on out-of-hospital cardiac arrest victims prior to ambulance arrival. Resuscitation 82, 1514–1518 (2011)

Tweeting about Diabetes and Diets – Content and Conversational Connections

Kim Holmberg[1,2], Kristina Eriksson-Backa[2,3], and Stefan Ek[2,3]

[1] Department of Organization Sciences, VU University Amsterdam, Amsterdam, Netherlands
[2] School of Business and Economics, Information Studies, Åbo Akademi University,
Turku, Finland
[3] Medical Research Center Oulu, Oulu, Finland
{kim.holmberg,krieriks,sek}@abo.fi

Abstract. The aim of this paper is to analyze 1) the semantic content of tweets discussing diabetes and diets, and 2) the conversational connections of those tweeting and those being mentioned in the tweets. The content analysis of the tweets aims at mapping what kinds of diets are mentioned in conversations about diabetes and in what context. Our data consists of 9,042 tweets containing the words "diabetes" and "diet". The findings indicate that analyzing Twitter conversations can be an efficient way to map public opinions about diabetes and diets. The results also showed that many private persons act as diabetes advocates spreading information and news about diabetes and diets. Surveying these topics can be useful for healthcare practitioners; as these are in contact with patients with diabetes, it is important that they are aware of both the most discussed topics and the most common information sources, who are often laymen.

Keywords: diabetes, diets, health, health communication, health information, health information dissemination, information sharing, social media, social networks, tweets, Twitter.

1 Introduction

The rapid increase of the worldwide prevalence of diabetes has been called epidemic [1], even a "silent pandemic" [2]. Estimates suggest that diabetes was the fifth leading cause of death globally in the year 2000 [3]. It has also been projected that from 2010 to 2030, there will be a 69% increase in numbers of adults with diabetes in developing countries and a 20% increase in developed countries, respectively [4]. In Finland, a good 8% of the adult population have diabetes, and an additional 9% of the population suffer from impaired glucose tolerance, i.e. prediabetes [5]. In the U.S., there are already as many as 79 million people with prediabetes, representing more than one-third of the adult population and half of people aged over 64 years [6]. Their risk of developing type 2 diabetes is estimated to be 4–12 times higher than it is for people with normal glucose tolerance [7]. The overall risk of dying among people with diabetes is at least double the risk of their peers without diabetes [3]. Attempts to tackle

K. Saranto et al. (Eds.): WIS 2014, CCIS 450, pp. 46–56, 2014.
© Springer International Publishing Switzerland 2014

this development are, hence, needed, and as communication plays a crucial role in influencing people's attitudes and behavior, the role of information and communication related to diabetes is an important topic. Online health communication that is dynamic, in contrast to static as traditional health-related web sites are, offers users with certain conditions an opportunity to benefit from social networks to learn about the condition, and to be supported by others with similar experiences [8]. Social networking tools offer the potential of supported learning, networking with peers, families and friends, as well as sharing problems, processes and outcomes with a global community [9]. Social networking sites can, furthermore, narrow online information to something that is relevant to specific users. It can even help to create what can be called a collective intelligence [10]. The aim of this paper is to analyze the semantic content of tweets discussing diabetes and diets, and the conversational connections of those tweeting and those being mentioned in the tweets.

2   Social Media and Health Information

It has been argued that social networks could become central to future health care delivery. Currently health information from social networks complements traditional sources but social networks have the potential to change patterns of health inequalities and access to health care [11]. Evermore researchers have started to show interest in health-related content on social media, especially as information sources for groups of patients [e.g., 9]. Shaw and Johnson [12] studied the online health information seeking behavior of a group of diabetics in the US, in order to see if they use social media and if they would be willing to use these sites to discuss health information. The 57 diabetics surveyed were quite active online users; 86% sought online health information, and 82% sought information about diabetes. Nearly 60% of the respondents did, furthermore, use sites such as Facebook or MySpace, 73% read online blogs, and about 50% watched YouTube, but less than 20% used Twitter. As many as 65% of the respondents, furthermore, said that they would be willing to discuss health information in an online environment such as chat rooms, discussion groups, or online support groups.

The contents of the shared information have interested several researchers. Greene et al. [8] conducted a content analysis of discussions about diabetes on Facebook in 2009 and found that most posts (66%) were information-providing and described users' personal experiences with diabetes management, whereas 29% of the posts tried to provide emotional support. Promotional posts that are often advertisements for "natural" products, was the third most common category (27%). According to Winston [13], Twitter can encourage members of, for example, communities of diabetics to share experiential knowledge, such as their health stories. Through the process of sharing information members of these so-called end-user communities learn from one another as well as have an opportunity to develop themselves. Clinical knowledge, on the other hand, is shared by e.g. hospitals and can include real time broadcasts of surgeries. Winston [13] conducted a case study of a juvenile diabetic and found that experiential knowledge was the type that was mainly tweeted. This included reports on daily events, practical guides on how to take a blood sugar count, and problems to maintain sports activities. Heaivilin et al. [14], on the other hand, investigated the contents of 1,000 tweets about dental pain from 7 non-consecutive days. The most common categories were general statements of dental pain (83%), actions taken in response to toothache (22%), and impact on daily life (15%). Scan-feld et al. [15] reported a content analysis of tweets in order to determine the main categories of content mentioning antibiotics and to explore cases of misunderstanding and misuse. They found that Twitter is a space for informal sharing of health informa-tion and advice. Most commonly antibiotics were mentioned in the category "general use", including tweets about taking antibiotics, followed by "advice and information", including references and links to news articles, with the category "side ef-fects/negative reactions" in third place. Misunderstandings were often connected to the belief that antibiotics would help in the case of colds. Twitter has, furthermore, interested researchers as a source for gathering of data about how an epidemic spreads, as was the case during the Influenza A H1N1 (swine flu) outbreak in 2009 [16-17].

One of the drawbacks of the amount of health information on the internet is that it can be inaccurate or misleading, and information on social networking sites does not necessarily form any exception. Despite of high ratings, a website can be scientifical-ly inaccurate [10]. The study by Weitzman et al. [18] on the quality and safety of diabetes-related social networks did, in fact, show varying quality, as only around half of the studied sites contained contents that were aligned with diabetes science or clin-ical practice recommendations. Twitter, as a particular type of social media, enables rapid, global communications between people with shared interests and information dissemination to a wide audience. Because the tweets are limited to a maximum of 140 characters the users do not need to put much effort in creating content and updates can be more frequent than for traditional blog posts. As such, Twitter has become a popular platform for conversations about health conditions, diseases, and medicines [e.g., 19] and it could, furthermore, provide an effective information chan-nel for practitioners to provide relevant information [9]. Twitter has a large potential of disseminating information through the networks of followers and the culture of retweeting, but this information can be both valid and invalid [15]. It has, in fact, been found that it is more common that health-related tweets link to news web sites, than to sites of government and public health authorities [16].

3   Aim and Methods

One of the most important factors associated with our well-being is our diet. This is even more important concerning people with diabetes, who usually need to apply restrictions to their diet. Diets can be sensitive to vagaries of fashion [20-21]; and as especially social networks spread information (and misinformation) rapidly and wide-ly, it is important to be aware of the nature of discussions about this matter. The aim of this paper is to analyze 1) the semantic content of tweets discussing diabetes and diets, and 2) the conversational connections of those tweeting and those being mentioned in the tweets. The content analysis of the tweets aims at mapping what kind of diets are mentioned in conversations about diabetes and in what context (e.g. diets that help and diets that do not help). By mapping the most frequent conversational connections of those involved in the diabetes conversations (i.e. those sending the tweets and those being mentioned in the tweets) we will use methods from social network analysis to explore a) the opinion leaders in the conversations and b) the sources mentioned in the messages.

Towards that goal a total of 607,905 tweets containing the word "diabetes" were collected via Twitter's API using Webometric Analyst (http://lexiurl.wlv.ac.uk/) between October 4 and November 6, 2013. These tweets were sent by 349,551 different tweeters. Of these tweets a total of 9,042 contained the word "diet". These tweets were sent by 6,116 different tweeters.

In order to analyze the semantic content of the tweets the frequently used noun phrases (i.e. word sequences of nouns and adjectives that end with a noun) were extracted from the tweets using VOSviewer [22] and the semantic word map created from the co-occurrences of the noun phrases was visualized with Gephi [23]. To focus on the most frequently discussed topics related to diabetes and diets we filtered the word map by including only the noun phrases that were mentioned 5 or more times and that were connected to other noun phrases at least twice. This left us with 266 nodes that were connected to each other through 497 edges. Using the built-in community detection algorithm in Gephi we visualized the local clusters in the map.

By conversational connections we mean pairs of authors of the tweets and usernames they mentioned in the tweets. These author-username pairs were extracted from the tweets with Webometric Analyst and converted into a network map. The network was visualized with Gephi and the built-in Force Atlas layout. Methods from social network analysis were used to analyze the conversational connections. Both indegree and outdegree were calculated for each node in the graph in order to map who were frequently initiating conversations (outdegree) and who were frequently mentioned (indegree) in the tweets.

4   Results

A total of 25 communities of tightly connected noun phrases were detected in the graph (Figure 1) using the built-in Laplacian community detection in Gephi. Because we chose to focus on the most frequently mentioned noun-phrases these 25 clusters represent the very core of the Twitter communications about diabetes and diets.

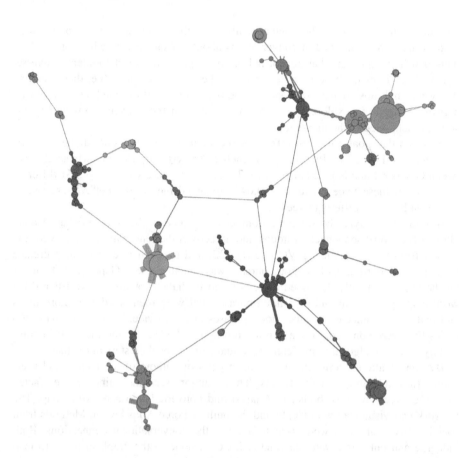

Fig. 1. Semantic map from the co-occurrences of the noun phrases in the tweets about diabetes and diets (modularity = 0,917)

A closer look at the clusters and connections between the noun phrases reveal for instance a connection between "gestational diabetes" and "carb diet" in the Twitter conversations (figure 2), however, the connection was created due to a frequently tweeted and retweeted article sent by @medpagetoday stating that:

Low Carb Diet Won't Help in Gestational Diabetes http://t.co/1loKmtqMLH @medpagetoday

"Carb diet" was mentioned in 192 tweets, and "low carb diet" was mentioned 222 times. Other diets mentioned include (in alphabetical order) bean diet (51 tweets), celeb diet (5), Cuban diet (19), fat diet (39), high fat diet (47), low calorie diet (56), super diet (11), and a certain "new diet" by an American media personality was mentioned 130 times.

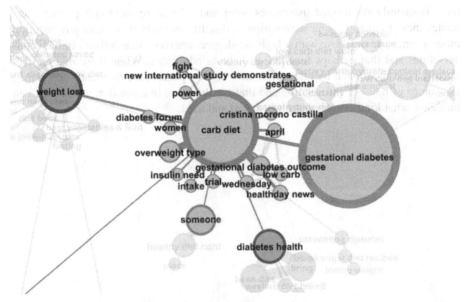

Fig. 2. Noun phrases connected to "carb diet"

Another example of frequently discussed topics is gastric bypass surgeries or bariatric surgeries:

Diabetes Improvements After Gastric Bypass Due to Diet: The finding is based on a prospective study of 10 pati... http://t.co/EMhQjUwClR

Content analysis of the tweets showed that the tweets frequently contained URLs as sources of information and news; a total of 5,941 URLs were included in the 9,042 tweets that were analyzed. Although analyzing the content of the webpages shared was beyond the scope of this research, it appears that at least some of the URLs were blog entries and other webpages containing diabetes news for which the author or owner of the website could not be verified. In some cases it was clear that the webpage functioned as an entry page to a commercial site and that it was perhaps also created to improve the ranking of the website in search engines by increasing the number of links to the website. Having said that, there were also some URLs to news and information provided by various diabetes organizations for which sources and affiliations could be verified.

The single most frequently retweeted tweet was a tweet with a tip from @droz. Slightly different versions of the tweet were retweeted almost 700 times:

@droz never too late to prevent diabete add teaspoon of vinegar to your diet daily to lower your blood sugar #oztip

The conversational connections were also mapped (Figure 3) and the in-degrees and out-degrees of the usernames were compared. This allowed us to map who the

most frequently mentioned usernames were and who were mentioning other usernames most frequently. Our assumption is that the tweeters that frequently mention
other usernames, i.e. those with a high out-degree, are those that actively initiate conversations and that perhaps function as diabetes advocates. While those that are frequently been mentioned by others, i.e. have high in-degree, are frequently mentioned
as sources of news or information and that are therefore in a position where they can
influence what kind of information is shared and used.

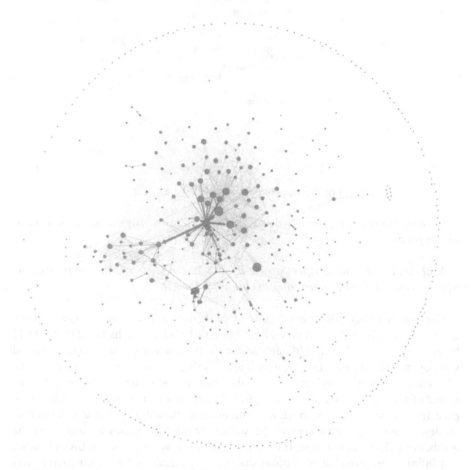

Fig. 3. Conversational connections in the diabetes communications on Twitter (node size
equals degree centrality, edge thickness equals number of connections (mentions) between the
tweeters)

The strongest connections are between @1Medical2News, an account tweeting and
retweeting breaking medical news, and accounts that belong to a company specialized
in medical technology (@EveryDayHealth, 366 co-mentions), a news sharing account
from a company specialized in medical technology (@diabetesfacts, 288 co-
mentions), and a UK based charity organization (@DiabetesUK, 200 co-mentions).

The Twitter accounts that were most frequently mentioned in the tweets, i.e. had the highest in-degree, were American Diabetes Association (in-degree = 82), Sanofi[1] US Diabetes (80), Diabetes Mine[2] (60), JDRF Juvenile Diabetes Research Foundation (57), and Diabetes Hands Foundation[3] (56). The out-degrees for the remaining usernames were less than 50. The two Twitter accounts with clearly highest out-degree (i.e. usernames that mentioned other usernames most frequently) were Divabetic (out-degree = 93), which is "a national nonprofit organization that empowers women affected with diabetes to stay healthy and positive about their diabetes self-care management", and 1Medical2News (89), an account tweeting breaking medical news and information. The out-degrees for the remaining usernames were less than 50.

We chose the usernames with an in-degree of 20 or higher (44 users) and the usernames with an out-degree of 20 or higher (47 users) for closer analysis and coded the usernames based on the type or role of the user (Table 1). Private persons were both frequently mentioned (38.6%) and frequently mentioning other usernames (53.2%). Among those with high in-degrees were more organizations, compared to those with high out-degrees, indicating how organizations of various types are frequently mentioned in tweets, perhaps as sources of information, but they are not that active at connecting with other users.

Table 1. Usernames with highest in-degrees and highest out-degrees coded by role

	Role of usernames with high in-degree	Role of usernames with high out-degree
company	13.6% (6)	12.8% (6)
magazine	4.5% (2)	2.1% (1)
news sharing	6.8% (3)	4.3% (2)
online community	4.5% (2)	6.4% (3)
organization	20.5% (9)	8.5% (4)
private person	38.6% (17)	53.2% (25)
research	9.1% (4)	6.4% (3)
other	2.3% (1)	6.4% (3)
	100.0% (44)	100.0% (47)

Overall there were some overlap between the usernames with high in-degree and usernames with high out-degree (r = 0.534).

---

[1] "Sanofi US is part of a leading global healthcare company that discovers, develops, produces and markets innovative therapies to help protect health and enhance people's lives." http://www.sanofi.us/

[2] "Diabetes newspaper with a personal twist." http://www.diabetesmine.com/about

[3] "Our mission is to bring together people touched by diabetes for positive change so that nobody living with this condition ever feels alone." http://diabeteshandsfoundation.org/

5   Discussion

Social media are ever more commonly used as sources for information related to health issues. One of the most alarming health threats today is diabetes [3], and hence diabetes and social media have started to attract the interest among the research community [8], [12-13]. This paper adds to the growing knowledge around this topic and presents results of a study on the semantic content of a total of 9,042 tweets discussing diabetes and diets between October 4 and November 6, 2013, as well as the conversational connections of those tweeting and those being mentioned in the tweets.

Content analysis has been used previously to analyze health-related content in Twitter conversations, including content related to diabetes [8], [14-16], but to the best of our knowledge, no one has previously studied related concepts concerning diet and diabetes in Twitter posts and presented them in semantic maps. Health-related tweets are often experiential, that is, the tweeters are tweeting about their own experiences of, for example, diabetes management [8] [13], dental pain [14], use of antibiotics [15], or smoking cessation [24]. In the case of the swine flu outbreak in 2009, however, personal experiences came second to the category resources, meaning tweets containing news or updates, possibly containing a link to an article [16]. In our study of diabetes and diets, the tweets were frequently of this resource type as roughly two thirds of the tweets contained a URL. It is somewhat alarming that many of these URLs appeared to be blogs and other news sites for which the author or the owner could not be verified, and hence, the information on these sites should be treated with caution. Yet, these URLs were frequently shared on Twitter without any discussion of the accuracy or reliability of the information on them. More research is, however, needed to find out what exactly the proportion of these somewhat questionable sites is in the diabetes discussion on Twitter.

The results showed that many private persons act as diabetes advocates spreading information and news about diabetes and diets. Also previous research has shown that the resources the tweets link to are not necessarily scientific. In the case of tweets about the swine flu, around 23% of all tweets linked to a news web site, whereas only 1.5% linked to sites of government and public health authorities [16]. Weitzman et al. [18], furthermore, reported that also many diabetes-related social network sites lack a link to, for example, a specific disease or professional association, which affects the quality of the contents. In the current study, however, the American Diabetes Association obtained the highest in-degree, that is, it was the Twitter account that was most frequently mentioned in the tweets.

Surveying Twitter for people's opinions has advantages: tweeting about experiences of health-related issues often happens in real-time, and the risk of recall bias is diminished. Users also represent a global community, and posting can be quite frequent, not the least by the increased use of mobile devices. People are also keen on sharing their experiences, perhaps because they find comfort in the fact that they are not alone on the matter, or possibly because they want to seek advice [14]. Despite the fact that Twitter users are not representative for the entire population [14] [16-17], and although some posts might be embellished or exaggerated [15], tweets can be a rich and relevant source of data [16-17].

It has been shown that diabetics frequently seek online health information and are willing to discuss health-related topics in social settings [12]. For healthcare practitioners knowledge about the topics that were found in the current study can be very useful; as these are in contact with patients with diabetes they need to be aware of people's opinions and beliefs, and also about the source people use to get their information (and misinformation) from. This is especially important as some tweets contain pure misunderstandings of, for example, the use of certain medications [15], and sometimes sensitive aspects of diabetes management that are not likely to be revealed to a doctor are discussed in social media, such as how you can extend your intake of alcohol [8]. A fair amount of the diabetes-related contents are, furthermore, promotional, often advertising products that are not approved in diabetes care [8] [18]. Lo and Parham [10] recommend that physicians promote the benefits of online information and minimize the risks and burdens of it, by guiding patients to use reliable websites, for example, and by not feeling threatened about the fact that patients might have sought information elsewhere. This recommendation can also be supported by the findings of this study.

6   Conclusions

The findings of this study indicate that analyzing Twitter conversations can be an efficient and cost-effective way to map as well as to instantly track short-term fluctuations in public opinions about diabetes and diets. It is important for health practitioners to be aware of both the most discussed topics and the most common information sources, who often are laymen. Because the discussions in social networks such as Twitter might have the potential to affect both the opinion and the behavior of their patients, this will help the practitioners to, for instance, be prepared to correct possible misunderstandings and cope with the possibility that their advice are questioned.

References

1. Bonow, R.O., Gheorghiade, M.D.: The Diabetes Epidemic: a National and Global Crisis. Am. J. Med. 116, 2S–10S (2004), doi:10.1016/j.amjmed.2003.10.014
2. Shaw, J., Tanamas, S.: Diabetes: the Silent Pandemic and its Impact on Australia. Baker IDI Heart and Diabetes Institute, Canberra (2012), http://www.healthinfonet.ecu.edu.au/key-resources/bibliography/?lid=22970 (retrieved on March 12, 2014)
3. Roglic, G., Unwin, N., Bennett, P.H., Mathers, C., Tuomilehto, J., Nag, S., Connolly, V., King, H.: The Burden of Mortality Attributable to Diabetes: Realistic Estimates for the Year 2000. Diabetes Care 28(9), 2130–2135 (2005)
4. Shaw, J.E., Sicree, R.A., Zimmet, P.Z.: Global Estimates of the Prevalence of Diabetes for 2010 and 2030. Diab. Res. Clin. Pract. 87, 4–14 (2010), doi:10.1016/j.diabres.2009.10.007
5. International Diabetes Federation: IDF Diabetes Atlas. International Diabetes Federation, Brussels (2009)
6. Bergman, M.: Inadequacies of Current Approaches to Prediabetes and Diabetes Prevention. Endocrine 44, 623–633 (2013)

7. Albright, A.L., Gregg, E.W.: Preventing Type 2 Diabetes in Communities across the U.S.: the National Diabetes Prevention Program. Am. J. Prev. Med. 44, S346–S351 (2013), doi:10.1016/j.amepre.2012.12.009

8. Greene, J.A., Chowdhury, N.K., Kilabuk, E., Shrank, W.H.: Online Social Networking by Patients with Diabetes: a Qualitative Evaluation of Communication with Facebook. J. Gen. Int. Med. 26, 287–292 (2010)

9. Pulman, A.: Twitter as a Tool for Delivering Improved Quality of Life for People with Chronic Conditions. J. Nurs. Healthc. Chronic Illn. 1, 245–252 (2009)

10. Lo, B., Parham, L.: The Impact of Web 2.0 on the Doctor-Patient Relationship. J. Law Med. Ethics 38, 17–26 (2010), doi:10.1111/j.1748-720X.2010.00462.x

11. Griffiths, F., Cave, J., Boardman, F., Ren, J., Pawlikowska, T., Ball, R., Clarke, A., Cohen, A.: Social Networks – the Future for Health Care Delivery. Soc. Sci. Med. 75, 2233–2241 (2012)

12. Shaw, R.J., Johnson, C.M.: Health Information Seeking and Social Media Use on the Internet among People with Diabetes. Online J. Public Health Inform. 3 (2011), doi:http://dx.doi.org/10.5210/ojphi.v3i1.3561

13. Winston, E.: What's this Twitter all About? An e-Patient's End-User Community (EUCY). Issues in Information Systems 11, 184–191 (2010), http://iacis.org/iis/2010/184-191_LV2010_1481.pdf (retrieved on March 31, 2014)

14. Heaivilin, N., Gerbert, B., Page, J.E., Gibbs, J.L.: Public Health Surveillance of Dental Pain via Twitter. J. Dent. Res. 90, 1047–1051 (2011), doi:10.1177/0022034511415273

15. Scanfeld, D., Scanfeld, V., Larson, E.: Dissemination of Health Information through Social Networks: Twitter and Antibiotics. Am. J. Infect. Control 38, 182–188 (2010)

16. Chew, C., Eysenbach, G.: Pandemics in the Age of Twitter: Content Analysis of Tweets During the 2009 H1N1 Outbreak. PLoS ONE 5, e14118 (2010), doi:10.1371/journal.pone.0014118

17. Signorini, A., Segre, A.M., Polgreen, P.M.: The Use of Twitter to Track Levels of Disease Activity and Public Concern in the U.S. During the Influenza A H1N1 Pandemic. PLoS ONE 6, e19467 (2011), doi:10.1371/journal.pone.0019467

18. Weitzman, E.R., Cole, E., Kaci, L., Mandl, K.D.: Social but Safe? Quality and Safety of Diabetes-Related Online Social Networks. J. Am. Med. Inform. Assoc. 18, 292–297 (2011), doi:10.1136/jamia.2010.009712

19. Prieto, V.M., Matos, S., Álvarez, M., Cacheda, F., Oliveira, J.L.: Twitter: a Good Place to Detect Health Conditions. PLoS ONE 9, e86191 (2014), doi:10.1371/journal.pone.0086191

20. Fakih, S., Hussainy, S., Marriott, J.: Women, Pharmacy and the World Wide Web: Could They Be the Answer to the Obesity Epidemic? Int. J. Pharm. Pract. 22, 103–165 (2014), doi:10.1111/ijpp.12020

21. Lee, S., Fowler, D., Yuan, J.: Characteristics of Healthy Foods as Perceived by College Students Utilizing University Foodservice. J. Foodserv. Bus. Res. 16, 169–182 (2013), doi:10.1080/15378020.2013.782239

22. Van Eck, N.J., Waltman, L.: Software Survey: VOSviewer, a Computer Program for Bibliometric Mapping. Scientometrics 84, 523–538 (2010)

23. Bastian, M., Heymann, S., Jacomy, M.: Gephi: an Open Source Software for Exploring and Manipulating Networks. In: Proceedings of the International AAAI Conference on Weblogs and Social Media (2009), http://gephi.org/publications/gephi-bastian-feb09.pdf (retrieved on February 11, 2014)

24. Prochaska, J.J., Pechmann, C., Kim, R., Leonhardt, J.M.: Twitter=Quitter? An Analysis of Twitter Quit Smoking Social Networks. Tob. Control 21, 447–449 (2012), doi:10.1136/tc.2010.042507

Documentation of the Clinical Phase of the Cardiac Rehabilitation Process in a Finnish University Hospital District

Lotta Kauhanen[1], Laura-Maria Murtola[1,2], Juho Heimonen[3,4], Tuija Leskinen[5], Kari Kalliokoski[5], Elina Raivo[1], Tapio Salakoski[3,4], and Sanna Salanterä[1,2]

[1] Department of Nursing Science, University of Turku, Finland
{anloka,lmemur,elina.k.raivo,sanna.salantera}@utu.fi
[2] Turku University Hospital, Turku, Finland
[3] Department of Information Technology, University of Turku, Finland
[4] TUCS - Turku Centre for Computer Science, Finland
{juaheim,tapio.salakoski}@utu.fi
[5] Turku PET Centre, University of Turku, Finland
{Tuija.Helena.Leskinen,Kari.Kalliokoski}@tyks.fi

Abstract. Cardiac rehabilitation (CR) is an essential part of the treatment and recovery process of cardiac patients by which mortality can be reduced. CR is documented in the patient's health records to ensure continuity of care. The aim of this study was to describe and evaluate the contents of the clinical phase documentation of CR according to the care notes of physical therapists and physiatrists. The data set used in this register-based study consisted of the electronic health records (EHR) of patients, with any type of cardiac problem admitted to a Finnish university hospital district between 2005 and 2009. The main findings indicate that 1) only a small part of the eligible patients' records include CR documentation 2) the patients with CR documentation are relatively old when compared to the age distribution of all cardiac patients ($p<0.001$), 3) the documentation does not systematically follow the national guidelines, 4) the evaluation of treatment is rarely documented, and 5) the most commonly documented therapy concerned walking- and breathing exercises.

Keywords: documentation, physical therapy, cardiac rehabilitation, electronic health records, patient safety, registry-based research.

1 Introduction

Cardiovascular diseases are a global burden by being among the most common conditions for premature death [1]. For example in Europe, cardiovascular diseases cause 47% of all deaths [2]. Patients with cardiac problems have also high post-discharge mortality and readmission rates [3] resulting in higher costs of care.

Cardiac rehabilitation (CR), including exercise-based intervention, reduces cardiac patient's all-cause mortality by 13% and cardiac mortality by 26% when compared to usual-care [4]. Therefore, CR has been recognized as an essential part of the treatment and recovery of cardiac patients before, during and after hospitalization [5].

K. Saranto et al. (Eds.): WIS 2014, CCIS 450, pp. 57–67, 2014.
© Springer International Publishing Switzerland 2014

CR is part of the hospitalization period in the Finnish specialized health care. CR should be documented in the patient's health records according to the Finnish legislation [6,7] and different physical therapists' guidelines [8,9]. High quality documentation is important to ensure the information transfer, continuity of care, legal security of patients and health care professionals, and also to evaluate the treatment progress and outcomes [10,11]. However, not all patients who have experienced a cardiac event are referred to CR [12]. A study conducted in 2007 in Finland revealed that only 10 % of patients who had experienced a cardiac event reported that they had received CR [12]. Therefore, in this study we explored the cardiac patients' electronic health records (EHR) that included physical therapy or physiatry documentation during the inpatient stay in specialized health care in one Finnish hospital district. The results of this study may be used in improving the CR documentation and CR information flow.

2   Literature Review

2.1   Cardiac Rehabilitation

CR means multi-disciplinary and comprehensive prevention and rehabilitation that consists of following components: patient assessment, physical activity counselling and exercise training, weight control management and nutritional counselling, lipid management, blood pressure monitoring, psychosocial management and smoking cessation [13]. CR consists of four phases which are I) the preoperative phase, II) the clinical phase, III) the outpatient rehabilitation phase and IV) the post-rehabilitation phase [14]. In this paper we will focus on the content of the physical therapy related documentation in the clinical phase of the CR.

Generally the goal of the clinical phase in the CR process is to increase the physical and physiological recovery of the patient after a cardiac event [13]. Cardiac patients should achieve or maintain functioning in activities of daily living, get knowledge and understanding of the disease and learn to cope with the symptoms. This can be achieved through mobilization, breathing exercises, functional exercises and counselling, which all are usually conducted by physical therapists [14]. Physical therapy is particularly important for surgical patients as it reduces the post-operational complications i.e. pulmonary complications [15].

The treatment for all patients with percutaneous coronary intervention, coronary artery bypass grafting, acute myocardial infarction, chronic stable angina pectoris, chronic heart failure, heart transplant, valvular surgery or arrhythmias should include CR that begins at the hospitalization period (phases I and II) and continues to the outpatient settings (phases III and IV) [16].

Physicians play a pivotal role to ameliorate the CR process as the patient's CR enrollment is highly associated to physicians' referrals [17,18,19]. However, it seems that on average only one third of the eligible patients are referred - resulting in highly underutilized CR programs [17], [19]. Therefore, more knowledge of the evidential benefits of CR programs and possibilities of the local outpatient CR programs need to be given to healthcare professionals.

To improve the allocation of CR to all eligible patients we need to get familiar with the existing processes. By analyzing patient records we can seek the strengths and/or pitfalls in the current documentation of CR and also get data of the patients receiving CR in the clinical phase. However, the results of an analysis of patients' records does not necessarily reflect on real-life situations or actual physical therapy or physiatry events, but they describe the stage of the documentation.

2.2   The Importance of Health Care Documentation

Well-executed documentation of patient care is an essential part of the patient safety [20] since poor information transfer and communication failures are a usual cause of errors and adverse events in patient care [21]. Documentation is governed and controlled by Finnish legislation [6,7] and international [8] and national guidelines [9]. The health care professionals should document all medical information that is relevant in patient care according to the Finnish legislation concerning patients' rights [6(12§)]. This documentation includes care organization and planning, patients' health related observations, conducted procedures and monitoring of the care [6,7(7§)]. The care of hospitalized patients should be continuously and chronologically documented into the patients' health records [7(14§)]. Accurate documentation improves communication between professionals and facilitates high quality care. However, both the documentation [11] and the structure [22] of EHRs needs improvements to better support the professionals.

According to the World Confederation for Physical Therapy, physical therapy documentation is a process that includes *"recording of all aspects of patient care including the results of the initial examination/assessment and evaluation, diagnosis, prognosis, plan of care/intervention/treatment, interventions/treatment, response to interventions/treatment, changes in patient/client status relative to the interventions/treatment, re-examination, and discharge/discontinuation of intervention and other patient management activities."* [8]. The Finnish Physical therapy association recommends that the electronic documentation should include these phases regardless of the method of implementation, the length of the process or the service provider. The implemented physical therapy should be documented on a specific sheet in the patient's health record that is intended only for physical therapy notes. [9]

EHRs are used throughout the health care sector to longitudinally document the health related information of an individual. These systems are used by a variety of health professionals e.g. physiotherapists, nurses and physicians, and one of the main purposes of these systems is to support the continuity of a patients care [23].

The association between the quality of the note's in EHRs and quality of care has not yet been widely studied [24]. However, some evidence that a weak information transfer is associated with errors in care exists [21]. Edwards et al. (2013) did not find a significant association between the quality of physician notes and the quality of care, but they found great deficiencies in the documentation, such as lack of documentation of the reason for visit, medication, and timing for follow-up [24]. It is also suggested that electronic documentation may help in preventing diagnostic errors and quality of care [25]. The variability in the documentation habits and the complexity of required data elements in the EHRs makes the quality measurement rather difficult [26].

In nursing documentation studies, the content of the documentation is the most used audit approach to evaluate documentation. The nursing process has been used in several studies as a theoretical framework for analysis. [11] A review of 77 studies indicated that the nursing process was inadequately reported in a number of studies. In addition, documentation flaws concern patient assessment, preferences, previous health behavior, knowledge needs, quality of life, psychological, social, cultural and spiritual aspects of care and patient education [11]. A study of CR documentation by Bergh et al. (2007) found that nurses rarely document patient education activities of the CR process [27]. In a small descriptive study of 20 physical therapy records in stroke rehabilitation a lack of information about environment and participation was found in documentation [28].

To our knowledge, no previous studies of the contents of physical therapists' CR documentation exists. Therefore, in this study, we aimed to explore the documentation related to physical therapy, written on a specific physical therapy sheet in the patients' EHRs, to find new ways to support the continuity of physical therapy during the cardiac rehabilitation process in Finnish health care.

3   The Study Aims

The aim of this novel study is to describe and evaluate the contents of the clinical phase documentation of CR from the care notes written on a specific physical therapy or physiatry sheets in the patients' EHRs. The study follows a retrospective register-based research design.

The study focuses on the following questions:
1. How many patients with primary cardiac diagnose have CR documentation in the physical therapy or physiatry sheets in the EHRs?
2. What are the cardiac patients' demographics (age, sex) who have CR documentation in the physical therapy or physiatry sheets in the EHRs?
3. Does the documentation of the given CR follow the national guidelines?
4. What are the contents of physical therapy documented in the EHRs?

4   Methodology

The analysis was performed at the level of care episodes. We used a data set consisting of the EHRs of patients admitted to a Finnish university hospital with any type of cardiac problem as a primary or secondary diagnosis during a period of 2005 to 2009. The permission to access and use the data for research purposes had been obtained from the Ethics Committee Hospital District of Southwest Finland (17.2.2009 §67) and the Medical director of the Hospital District of Southwest Finland (2/2009). The data were anonymised prior to handing it to the research group. The data were processed and quantitatively analyzed with scripts written in the

Python programming language specifically for this purpose. Statistical analyses were done using IBM SPSS Statistical software.

The information regarding the care episodes was extracted from summary notes, each of which specifically contains the care dates and the ICD-10 diagnosis codes [29]. The data of 187566 care episodes was first filtered to include only those episodes in which a cardiac diagnosis was the primary diagnosis (n=40363). Second, the selection was further filtered to obtain the episodes that also included at least one physical therapy or physiatry sheet (n=465). Third, the background demographics of the patients with a cardiac diagnose in the whole data and in the selected episodes were extracted from the register. The age distributions were compared using two-sample t-test and the sex distribution using chi-square test.

A random sample of 100 care episodes of the selected 465 was analyzed. A sample size was decided due to the pilot nature of this study. The physical therapy or physiatry sheets of the selected care episodes were read and manually analysed by a domain expert. The analysis was conducted by using a deductive content analysis. According to the previous studies [11], the physical therapy process was used as the theoretical framework for the analysis of the CR documentation.

5   Results

5.1   Descriptive Statistics

Care Episodes
The overall register-based data contained 187566 care episodes of 26882 patients (55.4 % males). Of these, 40363 episodes had a cardiac diagnosis as the primary diagnosis but only 465 of them additionally contained physical therapy or physiatry sheets (722 and 17 notes in total, respectively). Thus, only 1.2% of the care episodes with a cardiac diagnosis as the primary diagnosis included physical therapy or physiatry sheets. Overall, these episodes covered 2.2% of the patients having a primary cardiac diagnosis.

Patient Demographics
The relative frequencies of birth years of all the patients in the data (n=26882, 55,4% males), of the patients with primary cardiac diagnosis (n=18094, 58.2% males) and of the patients with primary cardiac diagnosis and CR notes (n=380, 55.8% males) are shown in Figure 1. From the patients who had physical therapy or physiatry sheets 63.7% were born in 1920's and 1930's being 70 to 80 years old at the time of therapy. The age distribution of the group of patients that had primary cardiac diagnose and CR notes were significantly different from the group of all patients with primary cardiac diagnose (p<0,001). The mean age difference between these two patient groups was 5,4 years. The interquartile range of birth years was 16 years (median 1933, min 1908, max 1983). The sex distribution did not differ significantly in within the group of patients that had primary cardiac diagnose and CR notes and group of all patients with primary cardiac diagnose.

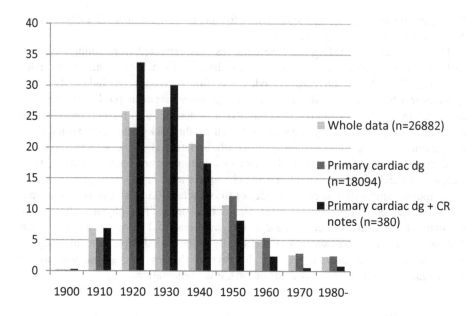

Fig. 1. Demographics, relative frequencies (f%) of birth years of all the patients in the data, of the patients with primary cardiac diagnosis and of the patients with primary cardiac diagnosis and CR notes

5.2   The Results of the Content Analysis

With the content analysis we wanted to explore the focus of physiotherapists practicing in CR through identifying the key elements in clinical physiotherapy documentation.

The results from the analysis of the random sample of 100 physical therapy and physiatry care episodes indicated that a written physical therapy referral from the attending physician were found in 81 care episodes, an oral referral documented by physical therapist were found in 6 care episodes, and no documentation about the referral were found in 13 care episodes (Table 1). The phases of the physical therapy process seen in the notes are illustrated in table 2, e.g., indicating that only in 35 care episodes the response to interventions or changes in patient status relative to the interventions was actually documented.

Table 1. The documentation of the physical therapy referral from the attending physician

The referral from the attending physician documented	The amount of care episodes (n=100)
A written referral	81%
No referral documented	13%
An oral request documented by PT	6%

Table 2. The phases of physical therapy process seen in the care notes

The phase of the physical therapy process	The amount of care episodes (n=100)
Prerequisites mentioned [a]	59%
Examination/assessment and treatment plan [b]	64%
Interventions/treatment documented [c*]	84%
Response to interventions/treatment or changes in patient status relative to the interventions/treatment	35%

[a] Yes also if referenced to look at the prerequisites from another sheet.

[b] At least one of the following must have been mentioned: examination, assessment, evaluation, observation, treatment objectives, methods or plan of care.

[c] What was done in the therapy session i.e. therapy methods, consultation, clinical tests.

[*] See table 3 for detailed contents.

The discharge/discontinuation of an intervention or other patient activities related to patient care were mentioned in 57/100 care episodes leaving 43 care episodes without a mention of the therapy continuum (Table 3). In 15 care episodes out of the 57 the physical therapy follow-up was mentioned, in 36 care episodes a given guidance (written material or oral discussion) was mentioned and in 6 care episodes there were documentation about both guidance and physical therapy continuum in another unit. The documentation about specific interventions or treatments concerned most often walking aid or other aid evaluation (57/100) and walking exercises (54/100). Breathing/coughing exercises were mentioned in 35/100 care episodes and sitting, standing and standing up exercises were mentioned in 31/100 care episodes. Muscular strength training exercise or active range of motion exercises were mentioned in 29/100 care episodes. Furthermore, the patients' own perceptions were documented relatively well, in 62 of 100 care episodes. (Table 3.)

Table 3. Interventions/treatment documented in physical therapy and physiatry care notes

Content of the interventions/treatment documentation	The amount of care episodes (n=100)
Patients' own perceptions documented (patient tells, wishes, wants, says)	62%
Walking aid evaluation or other aids mentioned	57%
The discharge/discontinuation of an intervention or other patient activities related to patient care	57%
Walking exercises	54%
Breathing/coughing exercises	35%
Sitting, standing and standing up exercises (including sitting or standing balance exercises)	31%

Table 3. (*continued*)

Muscular strength training exercise or active range of motion exercises	29%
Active or assistive stretching or joint mobility exercises	20%
Passive and assistive range of motion exercises including position therapy	13%
Stair climbing exercises	12%
6-minute walk test	8%
Relaxation exercises	5%
Cryotherapy	4%
Heat treatment	2%
Impulse electrotherapy	2%
Berg Balance Scale	1%

6   Discussion

The main findings of this study indicate that in a Finnish university hospital district in specialized health care 1) only a small part of the eligible patients' records include CR documentation, 2) the patients who have CR documentation are relatively old compared to the age distribution in all cardiac patients (p<0,001), 3) the documentation of the clinical phase of CR process does not systematically follow the national guidelines [9], since different practices occur on where and how CR is documented in the clinical phase, 4) the response to interventions/treatment and the effectiveness of CR is rarely documented (exiting only in 35% of the notes), and 5) the most commonly documented therapy contents were walking aid evaluation, walking- and breathing exercises.

Based on these findings, it seems that the existing documentation procedures do not support good quality documentation. The results show that 2.2% of the patients having a primary cardiac diagnosis had clinical phase CR documentation in physical therapy or physiatry sheets. However, the small amount (2.2%) does not necesserily equate to realistic amount of the patients that actually received physical therapy or physiatry consultation. Our hypothesis is that in most cases the physical therapy is documented in the daily nursing care notes under the title "physical therapy" to ensure a sufficient information transfer between the physical therapists and nursing staff. Thus, the goal of this approach is reasonable but the documentation outcome is not in accordance with the national documentation guidelines. In further studies, it is important to investigate also the daily nursing care notes to possibly achieve more accurate state of the clinical phase CR documentation.

Our results support the earlier literature that many deficiencies in the documentation in EHRs exists and further investigation in the area is warranted [11], [24], [27,28]. The results of our study are useful for the health care professionals conducting clinical phase in the CR process, and should therefore be noted among physical therapists, health care leaders, and other health care providers responsible for documentation in hospitals as well as researchers in the field of patient safety, documentation and CR.

Authors' Contributions. LK, LMM, JH, TL, KK, ER, TS and SS participated in the design of the study. The original manuscript was drafted by LK and reviewed and commented by LMM, JH, TL, KK, ER, TS and SS. LK, JH and TL conducted the data analyses.

Acknowledgements. The Academy of Finland is gratefully acknowledged for providing the funding for the IKITIK research project (140323/2010) which this project is part of.

References

1. World Health Organization. Global status report on noncommunicable disaeses 2010. Geneva, World Health Organization (2011a),
   `http://www.who.int/nmh/publications/ncd_report_full_en.pdf`
2. Nichols, M., Townsend, N., Luengo-Fernandez, R., Leal, J., Gray, A., Scarborough, P., Rayner, M.: European Cardiovascular Disease Statistics 2012. European Heart Network, Brussels, European Society of Cardiology, Sophia Antipolis (2012)
3. Ambrosy, A.P., Fonarow, G.C., Butler, J., Chioncel, O., Greene, S.J., Vaduganathan, M., Nodari, S., Lam, C.S., Sato, N., Shah, A.N., Gheorghiade, M.: The Global Health and Economic Burden of Hospitalizations for Heart Failure: Lessons Learned From Hospitalized Heart Failure Registries. J. Am. Coll. Cardiol. 63(12), 1123–1133 (2014)
4. Heran, B.S., Chen, J.M., Ebrahim, S., Moxham, T., Oldridge, N., Rees, K., Thompson, D.R., Taylor, R.S.: Exercise-based cardiac rehabilitation for coronary heart disease. Cochrane Database Syst. Rev. 7, CD001800 (2011)
5. Taylor, R.S., Brown, A., Ebrahim, S., Jolliffe, J., Noorani, H., Rees, K., Skidmore, B., Stone, J.A., Thompson, D.R., Oldridge, N.: Exercise-based rehabilitation for patients with coronary heart disease: systematic review and meta-analysis of randomized controlled trials. Am. J. Med. 116(10), 682–692 (2004)
6. Finlex 17.8.1992/785. Laki potilaan asemasta ja oikeuksista,
   `http://www.finlex.fi/fi/laki/ajantasa/1992/19920785`
7. Finlex 298/2009. Sosiaali- ja terveysministeriön asetus potilasasiakirjoista,
   `http://www.finlex.fi/fi/laki/alkup/2009/20090298`
8. World Confederation for Physical Therapy: WCPT guideline for records management: record keeping, storage, retrieval and disposal, London, UK (2011),
   `http://www.wcpt.org/guidelines/records-management`
9. Fysioterapiapalvelujen sähköinen dokumentointi - ohje rakenteiseen kirjaamiseen potilastietojärjestelmässä. Versio 1.0 (2012),
   `http://www.suomenfysioterapeutit.fi/index.php?option=`
   `com_content&view=article&id=293&Itemid=508`
10. Kolber, M., Lucado, A.M.: Risk management strategies in physical therapy: documentation to avoid malpractice. Int. J. Health Care Qual. Assur. Inc. Leadersh. Health Serv. 18(2-3), 123–130 (2005)
11. Wang, N., Hailey, D., Yu, P.: Quality of nursing documentation and approaches to its evaluation: a mixed-method systematic review. J. Adv. Nurs. 67(9), 1858–1875 (2011)

12. Mäkinen, A., Penttilä, U.R.: Sepelvaltimopotilaiden kuntoutus julkisessa terveydenhuollossa. Selvitys kuntoutuksen määrästä, sisällöstä ja järjestämistavoista. Suomen Sydänliiton julkaisuja 1 (2007), http://www.sydanliitto.fi/c/ document_library/get_file?uuid=03135813-392c-4251-ab8f-abde05c110e9&groupId=14302

13. European Association of Cardiovascular Prevention and Rehabilitation Committee for Science Guidelines; EACPR, Corrà, U., Piepoli, M.F., Carré, F., Heuschmann, P., Hoffmann, U., Verschuren, M., Halcox, J., Document Reviewers, Giannuzzi, P., Saner, H., Wood, D., Piepoli, M.F., Corrà, U., Benzer, W., Bjarnason-Wehrens, B., Dendale, P., Gaita, D., McGee, H., Mendes, M., Niebauer, J., Zwisler, A.D., Schmid, J.P.: Secondary prevention through cardiac rehabilitation: physical activity counselling and exercise training: key components of the position paper from the Cardiac Rehabilitation Section of the European Association of Cardiovascular Prevention and Rehabilitation. Eur. Heart J. 16, 1967–1974 (2010)

14. Achttien, R.J., Staal, J.B., van der Voort, S., Kemps, H.M., Koers, H., Jongert, M.W., Hendriks, E.J.: Exercise-based cardiac rehabilitation in patients with coronary heart disease: a practice guideline. Practice Recommendations Development Group. Neth. Heart J. 10, 429–438 (2013)

15. Hulzebos, E.H., Smit, Y., Helders, P.P., van Meeteren, N.L.: Preoperative physical therapy for elective cardiac surgery patients. Cochrane Database Syst. Rev. 11, CD010118 (2012)

16. Savage, P.D., Sanderson, B.K., Brown, T.M., Berra, K., Ades, P.A.: Clinical research in cardiac rehabilitation and secondary prevention: looking back and moving forward. Journal of Cardiopulmonary Rehabilitation and Prevention 31(6), 333–341 (2011)

17. Cortes, O., Arthur, H.M.: Determinants of referral to cardiac rehabilitation programs in patients with coronary artery disease: a systematic review. American Heart Journal 151(2), 249–256 (2006)

18. Arena, R., Williams, M., Forman, D.E., Cahalin, L.P., Coke, L., Myers, J., Hamm, L., Kris-Etherton, P., Humphrey, R., Bittner, V., Lavie, C.J.: Increasing referral and participation rates to outpatient cardiac rehabilitation: the valuable role of healthcare professionals in the inpatient and home health settings: a science advisory from the American Heart Association. Circulation 125(10), 1321–1329 (2012), American Heart Association Exercise, Cardiac Rehabilitation and Prevention Committee of the Council on Clinical Cardiology, Council on Epidemiology and Prevention, and Council on Nutrition, Physical Activity and Metabolism

19. Ghisi, G.L., Polyzotis, P., Oh, P., Pakosh, M., Grace, S.L.: Physician factors affecting cardiac rehabilitation referral and patient enrollment: a systematic review. Clinical Cardiology 36(6), 323–335 (2013)

20. Mansah, M., Griffiths, R., Fernandez, R., Chang, E., Thuy Tran, D.: Older Folks in Hospitals: The Contributing Factors and Recommendations for Incident Prevention. J. Patient Saf. (2014) [Epub ahead of print]

21. Wahr, J.A., Prager, R.L., Abernathy III, J.H., Martinez, E.A., Salas, E., Seifert, P.C., Groom, R.C., Spiess, B.D., Searles, B.E., Sundt III, T.M., Sanchez, J.A., Shappell, S.A., Culig, M.H., Lazzara, E.H., Fitzgerald, D.C., Thourani, V.H., Eghtesady, P., Ikonomidis, J.S., England, M.R., Sellke, F.W., Nussmeier, N.A.: Patient safety in the cardiac operating room: human factors and teamwork: a scientific statement from the American Heart Association. Circulation 128(10), 1139–1169 (2013), American Heart Association Council on Cardiovascular Surgery and Anesthesia, Council on Cardiovascular and Stroke Nursing, and Council on Quality of Care and Outcomes Research

22. Penoyer, D.A., Cortelyou-Ward, K.H., Noblin, A.M., Bullard, T., Talbert, S., Wilson, J., Schafhauser, B., Briscoe, J.G.: Use of electronic health record documentation by healthcare workers in an acute care hospital system. J. Healthc. Manag. 59(2), 130–144 (2014)

23. Häyrinen, K., Saranto, K., Nykänen, P.: Definition, structure, content, use and impacts of electronic health records: a review of the research literature. Int. J. Med. Inform. 77(5), 291–304 (2008)

24. Edwards, S.T., Neri, P.M., Volk, L.A., Schiff, G.D., Bates, D.W.: Association of note quality and quality of care: a cross-sectional study. BMJ Qual. Saf. 23(5), 406–413 (2013)

25. Schiff, G.D., Bates, D.W.: Can electronic clinical documentation help prevent diagnostic errors? N. Engl. J. Med. 362(12), 1066–1069 (2010)

26. Roth, C.P., Lim, Y.-W., Pevnick, J.M., et al.: The challenge of measuring quality of care from the electronic health record. Am. J. Med. Qual. 24, 385–394 (2009)

27. Bergh, A.L., Bergh, C.H., Friberg, F.: How do nurses record pedagogical activities? Nurses' documentation in patient records in a cardiac rehabilitation unit for patients who have undergone coronary artery bypass surgery. J. Clin. Nurs. 16(10), 1898–1907 (2007)

28. Gustavsen, M., Mengshoel, A.M.: Clinical physiotherapy documentation in stroke rehabilitation: an ICIDH-2 beta-2 based analysis. Disabil. Rehabil. 25(19), 1089–1096 (2003)

29. World Health Organization: International Statistical Classification of Diseases and Related Health Problems. 10th Revision, vol. 2. Instructional manual. 2010 Edition (2011b), http://apps.who.int/classifications/icd10/browse/2010/en

Special Features of Counselling Work Carried Out through Interactive TV

Sirppa Kinos, Sari Asteljoki, and Pia Suvivuo

Turku University of Applied Sciences, Turku, Finland
{sirppa.kinos,sari.asteljoki,pia.suvivuo}@turkuamk.fi.

Abstract. Objectives: The purpose of this article is to introduce the special features of professional counselling carried out through interactive TV. Interactive TV is one application of welfare technology. New innovations are needed in social and health care, because the number of elderly people is increasing and their service needs must be catered.

Methods: The main approach of this study is qualitative. The material was analysed by means of qualitative content analysis. The article is based on a survey carried out at Turku University of Applied Sciences. The survey was responded to by some of the students involved in the VIRTU project's transmissions (n=80). The survey consisted of a total of 25 questions. The article reports on four open-ended questions relating to the special features of counselling work.

Results: The special features of group counselling through interactive TV are particularly linked to the counsellor's role. The counsellor acts in an environment that differs from a physical, social and symbolic perspective.

Conclusions, practice implications: We present a model detailing the special features of counselling carried out through interactive TV and how they must be observed when providing personnel in the field with training in this.

Keywords: e-Health, safe living and working environments counseling.

1   Introduction

According to the National Knowledge Society Strategy [1], people's daily lives have been greatly influenced by the development of information and communications technology. The development of knowledge society has changed our way of perceiving the world, changed our idea of communality and opened new opportunities for the growth of productivity and efficiency. It has also strengthened equal opportunities and equality between different people and regions.

New innovations are needed in social and health care, because the number of elderly people is increasing and their service needs must be catered [2]. There have been doubts about the use of technological innovations. Technological applications have even been seen as the opposite of human care, but the attitudes of the elderly may change in a positive direction as they gain user experience [3]. It is important for the elderly to be part of the modern world and be capable of using modern information technology, particularly when they live in a rural area or have reduced functional capacity.

K. Saranto et al. (Eds.): WIS 2014, CCIS 450, pp. 68–77, 2014.

One of the opportunities provided by technology is interactive TV, which utilises videoconferencing technology. The term 'interactive TV' refers to a piece of equipment that, instead of one-way transmission, enables all participants in the transmission to interact both verbally and visually. The view on the screen can be adjusted. It may include several smaller screens at a time, depending on the number of people involved in the transmission.

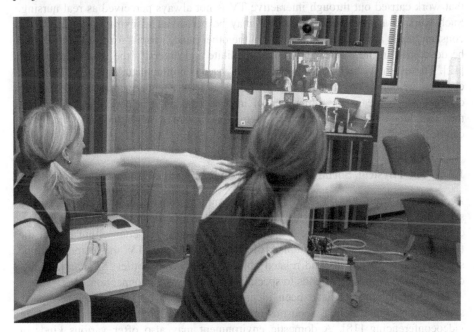

Fig. 1. Interactive TV

The purpose of this article is to introduce the special features of professional counselling carried out through interactive TV. Interactive TV has been used to a certain extent in the Finnish social and health service system. For example, the VIRTU project has developed and tested new innovations for the service needs of the elderly [4].

1.1   A New Kind of Tool and Orientation to Work

The terminology related to welfare technology and counselling through interactive TV is highly varied. Counselling through videoconferencing and similar equipment is called virtual counselling, interactive telerehabilitation [5], telecounselling or distance counselling [6]. It is also referred to as distance rehabilitation [7], telerehabilitation [8] and telemedicine. The above can be seen as part of gerontechnology [9]. The term 'virtual' is most often used to refer to communications over the Internet. However, it is probably useless to make a difference between the so-called real world and the virtual world, since they are phenomena that are interlinked in many ways [10].

Interactive TV, like many modern media applications, gives us the chance to overcome geographical obstacles. Counselling services are brought closer to the client, all the way home, without the client having to travel for the services [11]. The home is a safe and meaningful environment for rehabilitation and counselling through interactive TV.

In studies of the use of interactive TV in care for the elderly, it has been observed that work carried out through interactive TV is not always perceived as real nursing. Such work is a new phenomenon that may be perceived as extra work amidst the constant hustle and bustle of nursing. On the other hand, various forms of care should be developed in the future, and should facilitate and diversify the working methods [12]. The use of virtual technology requires various communication skills. This also changes the nature of clinical work [13]. Pressure for change increases resistance to change, which means the generation of internal resistance in people's minds when they feel they are faced with excessive requirements [14]. These challenges to change can be addressed by means of training.

1.2   The Physical, Social and Symbolic Environment of Counselling Activities

According to Kim (2000, 172–184), the environment consists of physical, social and symbolic elements [15]. From the perspective of the physical environment, counselling through interactive TV differs from face-to-face counselling in that the two parties are in separate locations [16] Through interactive TV, the recipient can be shown various documents and related objects, such as pill bottles. Similarly, clients can show their rashes or wounds to specialists over the video connection. [17]

Development targets have been identified relating to background noise, space, sound feedback and delay. Acoustics in a client's home have not been designed for videoconferencing [18]. A domestic environment may also offer various kinds of activities that may distract the client [19].

As a social environment, interactive TV offers a quick, easy and user-friendly technical solution for communality. Rehabilitation over a video connection is challenging if the client has physical, cognitive or speech problems [20]. The online environment also makes it easier to remain passive and withdrawn than face-to-face situations, in group situations in particular. Language and communications are a counsellor's most important tools. Interactive TV highlights the significance of verbal counselling, with gestures, expressions and other forms of non-verbal communication remaining more distant and more difficult to perceive. However, hints are also visually received from the group members' surroundings.

Constituents of the symbolic environment include experiences related to security, independence and autonomy. Skär and Söderberg [21] have found that technology increases the feeling of independence. Accordingly, the independence and autonomy of the elderly should be respected when utilising technology in their care [22]. On the other hand, technology may even increase the vulnerability of nursing and prevent the development of a confidential care relationship [23].

1.3   Counsellor's Role

Interactive TV brings its own challenges for interaction, even from the counsellor's point of view. It highlights the significance of some of the counsellor's skills, such as the clarity of verbal communication and dialogue skills.

Counselling is one of the key forms of professional interaction and an important method of client work [24]. The counsellor is responsible for guiding the group processes. The key group processes are communication, agreeing on the working guidelines, making decisions, handling problems and solving conflicts. In these tasks, the counsellor needs many kinds of skills, such as reaction (e.g. listening), interaction (e.g. setting limits) and operational skills (observing). Also important is non-verbal communication, such as gestures. [25]

The counsellor is responsible for planning and carrying out the counselling situations. The counsellor must also take care of the social and emotional side of the interaction. Knowledge of group phenomena and processes is important. The pedagogical tool is also significant. In counselling through videoconferencing equipment, manual counselling based on a physical touch is not possible. In addition, the counsellor must know how to act in the technical environment used. Experience and training increase knowledge, skills, enthusiasm and interest in the use of welfare technology. [26]

2   Methods

This article is based on a survey carried out at Turku University of Applied Sciences between 2 December 2011 and 31 May 2012. The survey was responded to by some of the students involved in the VIRTU project's transmissions, including 75 social and health care students and five hospitality management students. The student questionnaire (25 questions) was created by the VIRTU project's teacher workgroup. The students completed the questionnaire at the end of a course related to the VIRTU project. This article reports on four open-ended questions relating to the special features of counselling work carried out through interactive TV. Other parts of the survey were reported in the publication Active Ageing Online.

The clients in the VIRTU project's transmissions were old people living alone and family caregivers in the archipelago areas of the municipality of Naantali. Each transmission involved one to nine clients. The transmissions lasted about one hour and were carried out three days a week. More than a half of the students who responded to the survey were involved for the first time in VIRTU transmissions or similar activities at the time of the survey. One student had been involved more than 6 times, 30% have been involved in such transmissions 2–3 times and 13% 4–5 times.

While the main approach of this study is qualitative, the material is also quantified (frequency and percentage distributions). A qualitative approach emphasises the experiential nature of reality [27]. The material was analysed by means of qualitative content analysis, grouping the answers and arranging them by theme [29, 30].

3   Results

In this section, we describe the key results of the survey relating to the special features of counselling activities carried out through interactive TV as well as the challenges and opportunities brought by the technology.

3.1   Similarities and Differences between Counselling Performed through Interactive TV and Face-to-face Counselling

Most students (62 respondents, 78%) estimated that the essence of counselling is the same both virtually and face-to-face. Both methods are interactive: a personal connection is established with the client, and interaction between the counsellor and the client can be made to work. The client and the counsellor not only hear but also see each other, unlike over the phone, which facilitates discussion.

According to the students, the same issues and information can be handled with the client in the same way both face-to-face and in counselling through interactive TV. A clear way of speaking and clear instructions during the counselling were always seen as important, regardless of the counselling method and tools. Careful planning of the counselling situation, good knowledge of the target group and paying attention to each member of the group are also important in both counselling methods.

"Verbal expression and explanation are important in both cases. The same applies to paying attention to all participants and activating everyone. Meeting people and building community spirit also felt similar in the VIRTU transmission and close-contact counselling."

On the other hand, almost all students (77 respondents, 96%) mentioned several differences between interactive TV and face-to-face counselling.

A key issue mentioned by the students was the challenges brought to counselling by the technology and mastering it. Using the equipment requires certain skills that must be mastered by both the client and the student acting as the counsellor. Technical problems, such as interruptions in the audio and video connection or delay, may hamper the interaction and thus also the counselling.

"Virtual counselling relies on technology, so the risk of unsuccessful counselling is higher than in face-to-face situations. Some may find it easier to perform in front of a TV set than a live audience, while for others it's the other way around."

Different environments, such as the client's home environment, pose challenges to the counselling. Some clients may do their chores at the same time, which disturbs the counselling situation. The separate spaces create a feeling of distance.

The students also estimated that interaction is different. Gestures, facial expressions and non-verbal communication often go unnoticed in counselling through interactive TV. The students found it difficult to interpret expressions, gestures, feelings and moods. The lack of manual counselling may reduce the safety of exercise counselling. Counselling through interactive TV was considered more distant than face-to-face counselling. The students found both benefits and drawbacks in this.

"Face-to-face contact is more natural; feelings are conveyed more easily. Virtual counselling is naturally not as 'close' as face-to-face counselling, since the persons are not physically in the same space. Touching is also not possible virtually, as would be necessary to teach something hands-on, like injecting insulin."

In the students' opinion, counselling through interactive TV requires students to prepare more carefully for the counselling situation and understand the special nature of the counselling. In planning the counselling situation, attention must be paid to the challenges in using concrete examples, with the client unable to feel, smell or taste materials.

The students reckoned that counselling through interactive TV requires different counselling skills. The articulation must be clearer and the speech slower. The delays in the speech and text and their effects on the schedule must be taken into account, particularly in the event of large counselling groups. Assigning turns to speak is important to avoid overlapping speech, as is addressing the participants by their names. Eye contact cannot be used to show who should speak next.

3.2   Opportunities and Challenges

Challenges mentioned by the students (55 respondents, 69%) included developing the operation of the equipment such that the services can be used appropriately without their replacing face-to-face work with clients altogether. Another challenge mentioned was ensuring the technical expertise of both the professional staff and the clients.

The students assumed that the use of technology in social and health services will increase significantly in the future. They mainly consider this a very positive development, even though some of the respondents were critical of the issue.

The students pondered the question of whether equality is achieved; whether everyone has an equal chance to participate and whether all clients are capable of using technical equipment. The respondents had doubts about equality relating to the availability of the equipment. Besides, the designers of the service system must more boldly think about ways of better utilising interactive TV counselling and technology.

The functionality of technology and equipment as well as their development are concerned some of the most significant challenges in social and health services.

"Any technical problems will certainly pose a challenge to virtual counselling and the use of technology in my future work. A question springs to mind: Can technology ever be relied on one hundred per cent? New technology and the equipment it requires are fairly expensive."

Using the services requires technical know-how, which the students considered an essential part of professional skills in the future. Technical know-how and the related training needs pose a challenge to both professionals and clients. It was nevertheless regarded as a prerequisite for versatile professional skills and keeping up-to-date.

The students (59 respondents, 74%) said that interactive TV enables the services to become more efficient, the need for employee resources to decrease and customer services to improve as they become more diverse. Savings could be achieved in costs and other resources, such as working hours. Contacts with clients will become easier and more frequent. Interactive TV will increase the clients' feeling of security. The services may also improve the clients' social contacts, even international connections, thus increasing their social welfare.

"New kinds of networks can be created for clients who otherwise wouldn't necessarily have the chance to participate. Some simple tasks, such as control visits, could be handled virtually."

4   Discussion and Conclusion

Welfare technology, such as interactive TV, will play a key role in future client work in social, health and education services. To achieve this, new attitudes, knowledge and skills must be learned by clients, employees, students and teachers alike. All parties should be bold and not afraid to leave their comfort zones. The special features of counselling through interactive TV are illustrated in Figure 2. The figure can be used to help preparation and training for counselling work through interactive TV.

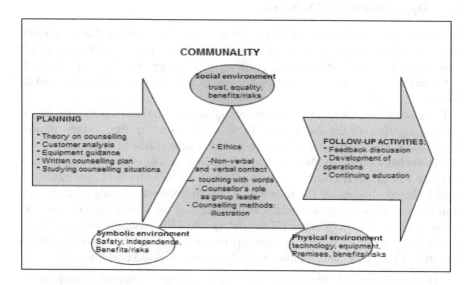

Fig. 2. Special features of counselling through interactive TV

In the planning of counselling through interactive TV, it is most important for the counsellor to get to know the client group and its special features (client analysis). Also important are the theoretical aspects of counselling, such as the basics of professional interaction and communications. On the basis of these, the person acting as the counsellor will prepare a written counselling plan including, according to the clients' needs, the objectives for counselling, the content and methods of counselling and the evaluation plan. It is also necessary to get to know the equipment and follow interactive TV transmissions, because otherwise it is difficult to perceive interactive TV as a special physical, social and symbolic environment.

In acting as a counsellor over interactive TV, the usual interaction methods and skills applied by a counsellor do not work as such from the social-communicative perspective. As regards the communicative and organisational role, the counsellor must plan and build the interaction, because only one group member can speak at a time. The counsellor must indicate who should speak next by saying the person's name.

Because looks and gestures are difficult to interpret, the counsellor is first and foremost a user of language, who constructs counselling situations by means of speech. Physical contact is not possible during the counselling, but some of it can be replaced with words. Author Reko Lundán wrote about touching with words. Words also allow us to get close to each other, and words turn into feelings. According to Lundán, this is the highest form of communication. [31]

The counsellor should also learn to manage social group processes in a manner that creates a confidential and equal atmosphere. Interactive TV is a special symbolic environment in which the rules and norms concerning interaction. From an ethical point of view, it must be borne in mind that clients participate in the transmission from their homes, which act as studios. The protection of privacy is challenging, since surprising events or visitors cannot be avoided.

In training for counselling through interactive TV, an important prerequisite for learning is to get feedback from clients participating in the group and have a feedback discussion between counsellors. The counsellors assess their own work and consider any development targets.

From the perspective of communality, the counsellor should bear in mind that interactive TV supports a very counsellor-centred model of group activities. The counsellor can encourage the group members to use interactive TV for personal contacts outside the transmissions.

In conclusion, it can be noted that the most important feature of interactive TV is the way it can build communality. Interactive TV makes it possible to overcome obstacles related to functional capacity and geography. This brings equality to the availability of the services. Interactive TV proves that, at its best, welfare technology enables human contact instead of replacing it.

References

1. National Knowledge Society Strategy 2007–2015. A renewing, human-centric and competitive Finland. Information Society Programme, Prime Minister's Office, Helsinki
2. Ahtiainen, M., Auranne, K.: Hyvinvointiteknologian määrittely ja yleisesittely [Definition and presentation of well-being technology]. In: Suhonen, L., Siikanen, T. (eds.) Hyvinvointiteknologia sosiaali- ja terveysalalla – hyöty vai haitta? [Well-being Technology in Social and Health Care – A Deficit or a Benefit?] A publication of Lahti University of Applied Sciences. Series C Artikkelikokoelmat, raportit ja muuta jankohtaiset julkaisut, part 26, pp. 9–20 (2007)
3. Sävenstedt, S., Sandman, P.O., Zinkmark, K.: The duality in using information and communication technology in elder care. Journal of Advanced Nursing 56(1), 17–25 (2006)

4. http://www.VIRTU.FI (retrieved on January 3, 2013)
5. Karppi, M.: Interactive telerehabilitation supporting convalescence of the elderly. Master's Thesis. University of Tampere, School of Health Sciences (2011)
6. Kolehmainen, P., Ikonen, J., Turunen, J.: Physical activity counselling for working age people via telecounselling. Mikkeli University of Applied Sciences (2012)
7. Russell, T.G.: Telerehabilitation: a coming age. Article in the Australian Journal of Physiotherapy 55, 5–6 (2009)
8. Hoenig, H., Sanford, J.A., Butterfield, T., Griffiths, P.C., Richardson, P., Hargraves, K.: Development of a teletechnology protocol for in-home rehabilitation. Article in the Journal of Rehabilitation Research and Development 43(2), 287–298 (2006)
9. Leikas, J.: Ageing, Technology and Ethics. Views on Research and Design of Human-Technology Interaction. VTT Technical Research Centre of Finland, VTT Working Papers 110 (2008)
10. Matikainen, J.: Verkko – ohjauksen väline vai arena? [Internet – a tool or an environment of counseling?]. In: Onnismaa, J., Pasanen, H., Spangar, T. (eds.) Ohjaus ammattina ja tieteenalana 3. Ohjauksen välineet [Counseling as a Profession and a Discipline 3. Tools for Counseling], pp. 125–139. PS-kustannus, Jyväskylä (2004)
11. Pilli-Sihvola, M.: Urasuunnitteluohjausta Internetissä [Career counseling on the Internet]. In: Onnismaa, J., Pasanen, H., Spangar, T. (eds.) Ohjaus ammattina ja tieteenalana 2. Ohjauksen toimintakentät [Counseling as a Profession and a Discipline 2. Environments of Counseling], pp. 34–43. PS-kustannus, Jyväskylä (2002)
12. Vuorio, E.: Asiantuntijoiden osaamisen kehittyminen ja työn muutos [Development of expertise and work]. In: Lehto, P., Leskelä, J. (eds.) Interaktiivinen HyvinvointiTV ja käyttäjälähtöiset e-palvelut [Interactive TV and Client centered e-services]. Final report of the Turvallinen Koti project. Laurea University of Applied Sciences, publication series 2011, B 44. Edita Prima Oy, Helsinki (2011)
13. Currell, R., Urquhart, C., Wainwright, P., Lewis, R.: Telemedicine versus face to face patient care: effects on professional practice and health care outcomes (Review). The Cochrane Collaboration. John Wiley & Sons Ltd. (2010)
14. Nurmi, H.: Onko virtuaalimaailmassa helpompi muuttua kuin tavallisessa? [Is changing easier in virtual life]? In: Ihanainen, P., Kalli, P., Kiviniemi, K. (eds.) Sosiaalinen media ja verkostoituminen [Social Media and Networking], pp. 11–24. Offset Oy, Saarijärvi (2010)
15. Kim, H.S.: The Nature of Theoretical Thinking in Nursing. Springer Publishing Company, New York (2000)
16. Vesterinen, R.: Etäkuntoutus –mahdollisuus kuntoutua kotona kaksisuuntaisen videoyhteyden avulla. Käytettävyystutkimus Innokusti-hankkeessa [Distant counseling – an option for rehabilitation at home by video negotiation equipment. Users' experiences]. Master's Thesis in Physiotherapy. University of Jyväskylä, Faculty of Sport and Health Sciences, Department of Health Sciences (2010)
17. Lehto, P., Leskelä, J.: Hankkeen arviointi ja vaikuttavuus [Evaluation and effect of the project]. In: Lehto, P., Leskelä, J. (eds.) Interaktiivinen hyvinvointi-TV ja käyttäjälähtöiset e-palvelut [Interactive TV and client centered e-services. Final report of the Safe Home project]. Laurea University of Applied Sciences, publication series 2011, B 44. Edita Prima Oy, Helsinki (2011)
18. Arvola, M., Nieminen, V.: Turvallinen Koti –hankkeen teknologiset ratkaisut [Tecnical solutions of the Safe Home project]. In: Lehto, P., Leskelä, J. (eds.) Interaktiivinen HyvinvointiTV ja käyttäjälähtöiset e-palvelut [Interactive TV and clinet centered e-services. Final report of the Safe Home project]. Laurea University of Applied Sciences, publication series 2011, B 44. Edita Prima Oy, Helsinki (2011)

19. Suvivuo, P., Asteljoki, S., Kuikkaniemi, A., Kinos, S.: Students' experiences of working on the VIRTU Channel. In: Karppi, M., Tuominen, H., Eskelinen, A., Santamäki-Fischer, R., Rasu, A. (eds.) Active Ageing Online: Interactive Distance Services for the Elderly on Baltic Islands – VIRTU Project 2010–2013. Reports 2013, 155. Turku University of Applied Sciences (2013)

20. Theodoros, D., Russell, T.: Telerehabilitation: Current perspectives. Studies in Health Technology and Informatics 131, 191–209 (2008)

21. Skär, L., Söderberg, S.: The Use of Information and Communication Technology to Meet Chronically Ill Patients' Needs when Living at Home. Open Nurs. J. 5, 74–78 (2011)

22. Zwijsen, S., Niemeijer, A., Hertogh, C.M.: Ethics of using assistive technology in the care for community-dwelling elderly people: An overview of the literature. Aging & Mental Health 15(4) (2011)

23. Harrefors, C., Axelsson, K., Savenstedt, S.: Using assistive technology services at differing levels of care: healthy older couples' perceptions. Journal of Advanced Nursing 66(7), 1523–1532 (2010)

24. Ruponen, R., Nummenmaa, A.R., Koivuluhta, M.: Ryhmäohjaus muutoksen mahdollisuuden maisemana [Group counseling as a tool for change]. In: Onnismaa, J., Pasanen, H., Spangar, T. (eds.) Ohjaus ammattina ja tieteenalana [Counseling as a Profession and a Discipline 1]. PS-kustannus, Jyväskylä (2000)

25. Peavy, R.V.: Sosiodynaaminen näkökulma ja ohjauksen käytäntö [Sosiodynanic counseling and practise]. In: Onnismaa, J., Pasanen, H., Spangar, T. (eds.) Ohjaus ammattina ja tieteenalana 3. Ohjauksen välineet [Counseling as a Profession and a Discipline 3. Tools for Counseling]. PS-kustannus, Jyväskylä (2004)

26. Välimäki, M., Suhonen, R., Koivunen, M., Alanen, S., Nenonen, H.: Hoitohenkilökunnan valmiudet hyödyntää informaatioteknologiaa potilasohjauksessa [Information technology competences of nursing staff in patient counseling]. Hoitotiede, 5, 19 (2007)

27. Foss, C., Ellefsen, B.: The value of combining qualitative and quantitative approaches in nursing research by means of method triangulation. Journal of Advanced Nursing 40(2), 242–248 (2002)

28. Tuomi, J., Sarajärvi, A.: Laadullinen tutkimus ja sisällön analyysi [Qualitative methods and content analysis]. Tammi, Helsinki (2006)

29. Hirsjärvi, S., Remes, P., Sajavaara, P.: Tutki ja kirjoita [Research and reporting], 15th, partially revised edition. Tammi, Helsinki (2009)

30. Eskola, J., Suoranta, J.: Johdatus laadulliseen tutkimukseen [Introduction to qualitative research]. Vastapaino, Tampere (2005)

31. Lundán, R., Lundán, T.: Viikkoja, kuukausia [Weeks, months]. WSOY, Helsinki (2006)

Evaluation of Intravenous Medication Errors
with Infusion Pumps

Eija Kivekäs[1,3], Kaisa Haatainen[1,2], Hannu Kokki[1,2], and Kaija Saranto[1]

[1] University of Eastern Finland, Kuopio, Finland
[2] Kuopio University Hospital, Kuopio, Finland
[3] Research Centre for Comparative Effectiveness and Patient Safety, Kuopio, Finland
eija.kivekas@uef.fi

Abstract. This paper presents the key issues of the use of intravenous infusion pumps to be able to further develop strategies that will improve patient safety and prevent medication errors. The study was conducted in four wards in a Finnish tertiary hospital. These units included medical intensive care unit, surgical intensive care unit, general medical unit and general surgical ward. Multi-disciplinary team, nurses and pharmacists, performed observations (N=492) on the units. The results indicated that errors were rated as A – B in the NCC MERP harm index. Lack of patient identification bands on some units and inadequate allergy documentation appeared as risk factors. Furthermore medication processes varied within the units especially in administering and documenting. In spite of the Electronic Patient Record system, several overlapping documentation forms were in use. Through this prevalence study, violation errors of hospital policy were found that could potentially place patients at risk.

Keywords: intravenous medication, intravenous administration, medication error, infusion pump, patient safety.

1 Introduction

Computerized patient infusion devices that include features for medication administration error prevention and data collection represent transformational clinical tools that can substantially decrease the rate of intravenous medication errors in hospitals [1]. Medication safety in hospitals depends on the successful execution of a complex system of scores of individual tasks, which are prescribing, preparing, dispensing, transcribing and monitoring the patient's response. Many of these tasks lend themselves to technologic tools. Patient safety is a matter of major concern that involves every health professional. Emerging technologies such as smart pumps can diminish medication errors as well as standardize and improve clinical practice with the subsequent benefits for patients. [1-4]

A technology provides medication error-reduction capabilities via programmed dose limit alerts with audio/visual feedback to staff regarding erroneous orders, improper dose calculations or programming errors. These devices have become

K. Saranto et al. (Eds.): WIS 2014, CCIS 450, pp. 78–87, 2014.

popular among acute care facilities and using smart pumps are very common in intensive care units but also in tertiary hospital wards. However, these devices have not always achieved their potential and important intravenous errors still persist. Rothschild et al. (2005) evaluated a very early version of pump and found that although smart intravenous pumps with decision support capabilities had the capacity to intercept many dangerous medication errors and allowed the detection of many errors that would have been extremely difficult to find through any other mechanism [5]. Manrique-Rodrigues et al. (2014) demonstrated that implementation of smart pumps proved effective in preventing infusion related programming errors from reaching patients [4].

HaiPro system is for organizational level reporting patient safety incidents in Finland. The main properties of HaiPro are: anonymity, confidentiality and freedom from sanctions. The HaiPro approach incorporates a system model that takes into consideration the features of natural human behavior and the pathway of divergent events development. The local incident reporting system is meant to prevent treatment adverse events through the improvement of operational procedures. At present, data is collected only at organization level and not send forward to or sent aggregated or analyzed on regional and national level [6].

1.1 Use of Infusion Pumps

The vast majority of patients who spend a few hours in a hospital encounter one of the most widely used medical technologies in healthcare is infusion pumps. Increasingly, computer-predefined smart pumps can be programmed to deliver controlled amounts of analgesics, antibiotics, insulin, chemotherapy drugs, nutrients, or other fluids. Smart pumps also can keep the electronic records of infusions, which are captured in the pumps' software. Infusion devices are used in homes and other healthcare settings as well. [2]

When smart pump work as intended, infusion pumps support the "five rights" of medication safety – right medication, right dose, right time, right route and right patient. In fact, infusion pumps provide important health benefits and reduce medical errors [7]. Technologies, such as computerized order entry, bar-coding and smart pumps and computerized adverse events monitoring, will undoubtedly play a key role in patient safety and institutions should be thinking seriously about implementing a number of these in clinical practice [8]. Smart intravenous infusion pumps have been developed to mitigate errors that occur at the administration stage [2].

Smart intravenous infusion pumps have customized drug libraries with standardized concentra-tions for commonly used drugs, which allow them to provide point-of-care decision support feedback for excessively high or low rates and doses. These devices enable programmed to provide soft alert feedback, which allows overrides and hard alerts that cannot be overridden. Drug libraries may be unit specific, with unique rules for individual clinical areas such as pediatrics, obstetrics and critical care [2,4]. While smart infusion pump alone may prevent pump programming errors, they cannot prevent giving the wrong drug or wrong concentration, or giving the drug to the wrong patient. Whereas, bar-coded medication administration (BCMA) coupled with an electronic medication administration record (eMAR) targets errors that occur at the drug dispensing, transcription and administration stages. BCMA provides point-of-care verification of the correct patient and medication. This medication system electronically connects the administration to the medication order when electronically linked to computerized provider order entry (CPOE) [2].

1.2   The Prevalence of Medication Errors Related to Infusion Pumps

According to the previous studies over 90% of intravenous medications had some type of error [9]. In Finland a study (2011) showed that 51% of 64.405 web-based incident reports concerned medication, the most common incidents were errors in documenting, dis-pensing and administering [10]. Husch et al. (2005) assessed the frequency of intra-venous medication errors and impact of potential smart infusion pump technology on the frequency of intravenous medication errors in the U.S. using a rapid assessment approach [11]. They observed 426 medications and of these, 285 (66.9%) had one or more errors associated with administration. Ohashi et al. (2013) study based on an observation sheet from Husch's study, key data elements required to capture all kinds of intravenous medication errors were identified [9,11].

Implementations of potentially transformative electronic health (eHealth) technologies are currently underway internationally, often with significant impact on national expenditure. Black et al. (2011) systematically reviewed the preexisting literature on eHealth technologies and their impact on the quality and safety of health care delivery [12]. They demonstrated that many of the clinical claims made about the most commonly deployed eHealth technologies cannot be substantiated by the empirical evidence. The paradox was that while the number of eHealth technologies in health care is growing, the understanding about technology is insufficient. They suggested that the methodology should be adopted multidisciplinary and thus to increase understanding a complex web of factors that may influence the results [12].

Hertzel and Sousa (2009) identified nine studies published from 2003-2008 that assessed the use of smart pumps for the prevention of medication errors [13]. The review summarized the study findings and identified lack of user compliance with soft alerts as an important factor that compromised the efficacy of smart pumps in the majority of studies. Poor caregiver compliance with the drug library and dosage limits may have explained the lack of advantage of smart pumps decision support in the Rothschild et al (2005) study also [5]. The infusion error rate decreased from 3.1 to 0.8 per 1000 doses from the pre-intervention, to the post-intervention period in Larsen et al. (2005) a retrospective before-after study on pediatric patients [14]. Larsen et al. (2005) compared medication infusion errors 12 months before and 12 months after adopting a new protocol using a combination of smart pumps, standard drug concentrations and human engineered (user-friendly) medication labels [14]. Adachi and Lodolce (2005) found only a small reduction in overall dosing errors, a larger reduction in pump-related errors [15]. Nine of the ten post-intervention pump programming errors occurred because users did not use the pump software. Eckel et al. (2006) reported a high frequency of programming where users bypassed the drug library when selecting a drug [16]. Both Eckel et al. (2006) and Field and Peterman

(2005) reported that users overrode of soft alerts quite often [17, 18, 19, 20]. In consequence, Institute for Safe Medication Practices (ISMP) has published a guideline for safe implementation and use of smart infusion pumps based on the literature review among other things [21].

Creation of safe and effective customized drug libraries is essential for the proper utilization of smart pumps. Institution must evaluate their clinical practice when determining what drugs and dosage limits to select for their library [21]. Drug libraries should at least include all high-alert drugs with standard concentrations as well as soft and hard stops to various dosage limits. Drug libraries must also be devoted to maintaining and updating constantly. Wireless communication technology in an organization's infrastructure allows easier adjustment or updating of drug libraries, which otherwise would require manually updating each pump separately [21].

This paper describes the preliminary results of a wider research project to identify the key issues of the use of intravenous pumps and to develop strategies that will improve the prevention of intravenous medication errors (before-after comparison). The types of intravenous medication errors within a medication process (including prescribing, transcribing, dispensing, administering and monitoring) are presented based on the results of the first observation phase.

2   Methods

2.1   Study Design

This study was conducted in four units in a Finnish tertiary hospital between February and March 2014. The study is a part of international research collaboration [3]. The proposed study will be conducted over three phases for a total of 36 months (2014-2016).

In first year (2014), the quality and quantity of reported adverse events were screened in order to have the baseline knowledge about the safety incidents in the units. An observational study was conducted by the investigators at multidisciplinary team. The investigators prospectively compared the medication, a dose, and infusion rate on the intravenous pump with the prescribed medication, doses, and rate in the medical record. Preventability with smart pump technology will be retrospectively determined based on a rigorous definition of currently available technology. Comparisons will be carried out across sites by overall rate and degree of variability among sites. Then, in second year (2014-2015), these results will be evaluated, and a consensus process including a face-to-face meeting with personnel and directors will take place to evaluate the types of events and to develop an intervention which will be implemented at multiple sites.   After a run-in period, the intervention will be tested in third year (2016) at the sites, and the data will be analyzed, and we will produce a report and a set of evidence-based recommendations.

2.2   Data Collection and Analysis

Observations of the intravenous medication administration processes at each of the four units were made over four days, eight hours per day. These units included medical ICU, surgical ICU, general medical intensive care unit (ICU) and general surgical ward. A survey was piloted in a maternity ward in January and observation instrument worked well. All epidural, patient controlled analgesia (PCA) and general use intravenous infusion pumps on inpatient care units were included in the investigation. To capture medica-tion errors, four to two observers (registered nurses and pharmacists) went to a ward and conducted observation on patients. This study was approved by the University of Eastern Finland Committee on Research Ethics.

On assigned inpatient units, using a prospective point prevalence approach, all data from intravenous medications at patient bedside were collected on the standardized form. Observers compared the infusing medication dose and infusion rate on the pump with the prescribed medication, a dose and rate in the medical record. All orders were obtained from both and handwritten paper-based medical records and all intravenous fluids were considered medication. Presence of correct patient identification band and name verification was recorded for each patient. Labeling of the infusing medication according to medication policy was assessed.

Table 1. Operational definitions of medication errors types [9]

Error Type	Definition
1. Wrong Dose	The same medication but the dose is different from the prescribed order.
2. Wrong Rate	A different rate is displayed on the pump from that prescribed in the medical record. Also refers to weight based doses calculated incorrectly including using a wrong weight.
3. Wrong Concentration	An amount of a medication in a unit of solution that is different from the prescribed order.
4. Wrong Medication	A different fluid/medication as documented on the IV bag label is being infused compared with the order in the medical record.
5. Known Allergy	Medication is prescribed/administered despite the patient had a known allergy to the drug.
6. Omitted Medication	The medication ordered was not administered to a patient.
7. Delay of Rate or Medication/Fluid Change	An order to change medication or rate not carried out within 4 hours of the written order per institution policy.
8. No Rate Documented on Label	Applies both to items sent from the pharmacy and floor stocked items per institution policy.
9. Incorrect Rate on Label	Rate documented on the medication label is different from that programmed into the pump. Applies both to items sent from the pharmacy and floor stocked items.
10. Patient Identification Error	Patient either has no ID band on wrist or information on the ID band is incorrect.
11. No Documented Order	Fluids/medications are being administered but no order is present in medical record. This includes failure to document a verbal order.

In order to confirm that an error was present, the observers had to agree that an error was made (Table 1). If an error was identified, that has the potential to cause harm, the staff nurse caring for that particular patient was informed so that he/she could correct it as warranted. Each error was rated by NCC MERP index (Table 2) [22]. Observers entered all data on the collection form.

Table 2. NCC MERP harm index (National Coordinating Council for Medication Error Reporting and Prevention 2001) [22]

(A) capacity to cause error
(B) an error occurred but did not reach the patient
(C) errors unlikely to cause harm despite reaching the patient
(D) errors that would have required increased monitoring to preclude harm
(E) errors likely to cause temporary harm
(F) errors that would have caused temporary harm and prolonged hospitalization
(G) errors which would have produced permanent harm
(H) errors that would have been life threatening
(I) errors that would likely have resulted in death

A number of factors collected for each participating wards, included the organizational level reporting of patient safety incidents (HaiPro), the institutional policies and procedures around medication administrations. The data from all the units, including the types of errors, were analyzed. This data was used as input to a meeting, at which interdisciplinary patient safety experts, including physicians, nurses, pharmacists and patient safety experts, reviewed current issues of intravenous infusion pump use and administration workflow. The multidisciplinary team will develop an intervention that may improve the safety of intravenous drug administration on the wards. Thus, the results and recommendations could be used in different clinical settings.

3   Results

3.1   Incidents Related to Medication Management

The HaiPro reports from 2011-2013 demonstrated that reporting had increased on each unit. Especially, the incidents of near missed have increased cases which illustrate that the preventative meaning of reporting has been emphasized. Most of incidents related medication or information management incidents. The majority of reported incidents were detected errors; recently the reports of near missed have increased (Figure 1).

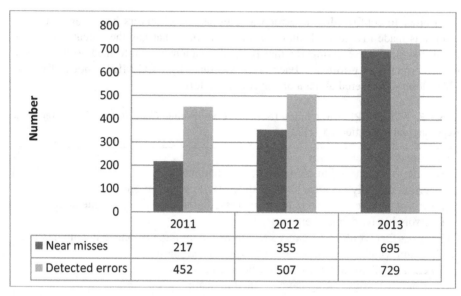

Fig. 1. Reported detected errors and near missed incidences (2011-2013) in the units

3.2   Type of Intravenous Medication Errors

The first measurement offered a diverse range variety of intravenous medication administra-tion adverse events. A few intravenous drug errors were identified during the observa-tion of 492 drug preparations and administrations. The most remarkable result was the review of medication processes which varied significantly across the units.

During the data collection period 137 inpatients in the four units were included in the study.   Over the data collection period 492 medications procedures were observed. There were 355 intravenous medication infusions and 137 fluids infusions. Infusion pumps were used in 56 percent of infusions, 26 percent of infusions was administered without pump. Fifteen percent of infusions were left at the patient's bedside discontinued.

The data consisted of observations in the four units: 18 patients and 29 infusions in medical ICU, 80 patients and 294 infusions in surgical ICU, 71 patients and 144 infusions in general medical unit (the department of oncology, outpatient clinic) and 25 patients and 25 infusions in surgical unit (cardiothoracic and vascular surgery). Generally, patients had one intravenous infusion. In the ICU patients had six or seven simultaneous infusions and in the department of oncology three or four simultaneous infusions respectively.

Violations of medication policies regarding labeling were the frequent error types. In hospital there is a label attached to each intravenous medication bag by nurses in the units.   Meanwhile a pharmacy label is attached by a pharmacist before dispensing medications from the pharmacy department. Missing information details of hospital labels varied between units. The most frequent type of missing information on a unit label was the name of a patient (76%) and the name of producer (nurse or pharmacist) was missing in 37 percent of 355 intravenous medication infusions.

Documenting medication orders and prescribing differed between units. Each prescription was found in an electronic patient record in some units. However, they used several and overlapping documentation forms and paper-based form to manage medication information. Considerable often missing information was the documentation of allergy. The highest score was 56 percent of observed patients (n=130) whose allergy was recorded to electronic patient record system. The rest of units documented less than 50 percent of patients' allergy. There were errors with regard to adherence of using a patient identification. There were units where every patient had an identification band and some wards did not provide any identification band nearly at all. The identification band was taken away before start an intravenous medication quite often.

Data collection in the four study units further indicated that errors were rated as A – B in the NCC MERP harm index. Indicating that capacity to cause an error or error occurred but did not reach the patient. Considering, in spite of the Electronic Patient Record system, several overlapping documentation forms were in use and medication processes varied significantly across the units. Through this prevalence study, the violation errors of hospital policy were found that could potentially place patients at risk.

4   Discussion

The results of this first phase of the intervention study showed the significance of this research project for the hospital to improve patient safety. The HaiPro incidents' statistics described the need to analyze medication management processes. Of all types of medication errors, medication administration errors are least likely to be noticed before they reach the patient [25]. A positive development of voluntary reporting of patient incidents and especially of near miss has increased in every year. These illustrate that their preventative meaning has been emphasized.

The main strength of an observation and medical chart review evaluation is that they directly look at the use of medical devices in clinical environments by actual users. Advantages of observation are obtaining data on authentic surroundings about what really happens in true-life [23, 24].

To prevent adverse events, there is a need to identify a measurement in order to be able to understand the problem. Studies of medication administration errors can be challenging and resource intensive as direct observation are generally required. However, methodological variations between studies exist and these can limit the interpretation of findings [25]. International research collaboration facilitates gathering of comparable data of intravenous medication errors. Several studies have suggested that mediation errors occurring in the administration phase of the medication process [4, 5, 9, 11]. According to these studies, the most frequent type of incidents occurring in hospitals and they are clearly frequent and have considerable potential for injury.

Central to the development of medical error reporting is a need for a controlled vocabulary and taxonomy. In response to reducing medication errors, the released medication error taxonomy [22]. The taxonomy provided us with a standard language and structure of medication error-related data for use in developing data-bases to analyze medication errors [26]. Brixey et al. (2002) found that an error involving an infusion pump was both a device use error and a medication error involving the use of a device. The NCC MERP taxonomy was designed for reporting a medication error. It lacks robustness and specificity for recording device error associated with a medication error. They noticed that one useful feature of the NCC MERP taxonomy in understanding medical errors is that it explicitly pays attention to the role of human factors and contributing systems factors [26].

In this study, intravenous medication had several types of errors. The most common error was lack of information on the label of a dose. This may increase the risk of administering wrong intravenous medications for a patient. Similar results are reported and they suggested that a hospital may need to update its labeling policy to suit current practices with various safety systems [9]. Previous studies have also demonstrated that the number and severity of medication errors had decreased [27, 9]. Ohashi et al. (2013) did not find any patient identification errors in their re-study; while patient identification error was quite common in our first observation study [9].

In this study the most remarkable result was the review of medication processes which varied significantly across the units. The first observations of intravenous medication errors identified the key issues around the use of infusion pumps or smart pumps. This will lead to the development of strategies to improve the prevention of intravenous medication errors. This study focused only one tertiary hospital. However, being in use all over in health care the safe use of infusion pumps is a shared challenge for health care organizations. The data was collected by a multidisciplinary team and all of the investigators were trained regarding the various types of errors. The support from the hospital management and their commitment to improve patient safety was a facilitator for the study.

References

1. Bates, D.W.: A National Study of Intravenous Medication Errors: Understanding How to Improve Intravenous Safety with Smart Pumps. Research Proposal. Brigham and Women's Hospital (2012)
2. Rothschild, J.M., Keohane, C.: The Role of Bar Coding and Smart Pumps in Safety. AHRQ WebM&M. Perspective on Safety (2008), http://webmm.ahrq.gov/perspective.aspx?perspectiveID=64 (accessed March 5, 2014)
3. Bates, D.W., Gawande, A.A.: Improving Safety with Information Technology. N. Engl. J. Med. 348, 2526–2534 (2003)
4. Manrique-Rodriguez, S., Sánchez-Galindo, A.C., de Lorenzo-Pi to, A., González-Vives, L., López-Herce, J., Carrillo-Álvarez, Á., Sanjurjo-Sáez, M., Fernández-Llamazares, C.M.: Implementation of Smart Pump Technology in a Paediatric Intensive Care Unit. Health Informatics Journal (February 4, 2014)
5. Rothscild, J.M., Keohane, C.A., Cook, E.F., Orav, J., Burdick, E., Thompson, S., Hayes, J., Bates, D.W.: A Controlled Trial of Smart Infusion Pumps to Improve Medication Safety in Critically Ill Patients. Crit. Care Med. 33(3), 533–540 (2005)
6. Doupi, P.: National Reporting Systems for Patient Safety Incidents. A Review of the Situation in Europe. National Institute for Health and Welfare (THL), Report 13/2009. Helsinki (2009)
7. AAMI/FDA. Infusing Patient Safety. Priority Issues From the AAMI/FDA Infusion Device Summit (2010)
8. Bates, D.W.: Using Information Technology to Reduce Rates of Medication Errors in Hospitals. BMJ 320, 788 (2000)

9. Ohashi, K., Dykes, P., McIntosh, K., Buckley, E., Wien, M., Bates, D.W.: Evaluation of Instravenous Medication Errors with Smart Infusion Pumps in an Academic Medical Center. In: Proceedins of the AMIA 2013 Annual Symposium, Washington, DC, US, November 16-20 (2013)

10. Ruuhilehto, K., Kaila, M., Keistinen, T., Kinnunen, M., Vuorenkoski, L., Wallenius, J.: HaiPro – What Was Learned From Patient Safety Incident in Finland Health Care Units in 2007 to 2009? Duodecim 127, 1033–1040 (2011)

11. Husch, M., Sullivan, C., Rooney, D., Barnard, C., Fotis, M., Clarke, J., Noskin, G.: Insights From the Sharp End of Intravenous Medication Errors: Implications for Infusion Pump Technology. Qual. Saf. Health Care 14(2), 80–86 (2005)

12. Black, A.D., Car, J., Pagliari, C., Anandan, C., Cresswell, K., Bokum, T., McKinstry, B., Procter, R., Majeed, A., Sheikh, A.: The Impact of eHealth on the Quality and Safety of Health Care: A Systematic Overview. PLoS Medicine (2011), http://www.plosmedicine.org/article/info%3Adoi%2F10.1371%2Fjournal.pmed.1000387 (accessed April 29, 2014)

13. Hertzel, C., Sousa, V.D.: The Use of Smart Pumps for Preventing Medication Errors. J. Infus. Nurs, 257–267 (2009)

14. Larsen, G.Y., Parker, H.B., Cash, J., O'Connell, M., Grant, M.C.: Standard Drug Concentrations and Smart-Pump Technology Reduce Continuous-medication-infusion Errors in Pediatric Patients. Pediatrics 116(1), 21–25 (2005)

15. Adachi, W., Lodolce, A.E.: Use of Failure Mode and Effects Analysis in Improving the Safety of i.v. Drug Administration. Am. J. Health Syst. Pharm. 1;62(9), 917–920 (2005)

16. Eckel, S.F., Anderson, P., Zimmerman, C.: User Satisfaction with an Intravenous Medication Safety System. Am. J. Health Syst. Pharm. 1;63(15), 1419–1423 (2006)

17. Fields, M., Peterman, J.: Intravenous Medication Safety System Averts High-risk Medication Errors and Provides Actionable Data. Nurs. Am. Q. 29(1), 78–87 (2005)

18. Schilling, M.B., Sandoval, S.: Impact of Intelligent Intravenous Infusion Pumps on Directing Care Toward Evidence-based Standards: A Retrospective Data Analysis. Hosp. Pract. 39(3), 113–121 (2011)

19. Fanikos, J., Fiumara, K., Baroletti, S., Luppi, C., Saniuk, C., Mehta, A., Silverman, J., Goldhaber, S.Z.: Impact of Smart Imfusion Technology on Admistration of Anticoagulants. Am. J. Cardiol. 1;99(7), 1002–1005 (2007)

20. AHRQ Making Health Care Safer II: An Updated Critical Analysis of the Evidence for Patient Safety Practices. Evidence Report/Technology Assessment Number 211 (2011)

21. ISMP Multiple Intravenous Infusions Phase 1a: Situation Scan Summary Report, Canada (2010)

22. National Coordinating Council for Medication Error Reporting. Prevention, NCC MERP (2001), http://www.nccmerp.org/ (accessed January 29, 2014)

23. Elias, B.L., Moss, J.A.: Smart Pump Technology. What We Have Learned. Computers, Informatics, Nursing 29(3), 184–190 (2011)

24. Sinivuo, R., Koivula, M., Kylmä, J.: Observation as a Data Collection Method in Clinical Context. Journal of Nursing Science 24(4), 291–301 (2012) (in Finnish)

25. McLeod, M.C., Barber, N., Franklin, B.D.: Methodological Variations and Their Effects on Reported Medication Administration Error Rates. BMJ. Qual. Saf. 22, 278–289 (2013)

26. Brixey, J., Johnson, T.R., Zhang, J.: Evaluating a Medical Error Taxonomy. In: AMIA 2002 Annual Symposium Proceeding (2000)

27. Keohane, C.A., Hayes, J., Saniuk, C., Rothschild, J.M., Bates, D.W.: Intravenous Medication Safety and Smart Infusion Systems. Lessons Learned and Future Opportunities. Journal of Infusion Nursing 28(5), 321–328 (2005)

Experiences on Telemedicine Solutions
for Diabetes Care – Case eMedic Project

Elina Kontio, Ursula Hyrkkänen, and Teppo Saarenpää

Turku University of Applied Sciences, Turku, Finland
{elina.kontio,ursula.hyrkkanen,teppo.saarenpaa}@turkuamk.fi

Abstract. Diabetes is one of the most common diseases in the world. The optimisation of diabetes treatment would mean remarkable savings in health care budgets. eHealth technology can provide new tools to increase healthcare access, improve care delivery systems, and support individuals in engaging in the treatment of their disease as well as provide new solutions for health care professionals. The aim of this paper is to describe the usability of self-management technological solutions in the eMedic project. A qualitative explorative study approach was applied. During the eMedic pilots on self-management, the usability of the devices and applications was assessed by using the System Usability Scale (SUS) questionnaire. The eMedic project shows that eHealth solutions in self-management can have a successful role in healthcare, but focus and effort must be put on the usability of the applications and technical solutions.

Keywords: System Usability Scale, Usability, Telemedicine, Diabetes Mellitus.

1 Introduction

Diabetes is one of the most common diseases in the world. Nowadays approximately 150 million people have diabetes worldwide, and the scenario is that this number may double by the year 2025 [1]. This increase will occur in developing countries and it will be significant both for the health care system and the economy. Diabetes mellitus is a metabolic disorder resulting from a defect in insulin secretion, insulin action, or both. A consequence of this is chronic hyperglycaemia with disturbances of carbohydrate, fat and protein metabolism. Long-term complications of diabetes mellitus include retinopathy, nephropathy and neuropathy. The risk of cardiovascular disease is increased. [2.] The optimisation of diabetes treatment would mean remarkable savings in health care budgets. eHealth technology can provide new tools to increase healthcare access, improve care delivery systems, and support individuals in engaging in the treatment of their disease as well as provide new solutions for health care professionals. However, there have been challenges in adapting eHealth services to daily work routines and converting eHealth pilots into everyday services. Within parts of the Baltic Sea region eHealth services have been adopted, but there is also an identified lack of services.

K. Saranto et al. (Eds.): WIS 2014, CCIS 450, pp. 88–93, 2014.

The use of technology in diabetes is growing, but the results are not clear. For example one systematic review [3], which provided a narrative report of 14 studies that looked at glycosylated haemoglobin A1c (HbA1c) levels, showed significant declines in HbA1c only in six studies. In addition, no significant differences were found post-intervention on studies that looked at changes in body weight, blood pressure, micro-albuminuria and renal function. At the same time, effects on lipids and depression were mixed. Finally, the interventions appeared to improve health-care utilisation with more foot exams and HbA1c monitoring but had no effect on hospital admissions.

In this paper, we introduce one eHealth project where new technological applications and monitoring tools for diabetes were implemented. The aim of this paper is to describe the usability of the self-management technological solutions in the eMedic project.

2   Background

The project eMedic – Developing new practices for teleconsultation and diabetes developed new technological applications and monitoring tools to increase the understanding of needs and requirements of eHealth services [4]. In the eMedic project we implemented telemedicine solutions with three telemedicine approaches: asynchronous, synchronous and telemonitoring. There were a total of nine pilots: four self-management pilots and five teleconsultation pilots. The self-management pilots were focused on diabetic patients' care process (three pilots) and on physical activity (one pilot). The teleconsultation pilots included experiments with diabetic foot care (four pilots) and home care for children (one pilot). In this paper we focus on diabetic patients' self-management pilots in Finland and Estonia.

The set of technology used for the diabetes patients' self-management pilots included:

- glucometers and blood pressure monitors with wireless data transfer (Bluetooth connection)
- Android smartphones with an application for a diabetes diary and the input of the necessary data for diabetes control
- a joint database / personal health record with web user interface (PHRbox) for the patient or entitled health care professional.

Measurements were transmitted to a smartphone via Bluetooth and the data from the phone was transferred automatically to the database with regular synchronisation. A patient and physician participating in the pilot used the same PHRbox for data collection, viewing and communication.

In the eMedic project we gave an education package for the patient and for the nurses and physicians. The aim of the education package was to expand nurse staff's knowledge and skills in the treatment of diabetes mellitus. The aim was also to provide support for professionals with new technological working methods. The education package included the introduction of new technology and support for the patient's self-treatment and motivation for care. There were five seminars for nurses and physicians during the project. The themes of the seminars concerned for example chronic wound care, hygiene/asepsis and wound care at home, complications of diabetes mellitus and lightening treatment of foot. The working counsellor visited the municipalities regularly for discussions about the implementation of the goals, the successes and challenges. The patients were trained individually during the implementation phase.

3   Methods

A qualitative explorative study approach was applied for assessing the user experiences and the usability of the new devices, applications and digital working processes. The usability of the devices and applications for self-management was assessed by using the System Usability Scale (SUS) questionnaire [5,6]. Usability can be defined as being a contextual property, meaning that usability should always be defined and measured in relation to specific settings [7,8,9,10]. Nielsen [7] stated that the two most important issues for usability are the users' tasks and their individual characteristics and differences. Therefore the SUS questionnaire was used during the user experience assessment procedures in most of the pilots. SUS analysis was carried out in all project countries (Finland, Estonia, Latvia and Sweden), but this paper concentrates only on Finnish and Estonian results. In both countries questionnaires were translated their respective languages but otherwise questionnaire form remained same. The users filled the questionnaire during focus group sessions, which were arranged after several months use experience of the wirelessly working glucometers, blood pressure monitors, smart phones and PHRbox. Participants for the focus group sessions were selected purposively representing different health care professionals from the participating health care centers as well as patients.

SUS was selected because it provides a high level subjective assessment of usability which can be used for comparing usability between the systems. SUS yields a single value on a range from 0 (negative) to 100 (positive) that can be used for comparing systems. SUS have been found highly reliable (alpha 0.91) and useful over a wide range of interface types [6].While a 100-point scale allows for relative judgments, there are different ways, how the numeric score could be translated into an absolute judgment of usability. In this study the descriptive adjectives tested by Bangor et al [6] have been applied. Table 1 presents the used adjective based interpretation of SUS results.

Table 1. Used adjective based interpretation of SUS points

SUS points	Interpretation
over 80.3	top 10%, excellent result
under 51	lowest 15%, poor result
68	average SUS result
over 80	Will most likely recommend the product to friends
under 67	Will most likely slander the product to friends
67–80	Passive, won't most likely either slander or recommend the product

4   Results

Population distribution and results from Finland and Estonia are described in table 2. In this testing, the analysis was made on two separate groups:

- Group 1, self-monitoring patients
- Group 2, self-monitoring physicians and nurses

Table 1. SUS scores from Finland and Estonia

Test group	Number of test persons		Average SUS score from tests	
	FIN	EST	FIN	EST
Group 1	1	1	45	45
Group 2	3	19	59	76.6

In the self-management pilots, health care personnel rated the perceived usability of the system above average (a score of 76.6) in Estonia, but in Finland below average (a score of 59). In Finland as well as in Estonia, the SUS scores of patients were below average, meaning concerns on the usability of the system.

All Finnish scores were below average meaning serious usability issues on the system. The self-monitoring patient results were particularly low. All test persons are likely to slander the system to other users. However some indication can be taken from the user comments in the interviews after the SUS questionnaire was filled. Below are some excerpts:

Group 1 Comments during the Interview

- Sending BP measurement from mobile phone is difficult – phone shows red
- BP measurement device does not give feedback
- Blood glucose meter is easier to use and more reliable
- Phone screen turns off by itself

- Measurement data are loaded to internet with 4–5h delay
- Accessing internet is easy since login information and link are saved to browser
- However help was needed when above mentioned information was saved to browser
- Mobile was difficult to use
- Battery drains quickly

Group 2 Comments during the Interview

- Often "Other" was only possible measuring moment to be set to blood pressure measurements
- Lunch and dinner times are not flexible on database
- Touch screen mobile is difficult to use
- Patient information is irregularly checked from the system
- System does not fit to most home care patients (unfamiliar technology and memory problems)

Group 1 SUS score on Estonia was very low and incidentally the same as in Finland. The Interview comments were not available from any Estonian groups but most likely similar user problems caused this value as in Finland. This should however be verified before any actions. The group 2 SUS score was high and well above average. That indicates that Estonian nurses are pleased with the self-monitoring system and actually the SUS scores of 40% of nurses rated in 80 or higher meaning that these users would recommend the system to friends and colleagues. The differences with Estonian and Finnish results in group 2 are notable and reasons for this should be further investigated. The difference could be explained with different processes in healthcare, for example, or with some other reasons but those are not discussed here.

5   Discussion

The eMedic project shows that eHealth solutions in self-management can have a successful role in healthcare, but focus and effort must be put on the usability of the applications and technical solutions. New developed systems should be integrated into present ones in such a way that they require no extra effort from users. If users experience a system as cumbersome, even if it at the same time is considered as useful, they will likely stop using the system after some time. The piloting period was very tight with only few users which probably might affect the results. Furthermore, it is important to understand that SUS does not show the issues that cause usability problems but it does indicate when such problems exist, as in the eMedic case. Other methods like Nielsen's heuristic evaluation would do that, but it is not covered here.

A common theme identified in the pilots was the desire for better system integration, easier data transfer and access to personal health records as well as easier processing of data in the personal health record. Furthermore, eMedic's results show that the actual care process has to be modified when eHealth solutions are implemented.

On the other hand, education and high motivation is equally expected from physicians as improvements in diabetes care can be achieved through intensive communication between the physicians and patients, at least for limited periods of time. Therefore, usability issues are extremely important in order to implement remote diabetes monitoring into everyday practice. User experiences (both patients' and physicians') should constantly be assessed and analysed in order to update such systems to the user's requirements.

References

1. WHO Media Centre,
   http://www.who.int/mediacentre/factsheets/fs138/en
2. American Diabetes Association. Diabetes Care 32(suppl. 1), S62–S67 (2009)
3. Jackson, C.L., Bolen, S., Brancati, F.L., Batts-Turner, M.L., Gary, T.L.: A systematic review of interactive computer-assisted technology in diabetes care. Interactive information technology in diabetes care. Journal of General Internal Medicine 21(2), 105–110 (2006)
4. eMedic – Developing new practices for teleconsultation and diabetes,
   http://julkaisut.turkuamk.fi/isbn9789522164780.pdf
5. Brooke, J.: SUS: a "quick and dirty" usabilityscale. In: Jordan, P.W., Thomas, B., Weerdmeester, B.A., McClelland, A.L. (eds.) Usability Evaluation in Industry. Taylor and Francis, London (1996)
6. Bangor, A., Kortum, P.T., Miller, J.T.: An Empirical Evaluation of the System Usability Scale. International Journal of Human-Computer Interaction 24(6), 574–594 (2008)
7. Nielsen, J.: Usability Engineering. Academic Press, Inc., San Diego (1993)
8. Shackel, B., Richardson, S. (eds.): Human Factors for Informatics Usability. Cambridge University Press, New York (1991)
9. Shneiderman, B.: Designing the User Interface: Strategies for Effective Human-Computer Interaction. Addison-Wesley, Reading (1987)
10. Bevan, N.: Usability is Quality of Use. In: Proc. HCI International 1995, pp. 349–354 (1995)

Problem Limiting the Public Domain -Rawls's Veil of Ignorance and Time

Jani S.S. Koskinen[1], Kai K. Kimppa[1], and Ville M.A. Kainu[2]

[1] Information System Science, University of Turku
[2] Business Law, Turku School of Economics, University of Turku
20014 Turun Yliopisto, Finland
{jasiko,kai.kimppa,vilkai}@utu.fi

Abstract. Information, ideas and new inventions are crucial parts of modern society. Accumulated knowledge is a huge possibility for mankind and information technology has especially made it possible to share resources with all mankind. Nevertheless, the current situation where strong intellectual property rights exists the public domain has been limited and thus the possibilities to use that knowledge is limited especially for people lacking adequate income or property. It seems that the current situation is not well justified because current intellectual property rights are against the two Principles of Justice presented by Rawls. In addition intellectual property rights are a source of inequity towards the people of the future and would not be implemented behind Veil of Ignorance which is the core way to define whether a society is just according to Rawls. This paper shows examples which emphasize the view that new legislation for intellectual property is needed.

Keywords: Veil of Ignorance, Rawls, Theory of Justice, Intellectual Property Rights, Public Domain, Ethics.

1 Introduction

Public domain and its limits have been topics of scientific debate and also targets of lobbying at the political level [1, 2]. This is understandable given the economical and practical significance of public domain in modern societies. Corporations' and people's opportunities to use information, software and tools are bound to the public and the private domain and how those domains are arranged and regulated. Different arguments can be found for various solutions and we argue that the position where the argumentation is created has major impact which solution is recommended for use. For example corporations have tended to emphasize the need for protection to guarantee that making new software and solutions remains profitable.

In this paper Rawls's Theory of Justice [3] is used as the basis for argumentation. The main focus is in the *Veil of Ignorance* which is a part of Rawls's starting position to define a just society which sees "justice as fairness." The Veil of Ignorance is crucial component of a hypothetical situation where one cannot know the position in which one ends up in the society and is developed by rational persons trying to create

K. Saranto et al. (Eds.): WIS 2014, CCIS 450, pp. 94–99, 2014.

a just society. Rawls argues that the outcome of that situation is a society so arranged that it secures the position of all of its members regardless of their natural abilities, which obviously cannot have been chosen by the persons themselves. On the two Principles of Justice Rawls defined the First Principle to achieve a fair distribution of wealth. The Second Principle is used to ensure that everyone has a fair chance to attain offices and positions in society [3].

Rawls's fair distribution of wealth is used for argumentation about public domain and it has strong arguments which support limitations for too strong private domain or even need for withdrawing the IPR's altogether [4]. But the main argument in this paper is that the Veil of Ignorance gives a new perspective to the topic. Behind the Veil of ignorance rational persons are creating a just society, but in many cases one factor forgotten in that argumentation is *time*. If we are defining a truly just society, behind the Veil of Ignorance we cannot know in what position and in which time we are in the society. Veil of Ignorance together with the Two Principles of Justices shows that current legislation and thus society is not fair in the context of IPR's and thus there is need for new laws.

2   Public Domain

Public domain is not defined clearly or without gaps [5]. Like Lessig [6] stated public domain is free but how it is free is a question which needs to be solved and there is a need for new crafted public domain. Jessica Litman's [7] definition for public domain is domain, which technically is the permission-free zone defined by the limits of copyright. Lessig [6] is stating – when referring the Litmans definition – that the effective public domain should be also a lawyer free zone. The current IPR system is so complicated and the danger of violating some IPR is making the situation such that one should always have a lawyer to tell one what to do when using potentially IPR protected materials. And even then there is a risk for getting sued in a court (at least in some countries). Still there is no register or system from which one could ask if something is copyrighted or may belong to public domain [6].

For reasons of clarity in this paper public domain is defined as the information and artefacts (software, books, technical solutions etc.) that are freely accessible and reusable by all interested groups and parties (and the lawyer problem aforementioned by Lessig is bypassed). Regardless of what is the exact definition of the public domain it is obvious that the public domain is nowadays limited with IPRs and it seems that the domain is constantly becoming more limited and narrow.

Boyle describes the situation where things originally in the public domain are taken into the private domain when a private party undertakes the piecemeal enclosure of the public domain via computers that have the power to turn unpatentable ideas into patentable machines [2]. For example moving one's fingers in a certain manner can be patented in certain environments, e.g. US patent # US20130185680 A1 'Unlocking a Device by Performing Gestures on an Unlock Image' which is a patent owned by Apple Inc. In such situations we are limiting the formerly public domain to be the property of some interest group and thus excluding others outside of that formerly free idea. Before that process had taken action, individuals were able to use those ideas freely. But people after that are excluded from using it – at least if they do not pay the price dictated by the possessor of the patent. Thus, *de facto* situation is that the public domain is firstly narrowing down and secondly blurred because the various legislations of intellectual property which makes it hard for layman to see does the immaterial object belong to public domain or does it have protection of intellectual property right and what kind that protection actually is.

3   Rawls and Reasons for Extending the Public Domain

Murphy analyses the compatibility of IPR's and Rawls's Principles of justice and presents arguments which reveals the conflicts between those [4]. In this paper we want to bring a new viewpoint to the discussion, based on Rawls's Theory of justice – the viewpoint of time. Behind the *Veil of ignorance*, there is a situation where the parties do not know certain kinds of facts which may be affecting the outcome of defining a just, a good society. Those facts are such which could be tempting a party to define rules in such a manner that they would serve the advantages of their own. Such are listed by Rawls of a person: *"his place in society, his class position and or social status; nor does he know his fortune in the distribution of natural assets and abilities, his intelligence and strength, and the like."* [3]. If we are thinking of time, we can easily see that it has great impact in whether the society is fair and just over the generations. Like Rawls's [3] description: *"I assume that the parties do not know the particular circumstances of their own society. That is, they do not know its economic or political situation, or the level of civilization and culture it has been able to achieve. The persons in the original position have no information as to which generation they belong"* shows the time has important and crucial place in Rawls way to define principles of just. Behind the Veil of Ignorance individuals do not know which time they will live on.

Even though Rawls [3] says that the treaty is made for all generations, and the persons making the deal cannot know which generation they belong to, this makes the argument unwieldingly theoretical, as the persons participating will not be members of any future generations. Even if rational decisions behind the Veil of Ignorance are presumed, we must remember that selfishness is also expected. Thus, the fate of future generations may not be considered (although it should) – as it would be an is-ought problem, from is (in this case the "purpose"[1] of evolution) does not follow ought (duty towards future generations), as the current generation might not share the idea that future generations would be 'selfishly' their concern. Moreover it is obvious that we cannot change the societies of the past – in light of present knowledge, which gives some relief for us – thus we must put our hearts in making the current situation and future as good as possible to avoid unjust scenarios at this point of time and hence forward. If we are limiting the public domain we are limiting the possibilities of future generations to use it as source of common good and thus we are conflicting

---

[1] ...Although it is of course clear that evolution has no *purpose*, per se, but only 'goes' to a direction that it happens to go due to environmental pressures.

with Rawls's principle of liberty *"Each person is to have an equal right to the most extensive total system of equal basic liberties compatible with a similar system of liberty for all"* [3]. With granting IPR's we are always taking liberties to use that target of IPR's – which were free for the people of the past – to become property of some and the right of others are limited..

In environmental and ecological research this aspect of time and duty towards future generations has been noticed and used as an argument for sustainable development of society [8]. Nevertheless, time argumentation is valid in defining fair public and private domain of intellectual property – even the idea that intellectual property is property is full of pitfalls – as well as ecological issues because both are dealing with same kind of problem – what we are leaving for the future generations. Like it is not fair to exploit the nature in such a way that the cost falls for the future generations to pay it is not justified to diminish the public domain and leave the consequences for others. Those who (including at least the future generation which lives during the time of an IPR) are not in a situation where there is a possibility to come up an idea or an invention protected by the granted IPR.

4 The Absurd World of Intellectual Property

Pharmaceutical development could be problematic if there would be no intellectual property rights (specifically patents) because the development of new drugs would be jeopardized if they would not have a clear way to make financial gain for drugs invented and tested (which can cost enormous amounts of money and take decades). So to ensure the development of new drugs or medical treatments a financial support model must be guaranteed. But what makes the drug issue especially interesting is that the patent is much shorter term right than most other intellectual property rights (especially copyright and trademark). One of the most absurd examples is the Disney copyright protection which has been extended every time it has been close to entering public domain [9]. Given that 20 years has been deemed sufficient IPR duration to recoup the development costs under patent, it seems somehow absurd that we protect fictional cartoon characters for around a hundred years and thus limit the public domain of the future time after time.

Regarding the situation behind the Veil of Ignorance we can apprehend that this situation where ever longer lasting protection has been given to intellectual property, consequently conditions where some parts of society have been able to freely exploit the ideas and inventions of previous generations yet at the same time limiting the rights of future generations, e.g. Ray Charles's 'I Got a Woman' and 'mashup' cases, have come about [2]. Those songs are good examples of problem of copyright and time. Ray Charles derived inspiration from musical works of others which was not under protection of copyright on that time. But after making those songs, he gained copyright over those melodies and thus those were driven away from public domain. The following quotation from Boyle [2] *"The freedoms Ray Charles says he used to create his song are denied to his successors until nearly a century after the song's release"* shows clearly the problem of fairness, if time is not considered as part to take account when defining principles of just society behind the Veil of Ignorance.

It may seem provocateur to state that that situation resembles cherry picking, but we claim that this is the actual situation or even more, it is about restricting others to even try to get cherries. Behind the Veil of ignorance, one cannot know to which time one is born and thus it is obvious that the aforementioned situation would not be agreed upon, because there is such misbalance between different generations. The unbalance on this issue is clear even the future generation most likely have some other advantages because work done by earlier generations. Nevertheless, the good done in one place is not justification to do bad in some other, especially when there is possibility to act justly.

By limiting the public domain we are, in fact, limiting freedom and opportunities of the weaker parties in society who are not able to obtain the benefits of those limitations. Hence the first principle of justice is violated in that unfair limitation and we favor the members of society who are already in a privileged status or position. Thus, we also limit the possibilities of future generations, a solution which is in conflict with original position behind the Veil of Ignorance where one cannot know the position (and time – in analogy, the difference is between three and four dimensional coordinates) in society. It cannot be fair to give privileges to any given generation at a cost to the future generations unless it strengthens the position of the weakest parties in the society – including future generations. This is especially problematic in light of the second principle: *"Social and economic inequalities are to be arranged so that they are both: (a) to the greatest benefit of the least advantaged, consistent with the just savings principle, and (b) attached to offices and positions open to all under conditions of fair equality of opportunity."* [3]. If we are limiting the access to intellectual property of the future generations the possibilities of the least advantages are limited because they most likely do not have possibility to buy or get the access to intellectual property — e.g. ideas and knowledge — which was free for past generations (see aforementioned example of Ray Charles). It seems unlikely to be a situation which is to the most benefit for the least advantaged parties of the (future) society.

The problem can be more readily understood with a comparison to the environmental issues. We cannot destroy the future to profit today – for example conduct exhaustive fishing – without violating the rights of the future generations. We can justify the use of natural resources if we give future generations a better basis to start and limit the harm that we cause. But we have to consider our actions towards a better future, because past time is gone and we cannot change it. We do not have a justification to harm nature if we have the possibility to avoid it. And if this is the case with environmental issues, what is the difference in limiting the public domain of future generations with unjustified (in light Rawls) IPRs?

Nevertheless, there has been developed different solutions (for immaterial rights) that bear closer similarity to fair and just society that Rawls defines in the Theory of Justice [1-2, 9-10]. To ensure the development of critical inventions – such as drugs, fusion power plants etc. – which need large financial investments we have a structure where income for those comes from governments and international (public) foundations. When thinking of how to encourage individuals to engage in intellectual work and how to secure an income from their work we can develop systems which allocate money to support those individuals – an argument which is used in the IPR discussion. But in the current system we are not actually supporting individuals. Instead, the current IPR-legislation protects corporations and few individuals which have been achieving an extraordinary position in the current system. When thinking of fair distribution of wealth we see the extreme distortion between current situation and a Rawlsian fair society. This is hardly benefitting the weakest part of society which is required by the first Principle of Justice in a just society by Rawls [3]. The current IPR-system is securing the needs of those who have and the cost is falling upon those who have not.

5   Conclusions and Discussion

When considering IPR's from a Rawlsian perspective, the consideration of time is supporting the need for different legislation for immaterial objects and artefacts. It is obvious that the current system is not fulfilling the principles of justice by Rawls. It is not fair towards future generation which are facing the shrinking area of public domain. This means that fair distribution of knowledge; information and innovation are sacrificed for the holders of IPR's. Future work must be done to find new ways to find the incentives for intellectual work which fulfils the justification in Rawlsian sense and for ensuring the great possibilities which information technology is offering for the whole mankind.

References

1. Hettinger, E.C.: Justifying Intellectual Property. Philosophy & Public Affairs 18(1), 31–52 (1989)
2. Boyle, J.: Public Domain: Enclosing the Commons of the Mind. Yale University Press (2008)
3. Rawls, J.A.: Theory of Justice, Revised edition, Cambridge. Belknap Press of Harvard University Press, Massachusetts (1999)
4. Murphy, D.: Are intellectual property rights compatible with Rawlsian principles of Justice? Ethics and Information Technology 14(2), 109–121 (2012)
5. Cohen, J.: Copyright, Commodification, and Culture: Locating the Public Domain. In: Guibault, L., Hugenholtz, P.B. (eds.) The Future of the Public Domain, pp. 121–166. Kluwer Law International (2006)
6. Lessig, L.: Re-crafting a Public Domain. Yale Journal of Law & the Humanities 18(3), 56–83 (2006)
7. Litman, J.: The public domain. Emory Law Journal 39(4), 964–1023 (1990)
8. Norton, B.: Intergenerational equity and environmental decisions: A model using Rawls' veil of ignorance. Ecological Economics 1(2), 137–159 (1989)
9. Lessig, L.: The Future of Ideas: The Fate of the Commons in a Connected World. Vintage Books, New York (2001)
10. Spinello, R.A.: Ethical Aspects of Information Technology. Prentice-Hall, Inc., Upper Saddle River (1995)

Utilising Social Media for Intervening and Predicting Future Health in Societies

Camilla Laaksonen[1], Harri Jalonen[2], and Jarkko Paavola[2]

[1] Turku University of Applied Sciences, Health and Well-Being, Turku, Finland
camilla.laaksonen@turkuamk.fi
[2] Turku University of Applied Sciences, Business, ICT and Life Sciences, Turku, Finland
{harri.jalonen,jarkko.paavola}@turkuamk.fi

Abstract. Background: The aims of this paper are to describe 1. systematic reviews describing the relation between social media and health and 2. previous research on utilising social media for predicting health on a population level. Method: A literature search utilising PubMed was performed in March 2014.

The inclusion criteria were that the article describes 1. the relation between social media and health or 2. the utilisation of social media in predicting health on a population level. Results: 11 systematic reviews and 4 articles were included in this review. The included articles were published between 2009–2014. There is a lack of knowledge about the relation and outcomes of social media and health. No systematic review on utilising social media to predict health on a population level was identified. Conclusions: Social media may carry crucial yet undiscovered means to predict and interfere in the health of populations. Future research, innovation and development in this area are highly recommended.

Keywords: Social media, public health, health promotion.

1 Introduction

Social media herein refers to a constellation of Internet-based applications that derive their value from the participation of users through directly creating original content, modifying existing material, contributing to a community dialogue and integrating various media together to create something unique [1]. Popular social media sites magnetise hundreds of users nowadays – the leading site is Facebook, which has well over a billion active users. Twitter, VK, Sina Weibo, to name a few other sites, have also reported rapid growth. A sophisticated guess is that in the OECD countries, two thirds of the population use social media more or less regularly. In fact, social media has integrated into the lives of people. Social media has brought with it 'media life', which Deuze [2] calls "the state where media has become so inseparable from us that we do not live with media, but in it" [3]. In a hyperconnected and networked society posts on Twitter may become a meme – a rapidly spreading and mutating piece of information [4].

K. Saranto et al. (Eds.): WIS 2014, CCIS 450, pp. 100–108, 2014.
© Springer International Publishing Switzerland 2014

In contrast to traditional mass communication, social media is an unregulated context which allows ordinary people to publish almost anything that come to their minds. Presumably social media carries several benefits as well as challenges for health and well-being on the individual, community and national but also on the continental and global levels. Social media has been suggested to be useful in the context of health promotion for purposes such as sharing information, developing positive brand pictures, expanding the reach of health promotion interventions to diverse audiences, supporting target group empowerment, engagement and participation. These features carry several benefits for health promoting but also for health contradictive purposes. [5-6].

Knowledge of how social media is related to health is still lacking but the body of knowledge in this field is rapidly increasing. It has been suggested that social media may have a central role in health related decisions as data in the social media may effect several phases of the decision making process. [7]. Researchers address serious concern regarding the emotional well-being of present day adolescents in general [8-10] and there have been suggestions that social media may increase and create new mental health problems, such as addiction to social networking, in certain populations [11].

The evidence addressing the addictive qualities of social networks are however scarce and social media is mostly used for common social purposes. It has been suggested that extravert personalities use social networking for social communication. Introverts however may use social networking sites for compensating social connections in the real world and this may lead to emotional problems [11]

Previous research suggests that social media may enable predicting health on an individual level but knowledge on how social media can be utilised to predict health on a population level and how potential early warning signs could be utilised for health promotion in populations is lacking. If social media enables predicting future health risks before these are identified in real life environments, it enables early, targeted health promotion interventions on the warning signs. Evidently this would crucially benefit the health and well-being of future individuals and societies. Capabilities to combine information from different sources in the Internet for monitoring and predicting flu outbreaks have been demonstrated by Google [12]. Estimates based on keyword searches match well to statistics collected from official sources. The aims of this paper are to describe 1. systematic reviews describing the relation between social media and health and 2. previous research on utilising social media for predicting health on a population level.

2   Methods

A literature search was performed in March 2014. The search covered one of the main health care field databases, PubMed. The inclusion criteria were that the article describes 1. the relation between social media and health or 2. the utilisation of social media in predicting health on a population level. At the first stage all search results were evaluated according to the title and the ones that fit the inclusion criteria were next evaluated by their abstracts.

Content analysis of the articles was performed according to the purpose of this paper. The aim, population, main results and outcomes of the included articles were extracted. The extracted data was synthesised to describe the present state of published research regarding the relation between social media and health and utilising social media for predicting health on a population level.

3   Results

The literature search on systematic reviews describing the relation between social media and health resulted in 51 titles. After evaluating the titles and abstracts, altogether 11 articles met the inclusion criteria and were included in this review. For the search describing the utilisation of social media in predicting health on a population level altogether 81 titles were identified. After evaluating the titles and abstracts four articles met the inclusion criteria.

3.1   Reviews Describing the Relation between Social Media and Health

Use of social media to promote healthy diet and exercise was evaluated by performing a systematic review including randomised controlled trials (RCT) on the topic. Several databases were searched for the time period 2000–2013. There were 22 studies that met the inclusion criteria. The results suggested high variation in interventions, outcomes and comparison groups and no significant changes in physical activity or significant differences between the intervention and control groups were identified. [13].

The impact of social media in online weight management was assessed by a systematic review including RCTs. Several databases were searched in March 2013. There were 517 identified citations and 20 articles met the inclusion criteria. Great variation in design and outcomes was identified. Message rooms and chat boards were most commonly included but effects on weight were rarely reported. Few studies have reported on the outcomes of web-based weight matter interventions and the impact is unknown. [14].

The impacts of health oriented social media informatics tools on health outcomes were assessed by a systematic review including RCTs on the topic. Only two articles of 600 met the inclusion criteria. According to the identified articles, social media interventions may improve pain control among patients with chronic pain and support weight loss among people trying to lose weight. More research was stated to be needed to confirm the preliminary findings on the effects of social media on health outcomes. The social component of a disease or a health problem may be an effective target for therapy, and socio-clinical interventions for health outcomes may be supported by social media. [15].

The potential roles of Internet surveillance in controlling and preventing the human H7N9 influenza outbreaks were assessed by examining daily posted and forwarded blogs on the Sina microblog website and Baidu Attention Index (BAI) using the keyword H7N9. The daily posted and forwarded number for H7N9 increased quickly during the three first days of the outbreaks (March 31st 0 posts vs. April 3rd 850 000 posts) and the amount of posts reminded high for five days. The researchers concluded that the first days of an epidemic outbreak are crucial for authorities to take action through Internet surveillance to prevent and control the epidemic, information, opinions and reactions. The researchers concluded that the Internet can be utilised as an effective tool to prevent and control public health emergencies. [16].

Vaccination attitudes were examined by tracking the debate on MySpace regarding the public's reaction to the human papilloma virus (HPV) vaccine. There were 303 blogs identified which met the inclusion criteria. Of these, about 50% were classified as positive, 40% negative and 10% ambivalent. According to the review, the public opinion and attitude toward the HPV vaccine was more positive than negative. Blog analysis was suggested to be a useful tool for officials to profile criticism and design appropriate education. Developing effective mechanisms to deliver and communicate information through social media to the general public was recommended. [17].

Internet based interventions to promote lifestyle among adults with type 2 diabetes (dm 2) were examined by searching the PubMed data base in January 2013. There were 2 803 papers identified but only nine met the inclusion criteria. The included papers suggested an improvement in diet, physical activity and glycaemic control when comparing web-based interventions to controls. Successful studies were theory-based, included interactive components, personalised feedback and peer support. Website utilisation declined over time. As a conclusion, web-based strategies provide a valuable option for self-management of dm 2. Future research was however recommended to target underserved populations suffering from dm 2, website utilisation patterns and long-term engagement. [18].

It was assessed whether diabetes applications have improved the self-management among patients with type 1 and 2 diabetes. The available applications supported self-management in nutrition, physical exercise, medication or insulin dosage and blood glucose testing. Other support tasks included different types of notifications or alerts, decision support, tagging input data and communication in the social media. The mobile applications seemed to have positive impacts on self-management but long-term research was missing. The conclusion was that more research is recommended to improve the usability and adoption of the new technology. [19].

A systematic review of social media sites on how the risks of diabetes and alcohol were communicated by people with type 1 diabetes (dm 1) in the social media was performed. There were 292 articles identified but only six met the inclusion criteria. The results show that social media was widely used for peer advice but professional advice was rarely identified. Inaccurate information was common. As a conclusion, the researchers stated that people with dm 1 use online resources to share information regarding diabetes and the use of alcohol. There is however a need for professional advice and there is a high risk of false knowledge that has to be taken into account in social media. [20].

Salient features between mobile applications for diabetes care and clinical guideline recommendations for diabetes self-management were assessed. There were 973 applications identified from which 137 met the inclusion criteria. Most common issues in the applications were nutrition, insulin or medical recording, information exchange or communication and weight management tools. A wide selection of different mobile applications for people with diabetes was identified. There were however gaps between general recommendations of diabetes self-management and the applications. Especially personalised diabetes-related education and sharing of information was lacking in the mobile applications. [21].

The ways that technology, including social media, has been utilised in decreasing health disparities and improving the health care access and outcomes of underserved populations were reviewed. There were 424 identified articles of which 125 met the inclusion criteria. The articles described 19 different types of underserved populations, introduced 30 different technologies and targeted 23 different health issues. The main result was that the technology targeting underserved populations need to be designed for the precise group and personalised. Technology may carry potential for reducing health disparities and improving health in underserved populations while designed for a specific group and personal needs. More research is however required in the field and the outcomes of the new technology need to be evaluated. [22].

The interaction between health and social media was reviewed. There were 514 identified publications that met the inclusion criteria and were classified into the following categories: commentaries and reviews (n=267), descriptive studies (n=231) and pilot intervention studies (n=34). Scarce empirical evidence on the interactions between health and social media and the effects of these interventions was found. The conclusion was that further research on the topic is highly recommended. [23].

3.2   Utilising Social Media in Predicting Health on the Population Level

Exploiting Twitter for public health monitoring was evaluated. The aim of the research was to identify hints and early warning signs on threats on public health and the usefulness of social media to monitor health on a population level. Data from Twitter, TV and radio was continuously and systematically collected using a list of key words. Sentences were automatically analysed and classified. The system was able to identify health issues in the social media. A minority of the signals referred to personal disease or symptoms but the majority of the signals to outbreaks in reality. The system detected a high amount of irrelevant data and needs future development to develop strategies for reducing false alarms. Automatic monitoring of the huge amount of data in the social media was however concluded to be less demanding than manual monitoring, and future development in the area was highly recommended. [24].

The potential of automatic prediction of suicide from social media variables was tested. The researchers tested suicide- and dysphoria-related weblog entries along with traditional, social, economic and meteorological predictor variables. Both social media variables strongly correlated with suicide frequency and two different types of background influences were identified. The social media variables may even be more effective predictors than the traditional economic (consumer price index and unemployment rate) predictors. The researchers concluded that social media may be of great value in forecasting and preventing suicides on population levels. [25].

In terms of vaccination related attitudes and perceptions of online social media users, the research suggested that information in the social media flows more effectively between users sharing the same sentiments and most communities are dominated either by positive or negative sentiments toward vaccines. Social media proved to be an effective channel to provide data regarding population perceptions and may provide effective tools for identifying target areas and groups for interventions as well as a source to analyse the effects of interventions. [26].

A framework for a set of public health informatics methods to analyse data in the internet was introduced by Eysenbach [27]. Infodemiology was defined as an area distributing and determining information in electronic medias, especially the Internet, with the aim of informing the population on health issues. The author proposes an expanded framework including basic metrics, such as information prevalence and incidents in social media and distinguishes supply-based applications, demand-based methods and active and passive infoveillance methods. The metrics and methods were suggested to be potentially useful for predicting health related issues but the need for further development and standardisation was addressed.

4   Discussion and Conclusion

Identified systematic reviews describing the relation between social media and health were published between 2011–2014. The aim of the identified reviews was to describe previously published research [13-15, 18, 22-23], blogs/sites [16-17, 20] or applications [19, 21]. The populations described in the articles were general adult population [13-17, 23], people with diabetes [18-21], unserved populations [22] and people with chronic pain [15]. Health related issues described in the reviews focused on a healthy diet, exercise and weight management [13-15], public health emergency control and vaccination [16-17], diabetes self-management [18-21], pain control [15], health promotion in general [23] and reducing health disparities [22]. A common conclusion of the reviews was that social media and new technology may carry potential for health outcomes but more research is needed to understand the relation between social media and health related issues as well as to evaluate the effects, especially the long-term outcomes.

The included articles on utilising social media to predict health in populations were published between 2009–2013. The articles described identifying early warning signs with regard to health status in populations [24], predicting national suicide incidents [25], vaccination control [26] and introducing a new framework of infoepidemiology to predict relevant health events in populations [27]. The results suggested that social media may carry the potential of predicting health related issues in populations but the main conclusion is that more knowledge about utilising social media for preventing population health related issues is highly needed.

The paper implicitly suggests that, in order to handle negative sentiments in terms of health issues, health providers should aim at the ability to map the seeds of negative sentiments as early as possible. This is because the value of negative emotion is the function of time. One possible approach to increase the ability to detect emotional-based weak signals is taking advantage of sentiment analysis [28-29]. Sentiment analysis, or opinion mining, refers herein to a computational study of sentiments, affects and emotions expressed in social media texts. Sentiment analysis is based on a very simple idea – texts are subjective and may express some personal feeling, view, emotion, or belief. Although a completely automated solution is nowhere in sight [28], it is expected that sentiment analysis provides health providers with a useful tool to improve their ability to detect symptoms of collective negative emotions, before they become an issue.

Although the area of sentiment analysis and opinion mining has recently enjoyed a huge burst of research activity, there has been an interest for quite a while. The foundation has been laid down in computer science, and factors behind this development include the rise of machine learning methods in natural language processing, efficient information retrieval, and the availability of datasets from the www and social media [30]. Some of the early works are Carbonell [31] and Wilks & Bien [32]. Since 2001, the amount of sentiment analysis publications starts to rise – for example Das & Chen [33], Tateishi, Ishiguro & Fukushima [34], and Tong [35] demonstrate the applicability of automated opinion analysis. This automated message processing is a necessity due to the nature of social media communications. The average number of tweets per day in Twitter is 58 million, and the same figure for Facebook status updates is 55 million. Even though searches could be limited to certain geographical areas by language selection, the number of messages is still far beyond what can be processed with manual analysis.

There are several limitations to this review that have to be considered. First, only few basic terms were used and only one database was searched. The aim of this review was however to get a general overview and motivate a systematic review and future research on the topic. Also the concept of social media was not clearly stated in the search resulting in the inclusion of research of very different types of technologies and web-based solutions.

As a conclusion of this preliminary review, knowledge is lacking about the relation between social media and health. No systematic review on utilising social media to predict health on population levels was found and the area of research is only in the beginning. Social media may carry crucial yet undiscovered means and possibilities to predict and interfere early with the health of populations. A systematic review on utilising social media to predict health in populations is highly recommended as well as future research, innovation and development in this area.

References

1. Kaplan, A.M., Haenlein, M.: Users of the world, unite! The challenges and opportunities of social media. Business Horizons 53, 59–68 (2010)
2. Deuze, M.: Media Life. Media Culture and Society 33(1), 137–148 (2011)
3. Karppi, T.: Disconnect.Me – User Engagement and Facebook, Doctoral Dissertations, Annales Universitatis Turkuensis, Ser. B Tom. 376, Humaniora, University of Turku (2014)

4. Hemsley, J., Mason, R.M.: Knowledge and knowledge management in the social media age. Journal of Organizational Computing and Electronic Commerce 23(1-2), 138–167 (2013)
5. Pujazon-Zazik, M., Park, J.M.: To Tweet or Not to Tweet: Gender Differences and Potential Positive and Negative Health Outcomes of Adolescents' Social Internet Use. American Journal of Men's Health 4(1), 77–85 (2010)
6. Seidenberg, A.B., Rodgers, E.J., Rees, V.W., Connolly, G.N.: Youth access, creation, and content of smokeless tobacco ("dip") videos in social media. Journal of Adolescent Health 50(4), 334–338 (2012)
7. Neiger, B.L., Thackeray, R., Van Wagenen, S.A., Hanson, C.L., West, J.H., Barnes, M.D., Fagen, M.C.: Use of social media in health promotion: purposes, key performance indicators, and evaluation metrics. Health Promot. Pract. (2), 159–164 (2012)
8. Sourander, A., Niemelä, S., Santalahti, P., Helenius, H., Piha, J.: Changes in psychiatric problems and service use among 8-year-old children: a 16-year population-based time-trend study. Journal of the American Academy of Child and Adolescent Psychiatry 47(3), 317–327 (2008)
9. Laaksonen, C., Aromaa, M., Heinonen, O.J., Koivusilta, L., Koski, P., Suominen, S., Vahlberg, T., Salanterä, S.: Health related quality of life in 10-year-old schoolchildren. Quality of Life Research 17, 1049–1054 (2008)
10. Laaksonen, C., Aromaa, M., Heinonen, O.J., Koivusilta, L., Koski, P., Suominen, S., Vahlberg, T., Salanterä, S.: The change in child self-assessed and parent proxy–assessed Health Related Quality of Life (HRQL) in early adolescence (age 10–12). Scandinavian Journal of Public Health 38, 9–16 (2010)
11. Kuss, D.J., Griffiths, M.D.: Online Social Networking and Addiction—A Review of the Psychological Literature. International Journal of Environment Research and Public Health 8(9), 3528–3552 (2011)
12. Google.org: Flu trends, http://www.google.org/flutrends/ (cited May 21, 2014)
13. Williams, G., Hamm, M.P., Shulhan, J., Vandermeer, B., Hartling, L.: Social media interventions for diet and exercise behaviours: a systematic review and meta-analysis of randomised controlled trials. BMJ Open 4(2), e003926 (2014)
14. Chang, T., Chopra, V., Zhang, C., Woolford, S.J.: The role of social media in online weight management: systematic review. J. Med. Internet Res. 15(11), e262 (2013)
15. Gibbons, M.C.: Personal health and consumer informatics. The impact of health oriented social media applications on health outcomes. Yearb Med. Inform. 8(1), 159–161 (2013)
16. Gu, H., Chen, B., Zhu, H., Jiang, T., Wang, X., Chen, L., Jiang, Z., Zheng, D., Jiang, J.: Importance of Internet surveillance in public health emergency control and prevention: evidence from a digital epidemiologic study during avian influenza A H7N9 outbreaks. J. Med. Internet Res. 17, 16(1), e20 (2014)
17. Keelan, J., Pavri, V., Balakrishnan, R., Wilson, K.: An analysis of the Human Papilloma Virus vaccine debate on MySpace blogs. Vaccine 28(6), 1535–1540 (2010)
18. Cotter, A.P., Durant, N., Agne, A.A., Cherrington, A.L.: Internet interventions to support lifestyle modification for diabetes management: A systematic review of the evidence. J. Diabetes Complications 28(2), 243–251 (2014)
19. El-Gayar, O., Timsina, P., Nawar, N., Eid, W.: Mobile applications for diabetes self-management: status and potential. J. Diabetes Sci. Technol. 7(1), 247–262 (2013)
20. Jones, E., Sinclair, J.M., Holt, R.I., Barnard, K.D.: Social networking and understanding alcohol-associated risk for people with type 1 diabetes: friend or foe? Diabetes Technol. Ther. 15(4), 308–314 (2013)

21. Chomutare, T., Fernandez-Luque, L., Arsand, E., Hartvigsen, G.: Features of mobile diabetes applications: review of the literature and analysis of current applications compared against evidence-based guidelines. J. Med. Internet Res. 13(3), e65 (2011)
22. Montague, E., Perchonok, J.: Health and wellness technology use by historically underserved health consumers: systematic review. J. Med. Internet Res. 14(3), e78 (2012)
23. Chou, W.Y., Prestin, A., Lyons, C., Wen, K.Y.: Web 2.0 for health promotion: reviewing the current evidence. Am. J. Public Health 103(1), e9–e18 (2013)
24. Denecke, K., Krieck, M., Otrusina, L., Smrz, P., Dolog, P., Nejdl, W., Velasco, E.: How to exploit twitter for public health monitoring? Methods Inf. Med. 52(4), 326–339 (2013)
25. Won, H.H., Myung, W., Song, G.Y., Lee, W.H., Kim, J.W., Carroll, B.J., Kim, D.K.: Predicting national suicide numbers with social media data. PLoS One 8(4), e61809 (2013)
26. Salathé, M., Khandelwal, S.: Assessing vaccination sentiments with online social media: implications for infectious disease dynamics and control. PLoS Comput. Biol. 7(10), e1002199 (2011)
27. Eysenbach, G.: Infodemiology and infoveillance: framework for an emerging set of public health informatics methods to analyze search, communication and publication behavior on the Internet. J. Med. Internet Res. 27, 11(1), e11 (2009)
28. Liu, B.: Sentiment Analysis and Subjectivity. In: Indurkhya, N., Damerau, F.J. (eds.) Handbook of Natural Language Processing. Chapman & Hall/CRC Press, Boca Raton, Florida (2010)
29. Thelwall, M., Buckley, K.: Topic-Based Sentiment Analysis for the Social Web: The Role of Mood and Issue-Related Words. Journal of the American Society for Information Society and Technology 64(8), 1608–1617 (2013)
30. Pang, B., Lillian, L.: Opinion Mining and Sentiment Analysis. Foundations and Trends in Information Retrieval 1-2(2), 1–135 (2008)
31. Carbonell, J.: Subjective Understanding: Computer Models of Belief Systems. PhD thesis, Yale (1979)
32. Wilks, Y., Bien, J.: Beliefs, points of view and multiple environments. In: Proceedings of the International NATO Symposium on Artificial and Human Intelligence, pp. 147–171. Elsevier North-Holland, Inc., USA (1984)
33. Das, S., Chen, M.: Yahoo! for Amazon: Extracting market sentiment from stock message boards. In: Proceedings of the Asia Pacific Finance Association Annual Conference, APFA (2001)
34. Tateishi, K., Ishiguro, Y., Fukushima, T.: Opinion information retrieval from the internet. Information Processing Society of Japan (IPSJ) SIG Notes 69(7), 75–82 (2001) (in Japanese) (Also cited as "A reputation search engine that gathers people's opinions from the Internet", IPSJ Technical Report NL-14411)
35. Tong, R.M.: An operational system for detecting and tracking opinions in on-line discussion. In: The Proceedings of the Workshop on Operational Text Classification, OTC (2001)

Practice-Oriented Safety Procedures in Work Environment with Visually and Hearing Impaired Colleagues

Riitta Lahtinen[1,2], Russ Palmer[2], and Stina Ojala[3]

[1] Communication Unit, Finnish Deafblind Association
[2] Intensive Special Education (ISE) Research Group, Department of Teacher Education,
University of Helsinki
[3] Department of Information Technology, University of Turku
riitta.lahtinen@kuurosokeat.fi, rpalmer2@tiscali.co.uk,
stina.ojala@utu.fi

Abstract. In work places where there are hearing and visually impaired colleagues, there are safety related issues that are not present in work environment where there are only hearing and sighted employees. For example all the premises and safe routes within have to be precisely memorised by all employees in case there is an emergency during the work day. In an ordinary work place annual safety rehearsals and fire drills are enough to remind all workers about the safe routes and procedures in an emergency, but for the visually and hearing impaired employees this is not enough, but for the dual-sensory impaired employee it might prove difficult just to realise what room he/she is in at a particular moment. This procedure is made easier by so-called body mapping, i.e. drawing a simplified floor plan of the room on the back or on the back of the hand of the worker [1, pp.136-138]. The body map includes the exits, the emergency exit should there be any, and safe routes to the exits. Sometimes, tactile maps can be provided for the same purpose too [2]. Another issue related to fire alarms is that the hearing impaired workers might not be aware of the fire alarm sound. Thus the information must be relayed to the colleagues using other methods. Currently, there is a specialised touch-based social quick message system [3], which is used in some international deafblind meetings and conferences, and it is also taught to hotel staff in venues of Finnish Deafblind Association AGMs.

Keywords: safety, sensory impairments, technical aids, haptics.

1 Introduction – Categorizing Different Safety Elements

Safety in working environments does not only apply to special emergency situations, but it is an essential part of daily working environment. This is especially poignant for visually or hearing impaired employers. To share a working environment with visually or hearing impaired colleagues requires type of collaboration between colleagues to be able to ensure a safe working environment every day for all employers. This is further pronounced when there are dual sensory impaired employers in the workplace.

K. Saranto et al. (Eds.): WIS 2014, CCIS 450, pp. 109–119, 2014.

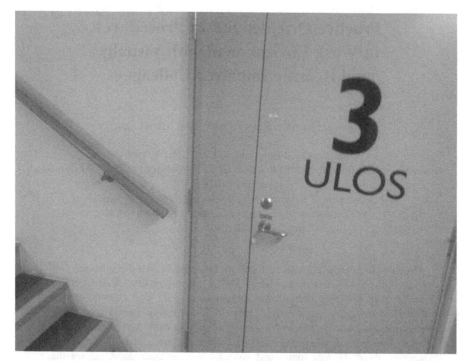

Fig. 1. Exit door. Please note large size number 3 as well as number three written in Braille on top of the door handle near to the handle itself. On the hand-rail there are three wooden buttons to denote third floor.

There are different categories of safety-related features: structures within the buildings, individual technical aids and person-to-person communication. The building-related safety issues must be considered already when designing a building, e.g. [4], as in that stage their inclusion will be most cost-efficient. Adding safety features later could prove expensive. This process of including safety-related issues for the sensory impaired in the building stage is called accessibility. The safety-related issues can be modest, such as using colour contrast in the walls denoting passageways, i.e. doors and elevators (Figures 1-3).

The colour contrasts in the walls are an example of everyday safety: the contrasts are there to enable the visually impaired workers to walk independently and safely from one place to another. This gives a person an opportunity to orientate oneself into the space; to orientate oneself where you are coming from, where the destination is and more specifically where one is along the route. From the previous example we note that safety is sometimes a "built-in" feature and as such, a very cost efficient part of the working environment safety. Another example of the everyday environment safety features could be different flooring materials: different materials distinguish passageways from staircases. In other words: the change in the flooring material pre-warns of the staircase in near vicinity. These two previous examples are designed for the visually impaired, but also people with normal vision can use them to be safe. At the very least it might make moving around more flexible.

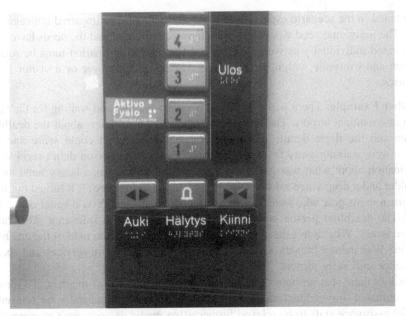

Fig. 2. Safety features in an elevator. Please note the bell button and raised symbol as well as raised exit floor buttons.

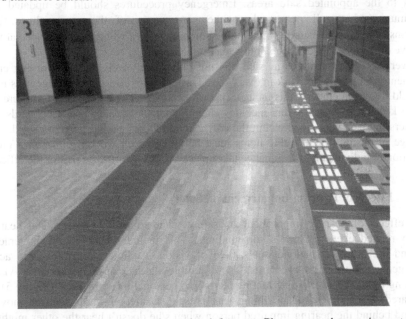

Fig. 3. General lobby area with safety related features. Please note changes in contrasts, different materials and tactile route markers that guide to the exits.

Not only hearing or visually impaired employers have to be trained but the hearing and sighted colleagues as well. The need for repeated and iterated process training is heightened in the scenario especially if there are dual-sensory impaired colleagues as well. The individual need wrt. safety are uttermost important and the needs have to be memorized individually as well. The general fire alarm information must be relayed to each and everyone within the premises, whether an employer or a visitor in the premises.

Another Example: There was a deafblind person travelling and waiting for the flight at an international airport. The special assistance personnel knew about the deafblind person and the flight details. For some reason the deafblind could sense and feel people were walking away from the departure lounge. The person didn't receive any information about what was going on. The first indication was a heavy hand on the shoulder and a deep voice asking: "Oi! What are you doing here?". It turned out to be a fireman in his gear who said: "There has been a bomb alert. You'd better come with me." The deafblind person was guided by the fireman to a safe area. This raises certain issues: Why didn't the special assistance personnel come to alert the deafblind person? Was there a breakdown in communication between fire services and special assistance staff at the airport?

Luckily there was no bomb, but it could have been a serious incident. To remedy this confusion any sudden emergency situation should automatically be relayed to special assistance staff to be relayed further using media devices, such as pagers etc. and staff should automatically pick up the people using special assistance and guide them to the appointed safe areas. Emergency procedures should be updated and communicated to all personnel so they are aware of these procedures. The responsibility of the visually impaired person is to have a white cane or a special vest to give the others a visual cue about visual impairment.

Everyday safety features as safety is not only about A&E but the working environment must be safe to work in every day. This is a joint effort: the passageways must be held free from clutter – this includes ladies' handbags, guide dogs etc., furniture has to be kept on its place – this includes chairs under tables after use. Cupboards and drawers must be kept close within the coffee room. Doors should be kept closed. Any change of position of movable items must be told to each worker, either in a group situation or individually if the change takes place in a less-worked-in part of the office.

1.1   Effects of Hearing Impairment on Safety

The effects of hearing impairment on safety relate to audible alarms and hearing safety-related events in one's surroundings. This includes e.g. others' movements around the premises beyond one's field of vision. Audible alarms relate to acute emergencies but also to fire drills. These audible alarms can be converted to visual flashing lights (Figure 4) or vibrating alerts into personal pager systems (Figure 5). In a shared office the mundane things can present a safety hazard, such as moving around behind the hearing impaired person when s/he doesn't hear the other might in a busy office cause bumping into each other. The more acute vision the hearing impaired person has, the easier it is to notice events in the peripheral field of vision despite the hearing loss [5, pp.487-492].

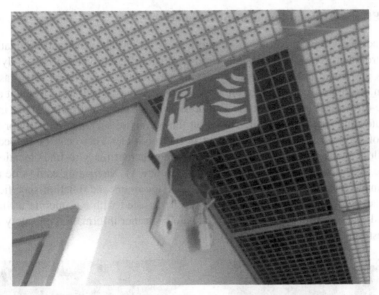

Fig. 4. A clear visual signal in the ceiling, if there is a general alert. There is also a loud siren type sound involved for the hearing impaired. This is also connected to employers' vibrating alert pagers.

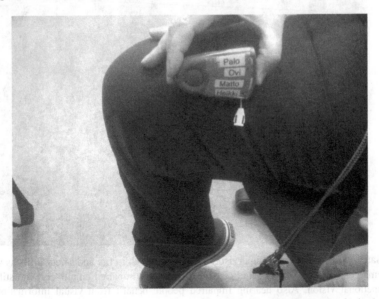

Fig. 5. The vibration alerting system carried by hearing impaired employers on the body. There are four different alerts, all with their own purpose. In this case they are: door, approaching person within office, a special alert for one of the colleagues and fire alarm. Fire alarm also alerts about general alerts in the building. The vibration is similar in all four scenarios, but the light display shows which one of the alerts it is.

1.2 Effects of Visual Impairment on Safety

The effects of visual impairment on safety relate to visual events and orientation in the environment. These can be categorised into two different types of issues: dynamic changes and static circumstances. The static circumstances are somewhat easier as they can be memorised and stored in the muscle memory as well as movement and/or distance-directional memory of the individual with visual impairment. These include safe routes and structure-specific issues on the premises, such as ramps, floor plans, design of staircases, furniture placement in the room etc. These can be helped with tactile floor plans (Figure 6) and Braille text in coherent (easy-to-find) locations on strategic places, such as doors and hand rails (Figure 1). Navigating using safe routes can be made easier with tactile route markers on the floors and function-specific floor materials (Figure 3). Navigating outside can be assisted with e.g. mobile navigation tools and crossing beacons with audio indicators (further information on safety issues on pedestrian crossing, please see [6]).

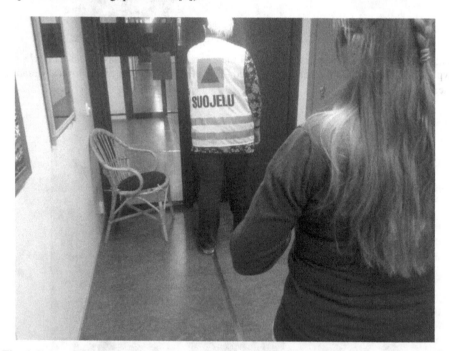

Fig. 6. Safety vest for the safety supervisor. This is used both in fire and safety drills as well as in real emergencies too. This is beneficial for the visually impaired employers who still have some functional vision. Also hearing impaired people benefit from visual information in a stressful and/or noisy situation.

Changes in the environment, which are not audible, present a continuous challenge for the visually impaired employee. These include people moving around in the office, especially if it's shared; changing places of the furniture, such as chair placement, opening doors into the corridor etc. A white cane helps to cope with these changing situations, which people with normal vision are not aware of, but which can present a safety hazard to the visually impaired employee. Usually though fire alarms are audible, so the visually impaired person is able to hear the alarm, it will only be a question of how to find the agreed evacuation point outside the work premises and a safe route to that agreed place.

1.3   Effects of Dual-Sensory Impairment on Safety

If there is a safety hazard such as a new item of furniture or an object that is placed in a room or other walkway this information should be relayed to all employees in appropriate way such as person to person or digital media format. This also includes hanging objects, such as flower pots on the walls or other objects on the eye level.

There are personal and individual needs for the lighting environment as when one person requires a dimmer lighting because of the glare for another person it might not be enough. That might be a safety issue that needs to adressed and some kind of compromise solution must be found.

2   Methods of Enhancing Safety in Work Environment

The importance of anticipation and preparedness for A&E cannot be exaggerated. This goes for all offices regardless of workforce; able-bodied or impaired. This should also be realized higher up in the organizational hierarchy, as it is not enough to the working staff to have regular drills and exercises, but also working time has to be allowed to be used for such exercises.

Exit floor. If a building is built on a slope, the entrance lobby might be situated on other floors than the ground one. This is one of the key elements to remember in the emergency situation, as the default exit floor is the ground floor. This particular building is designed for the visually-impaired [7], but as the building is built on a slope the exit floor is actually the third, which presents one possible safety hazard. As this is not a default as exit floor is usually the ground floor it adds up the memory load for the employees and visitors alike – and does so every day.

2.1   Safety Introduction Courses for New Employers

Not only the visually and hearing impaired new employers have to be introduced to the safety elements and their use in the working environment, but also the hearing and sighted employers have to be introduced to the new colleague's special safety-related needs, e.g. individual hearing and sight ability related to safety: what kind of safety support does this employer need. Within the same occasion the safety officer of the workplace and the new employer will be introduced to each other, but in more general terms, all of workforce needs to be acquainted with the safety related issues in a regular basis (Figure 7).

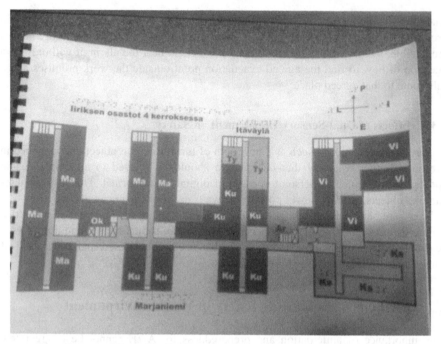

Fig. 7. Tactile floor plan map with Braille text

2.2   Everyday Working Safety

Methods of enhancing everyday working safety are quite mundane and apply for all situations, both at work and at home as well. The main safety feature in a work environment is to keep things in their places. There is also a need for keeping colleagues informed about changes in the environment as well as entering and leaving the room or office area [8].

This can be defined as object-location memory [9], which means, for example if one has a cup of hot coffee on the table and someone else comes along and moves the deafblind's coffee cup on the different location on the table the worker needs to inform where the new location is now. Otherwise the deafblind person who has a memory of the previous location will be confused. This could lead to accidents, i.e. knocking the coffee over.

2.3   Emergency Situations and Fire Drills

Fire drills are important for being prepared for emergencies. The importance is highlighted with hearing and/or sight impaired employees so that everybody can feel confident about safe routes, exits and getting out safely also in case of emergency. Fire drills include instructions, which are given most often in a spoken language as the insructors most often come from outside the company or association. In such a case the same information must be ensured also to the sign language users, possibly via interpreting. This includes not only signing in free space but also with restricted signing space and hands-on signing. For the deafblind employers there has to be tactile information available, both using tactile, hands-on signing but also written infor-mation in Braille. For the hearing impaired not using sign language there must be a text version available with the same information given in spoken language, in large print if needed.

The importance of tactile signing for the dual-sensory impaired is more poignant when there are lots of people and noise, it might be even more difficult to hear with hearing aids. Also if people are stressed and in a hurry they might not take notice of hearing impaired people needing to lipread. In a real emergency people sometimes panic, at least are more stressed, so it changes speech rate and also lip patterns, be-cause muscles become more tense [10]. Furthermore, the hearing impaired might not benefit from lip reading in a similar way as in calm situation as the person's own anxiety level also has an effect on the perception abilities of alternative communication methods. That is why tactile information might benefit hearing impaired people as well in addition to the visually impaired people.

Visual information in the building must be instructed, not only what they look like but also where to find them and especially if there are certain contrast details to note, such as a safety worker vest and visual fire alarms. Tactile information available must be guided to, so that the workers can find them by themselves, that is to know where the tactile information is. This also includes vibration alerting systems worn by employees. The system always has a special vibration for fire alarms. Different floor materials can be used to represent different functions in the premises. Safe routes must be kept free for safe passage. This includes also keeping routes to the tactile information free from advertisements, which sadly enough is often the case in shop-ping centres. It's no use having a tactile map if you cannot get to feel it because of the route being blocked with advertisement boards, so called A-boards.

There are two forms of touch-based emergency messages [11]. The first one is a pre-warning, a smaller version (x), it can be produced onto back, shoulder, upper arm and back of the hand. This would be used in a situation where further information is needed. The producer needs to stay in immediate vicinity of the deafblind or deaf-blinds in order to provide the further information or instructions when they are avail-able. The second, bigger version (X) is produced on the same body areas mentioned above. This means: "This is an emergency, everyone needs to clear the building via the nearest fire exit and proceed to the agreed meeting place out of harm's way." After reaching the meeting place, only then is there enough time to explain what was the emergency about and what has happened. One of the features of the emergency messages (x and X) is that they denote the fact that there is no time to discuss now, but the explanation will follow when emergency is over.

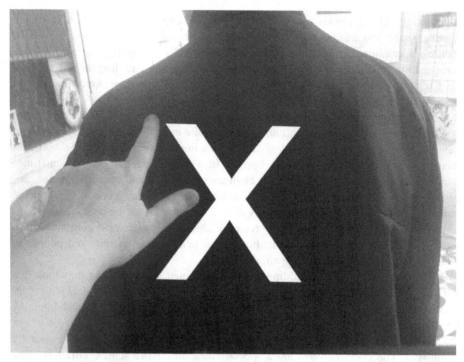

Fig. 8. Emergency message is produced onto a deafblind person's back as a default. Pressure must be felt clearly through clothing.

3   Discussion

Safety is for all employers regardless of hearing and visual status. That is the main reason why special concentration is needed both in everyday working situations as well as the heightened need in safety drills and especially in an emergency for the visually, hearing or dual-sensory impaired colleagues. It is a joint effort in making the working environment safe for all of the employers every day. In the case where an organization employs a person with a disability it is imperative that working practices and emergency procedures are evaluated and updated accordingly. Periodically there is a need to carry out safety checks and emergency practice drills. Then all employers are equally aware of the different disabilities and how they affect the person in an emergency situation. This ensures equality and constituency to all working practices. Accessibility procedures have to engulf also emergency policies to all workers with different disabilities.

References

1. Lahtinen, R.: Haptices and haptemes - A case study of developmental process in social-haptic communication of acquired deafblind people. Academic dissertation. University of Helsinki (2008)
2. Hirn, H.: Pre-maps: An educational programme for reading tactile maps. Academic dissertation. University of Helsinki (2009)
3. http://kuurosokeat.fi/quick_messages/index.php
4. Jokiniemi, J.: City for All Senses – Accessibility and Cross-Modality in the Built Environment. Academic dissertation. Helsinki University of Technology (2007)
5. Palmer, S.E.: Vision Science – Photons to Phenomenology. MIT (1999)
6. United Kingdom Department of Transport, Inclusive Mobility. A Guide to Best Practice on Access to Pedestrian and Transport Infrastructure. Section 3.12 (2002)
7. IIRIS Centre, Service and activity centre for the visually impaired. Visiting address: Marjaniementie 74, 00930 Helsinki, Finland (2006)
8. http://www.kuurosokeat.fi/kohtaaminen/index.php
9. http://sbfnl.stanford.edu/cs/bm/lm/bml_objectlocation.html
10. http://www.lipreading.net
11. http://kuurosokeat.fi/pikaviestit/video.php?video=1752

Revitalizing the Quantitative Understanding of the Digital Divide: An Uptake on the Digital Divide Indicators

Farooq Mubarak

University of Turku, Turku School of Economics, Turku, Finland
farmub@utu.fi

Abstract. Recent advances in ICT research have uncovered several facts regarding the nature of the digital divide. Following the renewed dimensions of the term, the need for universally accepted digital divide indicators has significantly heightened across the academic and policy discourses. Traditionally, researchers have subscribed to the belief that the digital divide is a mere separation between "have" and "have nots"; however, as the digital technology continues to experience innovation in the information age, digital divide is increasingly being understood as a multidimensional phenomena. The research to date has mostly focused on the qualitative rather than the quantitative nature of the digital divide. The few existent accounts of quantitative studies on the digital divide are often criticized for deploying unreliable data in their analysis. Inaccurate predictions significantly derail policymakers' abilities to form appropriate action plans in combating the digital divide. OECD and ITU have been hitting on front lines with their extensive research in ICT. This paper seeks to emphasize the quantitative understanding of the digital divide by reviewing the relevant literature and acknowledging the top indicators in the field. Apart from OECD and ITU, there is a general lack of research in determining the ICT indicators. Along with reviewing the relevant literature on latest ICT indicators, this study has documented twenty-nine significant ICT indicators and highlighted the need for future research into quantitative nature of the digital divide.

Keywords: information and communication technology (ICT), Digital divide, Digital divide indicators.

1   Introduction

The reality of unevenly distributed ICT landscape around the planet has encouraged debate on the topic of what is known as "digital divide". The traditional "twenty-eighty" rule in the discipline of marketing and sales also takes its riotous turn towards the digital divide. It is estimated that eighty percent of all Internet users worldwide are based in top twenty countries with high Internet bandwidth growth [1]. In the light of this fact, the digital divide emerges as an issue of serious concern across a range of academic and policy discourses.

K. Saranto et al. (Eds.): WIS 2014, CCIS 450, pp. 120–130, 2014.
© Springer International Publishing Switzerland 2014

The first serious discussions regarding the digital divide emerged during mid-1990s when US Department of Commerce published a report to create awareness about "have" and "have nots", concerning the access to digital technology. The pace of research in this area has accelerated in the last decade, witnessed by mounting literature on the topic. The term "digital divide" has been interpreted in various contexts in academia, resulting in a diverse and critical knowledge base on the topic. The definitions of the term vary in their complexity, however the frequently cited and what appears to be the most comprehensive definition is the one given by OECD (Organization for Economic Cooperation and Development). OECD defines digital divide as

The term digital divide refers to the gap between individuals, households, businesses and geographic areas at different socio-economic levels with regard both to their opportunities to access information and communication technologies and to their use of the Internet for a wide variety of activities [2].

Over the last decade there has been a dramatic increase in adoption of digital technologies worldwide, particularly in the developed world [3]. It appears that over time the digital divide has significantly reduced; nevertheless awareness about the issue has sparked interest across press, politics, and academia. As the debate continues to sharpen, new dimensions of the digital divide are unveiled, indicating that it is broadly a complex topic. It appears that parallel to the growth of new emerging technologies, challenges to accurately track and measure the digital disparities across planet have significantly increased.

Despite the digital divide has seen a reduction on the account of digital technology acquisition, the efficient usage of such technology is often an issue of concern in recent research. The study by Rahim, Pawanteh, & Salman [4] highlights this by noting that the digital divide is deepening and widening globally in terms of usage and skills required for operating ICTs. Following a review of research on digital divide across firms, Bach, Zoroja, and Vukšić [5] recommend that future research on digital divide across organizations should concentrate on appropriate action plans to minimize the digital gap. Nevertheless, appropriate policy formulation requires accurate quantitative and qualitative information upfront, a concern which is the call of present paper.

Considerable criticism has been levelled in the past research concerning the digital divide, owing to the fact that the digital divide is not only one divide but rather several divides. Therefore, some researchers [6, 7, 8] inspire that the digital divide is a confused theme in literature. Measurement of the digital divide then becomes a difficult task, due to the scarcity of data on a universally agreed standard measurement mechanism. The aim of this paper is to introduce concrete digital divide indicators to help create awareness about the measurement mechanism of the digital divide. While prior research has seen various attempts at describing and measuring the digital divide, this paper is unique in the sense that it revitalizes the quantitative understanding of the digital divide by noting the top twenty-nine indicators in the field till date.

2   Literature Review

2.1   Scarcity of Published Literature

There seems a scarcity of literature on the digital divide indicators. Even the most comprehensive quantitative studies on the topic such as [9] employed only five variables in measuring the digital divide across European Union. These variables included percentage of households with access to the Internet, percentage of households with a broadband connection, percentage of individuals who accessed the Internet at least once a week on average, percentage of individuals who have never used a computer, and percentage of individuals who ordered goods or services online for private use [9]. A small scale study [10] used social surveys to measure the digital divide in UK. Approaches of this kind carry with them various well known advantages like valuable input from the end-users; however considerably more information beyond social surveys is needed in performing such complex tasks.

The concept of the digital divide is grounded along the two main streams: efficient access to digital technologies, and the efficient usage of digital technologies. Earlier advances in defining the indicators to estimate the digital divide were mainly the parameters of technical nature regarding access to computers and Internet; later on research has established that the digital divide is also a human development concern [11]. Prior research has uncovered that both social factors such as motivation to learn and use ICT and technical factors such as infrastructure feasibility influence the usage of ICT. Thus, digital divide can be of a social or technical nature. It is in this belief that there are considerable differences among countries related to digitalization patterns.

In the context of the digital divide, literature often presents twin terms of technology penetration and technology adoption. It is worth noting the difference between these two terms. There has been no clear definition of "technology adoption" because of differences in types of technology and conditions under which people adopt those technologies [12]. Similarly, there is no clear definition of "technology penetration", however, as the name suggests, it is the technology access that is available in the market in a given location.

In some cases, technology penetration rates can be higher compared to the technology adoption rates and vice versa. For instance, China represents 25 % of the world Internet users by the year end 2011; however, Europe leads in mobile broadband penetration reaching 54% [13]. This indicates that China leads in technology adoption rates whereas Europe leads in technology penetration rates.

Cruz-Jesus, Oliveira, and Bacao [14] maintain that the use of indices instead of ICT-related indicators is becoming common in measuring the digital divide. Indicator is anything that indicates; whereas Indices are based on a weighted sum of different variables [15]. Thus, an index appears to be a measured scale which is derived from indicators. Nevertheless, indices based approach to measure the digital divide comes with its own challenges. Gesundheitswesen [16] highlights this by concluding that application of index measures may hide the effects of single indicator. It is therefore likely if the digital divide indicators are poorly understood, the resultant indices derived are bound to be questionable.

2.2   Groundbreaking Works by International Telecommunications Union and OECD

Comprehensive work on ICT indicators has been carried out by International Tele-communications (ITU), and Union and Organization for Cooperation and Economic Development (OECD). A recent official report highlights the importance of measuring and tracking the progress in ICT sector [17]. International Telecommunications Union has put forward significant proceedings in development of a standard index to measure the Information Society. The resultant index is referred to as "Digital Opportunity Index" or "ICT Development Index" which is based on 11 internationally agreed ICT indicators [1]. The index value ranges between 1 and 0, where 1 represents complete digital opportunity and 0 means no digital opportunity.

The vision of OECD is to embody best management practices with the goals of developing effective policy choices for governments around the globe [18]. OECD has emerged as a research-oriented think tank for its member countries by entering the fields of studies in science, technology, and economics [19]. OECD has undertaken intensive work to determine the key ICT indicators drawn from various publications and own research [20]. However, some indicators mentioned by OECD are meant solely for the OECD region.

United Nations Conference on Trade and Development [21] has released a manual regarding statistics on the information economy. The manual stresses the business usage of ICT as a distinctive characteristic of an information economy. Therefore, the business usage of ICT has appeared in various forms as key indicators of the digital divide, which are also reflected in the table 1.

Table 1 represents the top ICT indicators based on the data from the above mentioned organizations. It is evident from the Table 1 that the same indicator is often repeated with minor alterations depending upon the nature, type, place of access, and usage. For instance, one of the most important ICT indicators "Internet" has appeared in different forms based on the type, speed, intended usage, and area of access. This categorization helps in determining the actual digital divide from various perspectives.

Table 1. The digital divide indicators (Based on data from ITU [22] and OECD [23])

Number	Indicators of the digital divide	Source of the indicator
ICT indicators by infrastructure and access		
	Computers per 100 inhabitants	OECD
	Fixed telephone lines per 100 inhabitants	ITU
	Percentage of mobile phone users	ITU
	International Internet bandwidth per inhabitant	ITU
	Percentage of population covered by mobile cellular telephony	ITU
	Percentage of Internet users	ITU
	Percentage of localities with public Internet access centers (PIACs) by number of inhabitants	ITU
	Percentage of mobile broadband users	ITU
	Percentage of broadband users	ITU

Table 1. (*continued*)

ICT indicators by access and usage	
Percentage of individuals who used a computer (from any location) in the last 12 months	ITU
Percentage of individuals who used Internet (from any location) in the last 12 months	ITU
Percentage of households with Internet access at home	ITU
Households with access to a home computer	OECD
ICT indicators by businesses	
Percentage of businesses receiving orders over the Internet	ITU
Percentage of businesses placing orders over the Internet	ITU
Percentage of businesses using computers	ITU
Percentage of businesses using the Internet	ITU
Percentage of employees using computers	ITU
Percentage of employees using Internet	ITU
Percentage of businesses with an Intranet	ITU
ICT indicators by trade in ICT goods	
Trade in ICT goods	OECD
ICT goods import as a percentage of total import	ITU
ICT goods exports as a percentage of total exports	ITU
ICT indicators by education	
Percentage of ICT-qualified teachers in schools	ITU
Percentage of schools with a radio used for educational purposes	ITU
Percentage of schools with a televisions used for educational purposes	ITU
Percentage of learners who have access to Internet at school	ITU
Percentage of schools with electricity	ITU
Learners-to-computer ratio in schools with computer-assisted instruction	ITU

While most of the indicators often encompass the digital technologies, surprisingly electricity is now also considered a key factor in explaining the digital divide. Chinn and Fairlie [24] found that access to electricity is an important indicator in determining the digital divide. This indicator explains itself well in least developed countries, which are without continuous and reliable supply of electricity. Therefore, even the donation of computers alone does not tend to overcome the digital divide in areas with energy crises.

Percentage of computers in a given territory has traditionally been the most common indicator of the digital divide. Collecting data on computers is often derived from data on computer shipments in a given country. Since, old computers are replaced by new computers within years; therefore, accurate estimate on this indicator is a challenge. Furthermore, desktop computer appears to be old fashioned with the introduction of tablet computers, innovative laptop computers, and smart phones. For this reason, data from computer sales for the last five years is considered as a base measure.

Percentage of Internet subscribers is second most common indicator of the digital divide, often in line with the percentage of computers. An internet subscriber pays for using a defined or undefined amount of internet for a given period of time. In developed countries, this statistic can easily be obtained from cellular and Internet services providers. However, in developing countries one subscribed line is often shared among a group through illicit means. Data thus obtained from telecommunication authorities does not seem to represent actual figures in developing countries. A possible solution could either be taking into account the margin of error, or sampling the phenomenon of interest.

Traditionally, the percentage of fixed telephone lines in a given area has been an important ICT indictor. However, fixed telephone lines subscriptions are declining with the introduction of cellular phones and the cutting edge wireless alternatives. In the current age, it appears true for both developed and developing nations, with lower adoption rates in the later. It is likely that the fixed telephone lines be taken over by wireless technology in the near future. In technical terms, there is still a digital divide between two individuals, if one possesses state of the art wireless telephone system and the other traditional fixed line telephone. Differences such as these should be accounted or at least acknowledged while attempting to measure the digital divide.

Percentage of broadband subscribers is taken as a key indicator to measure the digital divide, particularly in the developed regions. Broadband is a high speed wireless Internet connection with speeds ranging from 256 Kbits/s to 100 Mbps. Broadband Internet seems to replace traditional wire based Internet connection at a steady rate. This statistic is measured irrespective of the device used to connect to the broadband Internet. Percentage of broadband subscribers in a given population is obtained by dividing the number of broadband subscribers by the given population and multiplying the result by 100.

Percentage of population covered by mobile cellular telephony refers to the percentage of inhabitants in a given geographical territory which that live within the areas covered by cellular signals. This statistic is measured irrespective of whether the inhabitants choose to use cellular services or not. In developed regions, this percentage is declining owing to the increased expansion of cellular area of coverage. In almost all countries, a number of remote villages and areas are always without mobile cellular coverage. This statistic is easy to calculate if the correct census of population and data from cellular companies is available.

Percentage of radio and television sets in use has been a historical indicator to measure the digital divide. The major limitation with this indicator would be in the case of developing regions, where accurate data collection on these indicators is a huge task. Sales of radio sets appear to decline as now the same is integrated into variety of smart phones and similar digital entertainment devices. This statistic is measured by dividing the number of radio and television sets in use by total population and multiplying the result by 100.

Some indicators such as percentage of households with radios, televisions, cellular phones appear similar to the percentage of radio, television, and cellular phones users; however, the difference is that percentage of households with digital devices is measured regardless if these devices are used or not, keeping in mind that the devices must at least be in working order or expected to be in working order soon.

Another set of indicators refers to whether a computer or Internet has been used in any given location during last 12 months. Data on this indicator is obtained through a survey. This statistic is measured by dividing the total number of in-scope individuals who used computer or Internet in the last 12 months by total number of in-scope individuals. This statistic thus measures those individuals also who did not possess ICTs but used the ICTs.

3   Discussion

Emergent inequalities in access and utilization of digital technologies across the globe have fostered debate on the topic of what is known as "digital divide". ICT has been a recurring theme in discussions across academia and press. In an official report of National Telecommunications Union, McConnaughey, Lader, and Chin [25] presented poverty as the principal factor responsible for the digital divide. The bitter standoff between poverty and the digital divide continues in the modern age, leaving millions of individuals excluded from the digital sphere globally. During late 1990s and the subsequent earlier years, it was believed that eradication of poverty shall eliminate the digital divide. The major indicators of the digital divide used to be percentages of computer, Internet, and telephone users for a given territory. Poverty and income disparities were considered to be the dominant factors in explaining the digital divide.

The research into the digital divide stimulated in the last decade, and ample literature was published across press, politics, and academic lines. Majority of the studies concentrated on describing the qualitative nature of the digital divide that took various forms with the continuous introduction of new digital technologies. Soon the digital divide was no longer a division between "have" and "have nots" only; instead the concept would break along a multiple range of fronts encompassing possession, ability to operate ICTs, motivation, gender, and cultural factors. While the advances on understanding digital divide unpacked several complexities, science seems to have forgotten the need of exploring the emerging indicators of the digital divide.

There is a scarcity of published literature solely on the topic of digital divide indicators. Quantitative studies on the digital divide have encompassed a variety of different ICT indicators, sometimes unique newborn indices; there has been no standard universally agreed measurement mechanism for the digital divide. The controversial methodology to measure the digital divide yields biased results and speculations which are inappropriate for accurate policy formulation. It is possible to hypothesize that measurement of the digital divide shall remain disputed and unreliable unless solid work is done on the ICT indicators that shall become universally acknowledged. International Telecommunications Union felt the need of determining the internationally agreed core ICT indicators to harmonize the research in this area. Equally important to note is the massive work of OECD in the arena of ICT, a task which has occupied OECD for several years in a row.

One of the most significant and common indicators of ICT is percentage of computers in a given area. However, latest innovative smart computers such as tablets are steadily substituting the traditional desktop computers. Nevertheless, the rates of replacing old computers by new ones vary in developing and developed countries. To eliminate the risk of data biases, the territory where this indicator needs to be measured may be divided into a certain number of fragments. From each fragment, a sample can be drawn estimating the presence of computers. Later on, the mean value can be taken into account for actual measurement of the indicator.

Sampling method applies to a series of other indicators of the digital divide as well where accurate data extraction is a rigorous challenge. This is especially true for villages and remote areas. Internet lines are often illegitimately shared among individuals and groups in the developing countries. Telephone and internet providers can provide data only for the actual subscribers of the data line. Sampling method can therefore help in obtaining data values which are true representatives of actual figures.

The set of indicators discussed indicate some holes in most of the recently quantified studies on the digital divide. A considerable number of studies stick to a few ICT indicators in their quantitative analysis, overlooking several other important ICT indicators. The need for a standard measurement mechanism based on these and any future possible indicators is also apparent. The quantitative studies on the digital divide shall continue to suffer from serious limitations of data manipulation, unless a universally agreed mechanism is formed. However, the measurement mechanism does not seem to offer the solution alone; solid steps must be taken by governments to ensure the data reliability, particularly in the developing regions.

It can be conceivably hypothesized that research on quantification of the digital divide without a reliable input of data does not tend to eliminate the economic challenges posed by the digital divide. Results from various quantitative studies on the digital divide seriously impede the correct policy formulations to combat the digital divide. The battle against the digital divide can be a slippery slope to walk on for the policy makers without the correct quantified information regarding the digital divide.

4   Conclusions

4.1   Summary of Findings

This paper has given an account of the emerging need for universally accepted digital divide indicators. In line with the aim of this research, the purpose was to enhance the quantitative understanding of the digital divide by exploring the digital divide indicators and presenting them in easily digestible chunks of information that can be used for measuring the digital divide. Numerous factors are responsible for how the ICT landscape is distributed across the planet. These factors when explored through extensive research take the form of structured digital divide indicators. The existing literature on the digital divide lacks a thorough work on the digital divide indicators with the exceptions of the work of International Telecommunications Union and OECD. The present study is one of its kind in creating awareness about the digital divide indicators.

The issue of the digital divide has caught the attention across a wide range of press and policy discourses, given its serious consequences on a global level. Although extensive research has been carried out on the digital divide, most studies have only focused on qualitative aspects. An array of studies has taken uptake on quantifying the digital divide; however, the experimental data are rather controversial, and there is no general agreement about a universal measurement system. Most of the quantitative studies on the digital divide are targeted on a specific geographical area. Few studies exist which set out to quantify the digital divide across a wide range of countries; however they relied too heavily on few ICT indicators. There seems a risk that controversial data and measures to quantify the digital divide shall fuel widespread speculations about the results far from the reality.

Beyond doubt, poverty appears to be a leading cause of the digital divide as advocated by number of worldwide organizations. Human rights watch dogs keep on releasing the statistics that show striking differences between wealthy and poor nations, on the accounts of poverty. Owing to the various known troubles in getting the real statistics, the majority of poor masses in developing and underdeveloped regions dwell in such indescribable states that even the official figures pale in comparison. It is, therefore, self-explanatory that poverty alone explains a major share of the digital divide pie. Most of the research has, however, forgotten to take into account various other indicators of the digital divide, which ultimately became the subject matter of the present paper.

The most common indicators of the digital divide appear to be the percentage of computer and internet users in a given geographical territory. This statistic is easier to obtain in developed countries than in the developing countries, given that the developed countries have good statistical data management systems in use. Currently, rigorous sampling method seems a feasible solution to obtain a data set from developing regions rather than relying on single large-scale survey.

Market forces shall eventually bring the costs of digital equipment down; it might take considerable time for developing countries to encompass better data management systems. The global political temperature would keep on rising as long as the digital divide persists and poses threats to the world economy. Considerably more work will need to be done to determine a standard framework which shall offer reliable insights into the quantitative nature of the digital divide, as it exists, rather than what is usually perceived.

4.2   Limitations

A number of caveats need to be noted regarding the present study. Although, some most important indicators were discussed in detail, the current study was unable to analyze all the indicators presented in the literature review. The present research was not designed specifically to evaluate all the factors related to the employment of the digital divide indicators in some useful formula for measurement. A reasonable approach could have been to discuss the evens and odds of each indicator with respect to their suitability in developed and developing countries. These were some issues that fell outside the scope of the present study; nevertheless, they are worthy areas for future research.

4.3   Future Directions

Further investigation and experimentation into determining the statistics related to digital divide indicators is strongly recommended. A detailed analysis of the digital divide indicators with respect to developing and developed countries could be helpful in measuring the digital divide in particular regions. More broadly, research is also needed to determine the most concrete ways of extracting the reliable data from the developing countries. A reasonable approach to tackle the issue of data nuances in developing countries could be large randomized controlled trials. The emergent need to work on the universally agreed digital divide measurement mechanism should fuel the future research in this area.

References

1. International Telecommunications Union, World Information Society Report (2007), http://www.itu.int/osg/spu/publications/worldinformationsoci ety/2007/ (retrieved on January 27, 2014)
2. Organisation for Economic Co-operation and Development, Understanding the Digital Divide, OECD Publications, pp. 1–32 (2001), http://www.oecd.org/ internet/ieconomy/1888451.pdf (retrieved on January 11, 2014)
3. Doong, S.H., Ho, S.-C.: The impact of ICT development on the global digital divide. Electronic Commerce Research and Applications 11(5), 518–533 (2012)
4. Gesundheitswesen. Single indicator or index? Comparison of measures of social differentiation. Pubmed. 70(5), 281–288 (2008)
5. Rahim, S.A., Pawanteh, L., Salman, A.: Digital Inclusion: The Way Forward for Equality in a Multiethnic Society. Innovation Journal 16(3), 1–12 (2011)
6. Bach, P.M., Zoroja, J., Vukšić, B.V.: Determinants of firms' digital divide: A review of recent research. Procedia Technology, 120–128 (2013)
7. Butcher, M.P.: At the foundations of information justice. Ethics and Information Technology 11(1), 57–69 (2009)
8. Hilbert, M.: The end justifies the definition: The manifold outlooks on the digital divide and their practical usefulness for policy-making. Telecommunications Policy 35(8), 715–736 (2011)
9. Van Dijk, J.A.G.M.: Digital divide research, achievements and shortcomings. Poetics 3(4-5), 221–235 (2006)
10. Vicente, M.R., López, A.J.: Assessing the regional digital divide across the European Union-27. Telecommunications Policy 35(3), 220–237 (2011)
11. Stewart, J.: The Digital divide in the UK: A review of quantitative Indicators and Public Policies. In: Proceedings of the International Conference Stepping Stones Into the Digital World, pp. 21–22 (2000)
12. Santoyo, S.A.: Estimation and Characterization of the Digital Divide, Round Table on Developing Countries Access to Scientific Knowledge, The Abdus Salam ICTP, Trieste, Italy, pp. 21–24 (2003)
13. Bridges To Technology, What is Technology Adoption? 2005 Bridges to Technology Corp. 21 (2005), http://www.bridges-to-technology.com/page21.html (retrieved on January 27, 2014)

14. Li, Y., Ranieri, M.: Educational and social correlates of the digital divide for rural and urban children: A study on primary school students in a provincial city of China. Computers & Education 60(1), 197–209 (2013)

15. Cruz-Jesus, F., Oliveira, T., Bacao, F.: Digital divide across the European Union. Information & Management 49(6), 278–291 (2012)

16. Cross Validated, What is the difference among Indicator, Index, Variable and Measure? StackExchange (2013), http://stats.stackexchange.com/questions/74377/what-is-the-difference-among-indicator-index-variable-and-measure (retrieved on February 25, 2014)

17. Gesundheitswesen. Single indicator or index? Comparison of measures of social differentiation. Pubmed 70(5), 281–288 (2008)

18. International Telecommunications Union, Measuring the Information Society (2013), http://www.itu.int/en/ITU-D/Statistics/Documents/publications/mis2013/MIS2013_without_Annex_4.pdf (retrieved on January 28, 2014)

19. Organisation for Economic Co-operation and Development, OECD 50th anniversary vision statement. OECD Publications, pp. 1–3 (2011), http://www.oecd.org/mcm/48064973.pdf (retrieved on February 28, 2014)

20. Stewart, J.: The Digital divide in the UK: A review of quantitative Indicators and Public Policies. In: Proceedings of the International Conference on Stepping Stones Into the Digital World, pp. 21–22 (2000)

21. Godin, B.: The New Economy: what the concept owes to the OECD. Research Policy 33(5), 679–690 (2004)

22. Organisation for Economic Co-operation and Development, Key ICT Indicators, OECD (2012), http://www.oecd.org/sti/broadband/oecdkeyictindicators.htm (retrieved on March 01, 2014)

23. UNCTAD (United Nations Conference on Trade and Development), Manual for the Production of Statistics on the Information Economy, Revised Edition, Geneva (2009), http://new.unctad.org/templates/Page____885.aspx (retrieved on January 27, 2014)

24. International Telecommunications Union, Core ICT Indicators (2010), http://www.itu.int/dms_pub/itu-d/opb/ind/D-IND-ICT_CORE-2010-PDF-E.pdf (retrieved on January 17, 2014)

25. Organisation for Economic Co-operation and Development, Key ICT Indicators, OECD (2013), http://www.oecd.org/internet/broadband/oecdkeyictindicators.htm (retrieved on January 17, 2014)

26. Chinn, D.M., Fairlie, W.R.: The Determinants of the Global Digital Divide: A Cross-Country Analysis of Computer and Internet Penetration, Discussion Paper Series, IZA DP No. 1305, pp. 1–28 (2004)

27. McConnaughey, J., Lader, W., Chin, R.: Falling through the net II: new data on the digital divide, National Telecommunications and Information Administration. Department of Commerce, US Government, Washington, DC (1998)

Information Management Efforts in Improving Patient Safety in Critical Care - A Review of the Literature

Laura-Maria Murtola[1,2], Heljä Lundgrén-Laine[1,2], and Sanna Salanterä[1,2]

[1] University of Turku, Turku, Finland
[2] Turku University Hospital, Turku, Finland
{lmemur,hklula,sansala}@utu.fi

Abstract. Patient safety is the responsibility of all professionals involved in the provision of health care services. The risk of harm is increased in the critical care setting due to complex care needs and frequent procedures. Information management is a contributing factor to a large number of incidents in the critical care setting. The aim of this study was to explore the current research of efforts in improving patient safety in the critical care environment. An integrative literature review was conducted and four databases (Cinahl, Pubmed, Scopus, and Web of Science) were searched. A total of 19 articles were included in the review. A theoretical framework of information management in decision-making in hospitals was used to guide the analysis. The results indicate that most research from a patient safety perspective focuses on means to improve information management on clinical level decision-making and that managerial information management remains vaguely explored.

Keywords: Patient safety, critical care, nursing, information management, decision-making.

1 Introduction

Patient safety is defined as "the absence of preventable harm to a patient during the process of health care" [1]. Ensuring patient safety is a multidisciplinary responsibility for all professionals involved in the provision of health care services through the reduction of the risk of unnecessary harm to the acceptable minimum [2]. There are areas in the health care setting where the risk for harm is increased. One such area is the critical care setting. Critical illness increases the risk for clinical error due to the complex and life-threatening health problems of the patients and the necessary and frequently performed procedures, which are conducted to support the patients' vital functions [3]. Unintentional events that compromise patient safety may occur in 38.8% per 100 patient days in the intensive care unit [4].

Care of critically ill patients is a collaborative task conducted by professionals from different disciplines and different specialties. This multiprofessional team consisting of medical, nursing and allied health professionals monitor and support the patients with failing vital organs in order to perform diagnostic procedures and medical or surgical therapies or procedures to improve the patient's condition [5].

K. Saranto et al. (Eds.): WIS 2014, CCIS 450, pp. 131–143, 2014.

Critical care medicine is responsible for the medical treatment of critically ill patients [6]. Critical care nursing is the specialty within nursing, which strives to ensure that acutely and critically ill patients and their families receive optimal care in relation to their life-threatening health problems [7].

Information management in the health care setting is a critical point with impact on patient safety. Communication between different professionals is a vital task in the coordination of critical care services both within a unit and beyond. Information management and communication problems are factors often responsible for errors, and good communication is vital for patient safety [8]. Teamwork issues account for 32% of incidents in the intensive care unit including difficulties with both verbal and written information [9]. There is a need to improve information management in critical care to ensure patient safety. The aim of this study is to describe current research of information management efforts in improving patient safety in critical care.

2   Theoretical Framework

Managerial decision-making in health care organizations is portrayed to occur on three different levels: strategic, tactical and operational levels. Information is managed in three different ways on each of these levels: vertically, laterally and longitudinally, according to the descriptive model of decision-making levels and information management in hospitals [10]. In this model, the strategic decision-making refers to long-term goals, the tactical decision-making to short term goals and the operational decision-making to daily goals. Moreover, the vertical information management refers to information, which is communicated top down and bottom up in the organizational hierarchy e.g. information about the adequacy of human and material resources to meet patients care needs. The lateral information management refers to information, which is communicated across different areas on the same level within the organization e.g. information about available patient beds in the hospital, and the longitudinal information management refers to information, which is in continuous transformation e.g. information about a patient's blood pressure.

As stated, this model describes information management on different levels of decision-making in the hospital from a managerial perspective. This refers to the decision-making conducted by the professionals responsible for the care coordination, such as the nurse managers, the medical directors and the shift leaders. The managerial decisions often concern the allocation of available resources to meet with the patients' care needs. However, evaluating managerial decision-making is not enough when patient safety is concerned, and therefore, we need to add clinical decision-making into the model. Clinical decision-making is the basis for all health care related organizational purposes and daily functions. Clinical decision-making is conducted by different professionals e.g. nurses, physicians and allied health staff, when they assess the patients' health related problems, plan and conduct needed interventions and evaluate the outcome in relation to a specific patients' care. Therefore, in this paper we have added a clinical level of decision-making into this descriptive model presented earlier [10], as illustrated in Figure 1.

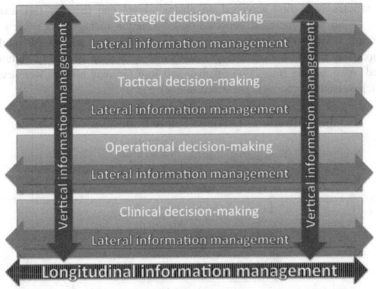

Fig. 1. Descriptive model of information management on the different decision-making levels in the hospital

3   Methods

An integrative literature review was chosen as research design. The search was conducted in four databases: Cinahl, Pubmed, Scopus and Web of Science. Database specific search terms were used when possible, and free text terms were used when searching with article titles. All searches were limited to peer reviewed journals. No temporal restrictions or language restrictions were used at this stage. The search resulted in 425 articles. The search is described in Table 1. This review does not require an ethical statement.

Table 1. Description of database search

Database	Search terms and limitations	Results
Cinahl	((MH "Critical Care") AND (MH "Patient Safety")) OR (TITLE("patient safety" AND "critical care")) Limitation: Peer reviewed	232
Pubmed	("Critical Care"[Mesh] AND "Patient Safety"[Mesh]) OR (TITLE(("critical care" OR "intensive care") AND "patient safety")) Limitation: Peer reviewed	148
Scopus	TITLE("patient safety" AND "critical care") Limitation: Subject area: Health Sciences Limitation: Document types: article or review	22
Web of Science	TITLE("critical care" AND "patient safety") Limitation: Document types: article or review	23
	In total	**425**

The articles were first screened on abstract level and then on full text level. Articles, which were included, reported on information management related studies with efforts to improve patient safety in the critical care setting for adults. No restriction was made on study design. Studies that focused on safety culture were excluded. Also, at this stage, two Spanish and four German articles were excluded. The article selection process is presented in Figure 2.

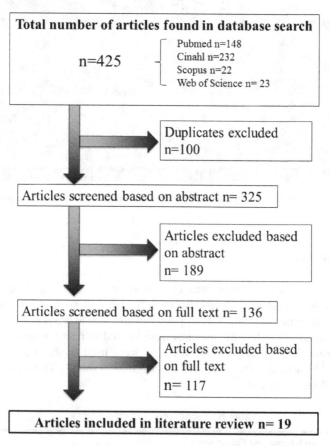

Fig. 2. Flowchart of article selection process

Data was extracted from the selected articles with two separate templates, depending on the study design. One of these templates was for exploratory studies and the other one for explanatory studies. The template for the exploratory studies included the following topics: authors, country and year of publication, purpose of study, methods, and results concerning information management issues connected to patient safety. The template for the explanatory studies included the following topics: authors, country and year of publication, purpose, study design and setting, intervention, and results concerning the impact of the intervention on information management to improve patient safety.

The quality of the studies was evaluated with an instrument developed by Kmet et al. [11]. This instrument consists of a qualitative and a quantitative quality evaluation template. The qualitative evaluation template comprises 10 criteria and the quantitative evaluation template 14 criteria to be scored. There are four scoring options for both of the templates: yes, partially, no and not applicable (for some criteria). A total score was calculated for all the studies by summing the evaluation score and dividing it with the total possible score. Criteria that were not applicable were excluded from the total possible scores. Hence, a higher total score indicates a better quality study.

4   Results

In total, 19 articles were included in the literature review. Nine studies were literature reviews, one study was a systematic literature review, four studies were explanatory intervention research reports, three studies were prospective observational studies and one study was a retrospective register study. Fifteen of the included articles were from the USA, three from Australia and one from Canada. The articles included in this review were published as follows: six in 2013, two each year in 2005, 2007, 2011 and 2012, and one each year in 2002, 2006, 2009 and 2010.

Most of the studies were descriptive literature reviews combining different quality improvement efforts in the critical care setting to improve patient safety. Three of the intervention studies evaluated a paper-based incident reporting systems and the fourth intervention study evaluated the impact of a structured checklist on communication between professionals. Only one systematic review was found, which evaluated the impact of the application of safety checklists. The exploratory studies are presented in Table 2 and the explanatory studies in Table 3.

Table 2. Exploratory research of information management efforts to improve patient safety

Author, Year & Country	Purpose	Methods	Information management issues connected to patient safety
[12] Frith 2013 USA	To explore research of medication errors and prevention of these errors in intensive care units (ICUs).	Literature review	Computerized provider order entry systems are implemented to reduce medication-prescribing errors. Education to improve nurses' knowledge about medication to reduce knowledge based errors. Bar code medication administration to reduce medication administration errors.
[13] Goran 2012 USA	To determine the relationship between tele-ICU use, and quality measures and patient outcomes.	Literature review	Tele-ICU systems have shown to improve clinical indicators of quality, reduce care costs, and furthermore, decrease mortality and length of stay.

Table 2. (*continued*)

[14] *Harder* *&* *Marc* *2013* *USA*	To review research on problems and solutions of work processes, technology and environmental/ infrastructure factors that impact on care delivery and patient outcomes.	Literature review	Structured handover tools e.g. (SBAR) may improve communication between clinicians and improve patient care continuity. Staffing models and workload indexes have been adopted to manage nursing resources for appropriate skill mix to meet care needs. Electronic health records (EHRs) may improve patients health related information management, but badly designed EHRs and bad access may increase charting time and the risk of forgetting to chart information. Patient monitoring systems are developed to aid clinicians in monitoring a patient's condition, but these systems give false alarms, which may result in omission of a real alarm. Patients' rooms with glass walls around workstations enable the clinicians to monitor the patients' conditions better. Clinicians need easy access to computers within and outside the patients' rooms.
[15] *Herasevi* *ch* *et al.* *2013* *USA*	Not specified	Literature review	EHRs are suggested to be adoptable for development of rule-based decision support systems for clinicians in the future. False alarms and insignificant positive alarms should be avoided in these systems.
[16] *Hewson-* *Conroy* *et al.* *2010* *Australia*	To outline quality and safety initiatives, to identify evidence-based processes of care applicable to the general adult ICU, and to summarise the research on quality improvement strategies.	Integrative literature review	The use of checklists to improve patient safety is on the increase. Checklists are implemented to improve staff education, uncover errors, assess commitment to safety standards and evidence-based care, increase knowledge of patient-centred care and augment to assess practices on clinical rounds.
[17] *Khunlert* *kit &* *Carayon* *2013* *USA*	To identify aspects of tele-ICU, which contribute to care processes and patient outcomes.	Cross-sectional qualitative study	Tele-ICU was experienced to 1) provide resources that may reduce mortality and length of stay, 2) function as trigger to improve evidence-based care, 3) support medication management and improve medication safety, 4) aid with camera to reduce risk of incidents, but also 5) maybe lead to medication errors when lack of patient-related information and 6) have no impact if the technology is not accepted.
[18] *Kruger* *&* *Tremper* *2011* *USA*	To discuss aspects, limitations and problems of a "human-in-the-loop" methodology in the medical domain, and to describe a system developed to address future care.	Not specified review	Reports aspects of future research that needs to address questions to reduce information overload in clinical work, e.g. frequent false alarms lead to the omission of true alarms by clinicians. Integrating real-time information displays are suggested to aid information management. EHRs could be used for integrated patient monitoring and artificial intelligence to support clinicians in information management and decision-making to improve patient outcomes.

Table 2. (*continued*)

[19] **Shake** **et al.** **2013** **USA**	To offer a framework of the latest advances influencing on the open-heart surgery patient, in order to enable the implementation of guidelines, protocols, checklists, and initiatives that improve patient safety.	Literature review	Written protocols, checklists and daily goal sheets have shown to reduce the risk of error by combining information for the professional to ensure important steps in the cardiac surgery care process.
[20] **Sherwood** **et al.** **2002** **USA**	To investigate the adaptation of an aviation model into the health care setting and to suggest a value-based teamwork approach to improve patient safety in critical care.	Literature review	A teamwork behaviour model, adapted from aviation, is suggested to have the potential to develop and change teamwork behaviour to reduce error in the critical care setting.
[21] **Simpson** **et al.** **2007** **USA**	To develop and refine an ICU Quality Improvement Checklist.	Prospective quality improvement project	A quality checklist is presented for the evaluation of the quality of patient care on a daily basis. Information collected with the checklist may furthermore be used for the continuous monitoring of the quality of provided care and to improve future care.
[22] **Taylor** **2005** **USA**	Not specified	Not specified review	The author argues that handheld devices i.e. personal digital assistants may improve access to information, which improves patient safety in the critical care setting.
[23] **Thomas** **et al.** **2013** **Australia**	To examine the characteristics, contributing factors and recovery processes of errors associated with clinical handover in the acute care setting.	Register research	The most common flaws in the clinical handover process concerned patient transfer without a proper handover (28.8%), absent or flawed critical information about the patient's condition (19.2%) and absent or flawed information about the patient's care plan (14.2%). A minimum standard and standardisation of handover with checklists and handover templates is suggested to improve communication and patient safety.
[24] **Vardama** **n** **et al.** **2012** **USA**	To explore the implementation of the structured handover tool (SBAR) and to investigate the potential impact of it on the nurses daily experiences.	Case-study	The structured handover tool (SBAR) may improve communication between professionals, and furthermore, support professionals with schematic formation to support decision-making, development of legitimacy and social capital for novel professionals, and also reinforce contemporary practices by standardising health care services.
[25] **Winters** **&** **Dorman** **2006** **USA**	To explore patient-safety initiatives in intensive care in the USA.	Literature review	Information management means exist to improve patient safety in the ICU e.g. the Comprehensive Unit-based Safety Program (CUSP), "bundles" that help integrate evidence-based knowledge into clinical work, and daily goal sheets to improve interdisciplinary communication. These sheets functions as a way of recording a patients care plan and also as a reminder to perform planned procedures.

Table 3. Explanatory research of information management efforts to improve patient safety

Author, year &	Purpose	Design and setting	Intervention	Impact of intervention on information management
[26] Haris et al. 2007 USA	To increase patient safety event reporting in three ICUs with a card-based system and to compare and evaluate differences in reporting among healthcare workers across these ICUs.	Prospective, single-centre, interventional study conducted in a medical ICU (19 beds), surgical ICU (24 beds) and cardiothoracic ICU (17 beds) of a 1,371-bed urban teaching hospital.	Card-based reporting program (SAFE) to enhance voluntary and anonymous reporting of medical errors and patient safety issues.	The card-based reporting system increased reporting significantly when compared with the usual Web-based reporting system from 20.4 reports/1000 patient days to 41.7 reports/1000 patient days. Results also revealed differences in reporting by different professionals and units.
[27] Ilan et al. 2011 Canada	To increase reporting of patient safety events and also to enhance analysis and responsive action of the reports.	Prospective intervention design in 2 ICUs (21-bed and 18-bed) of a tertiary 456-bed hospital.	Paper-based reporting tool (SAFE) available to staff in critical care settings.	Reporting rates increased significantly from 10.3 reports/1000 patient days to 34.5 reports/1000 patient days. There were differences in reporting between professionals and units.
[28] Ko et al. 2011 Australia	To explore if safety checklists applied by medical care teams improve patient safety when compared to not using a checklist.	Systematic review	The application of a safety checklist that addressed safety issues, by medical care teams (including a medical clinician or a surgeon).	The results suggest benefits of using safety checklists to improve patient safety. However, there is a high risk of bias due to the moderate quality of the studies.
[29] Nast et al. 2005 USA	To evaluate a new way of reporting and classifying patient safety events and to increase reporting, and to identify patient safety priorities.	Prospective, single-centre, interventional study in a cardiothoracic ICU (17-bed) and a post anaesthesia care unit (9-bed) of a 1,371-bed urban teaching hospital.	A patient safety event reporting system (SAFE) available for all health care professionals.	The new reporting system increased reporting significantly from 8.5 reports/1000 patient days to 25.3 reports/1000 patient days in the cardiothoracic ICU. A difference in reporting between professionals existed.
[30] Stahl et al. 2009 USA	To 1) study how critical information degrades and how it is lost during 24h, and 2) to explore if a structured handoff checklist inhibits information loss.	Prospective cohort study in a trauma and surgical ICU.	Structured ICU handoff checklist used by trauma team members.	Critical care related information reduced during 24h in the ICU due to communication problems. A structured handoff checklist reduced the lost information from 20.1% to 3.6%.

The most studied topics found were structured communication (e.g. clinical handover) and checklists. Several studies indicated supporting evidence for the use of structured handover [14], [23], [24], [30], checklists [16], [19], [21], [28] and patient safety reporting systems [26, 27, 29]. These safety reporting systems were designed to function as continuous quality improvement systems, which indicate areas in need of development. Also, structured care sheets were used for interdisciplinary communication, which recorded the patients care plan for the day, and additionally, functioned as a reminder for the professionals to perform planned procedures [25] in addition to other clinical electronic decision support systems [15], [18], [22]. Furthermore, one study focused on future aspects of research and the potential of artificial intelligence to support clinical decision-making [18].

Evaluating the quality of the different studies was difficult due to the variety of the study designs. A description of the used data collection methods that were reported in the reviews is presented in Table 4. A large risk of bias existed with most of the review findings as only the systematic review by Ko et al. [28], an integrative review by Hewson-Conroy et al. [16] and the review by Firth [12] described the data collection process at all. The qualitative and the quantitative original studies were evaluated with a quality assessment instrument developed by Kmet et al. [11]. Based on these evaluations, there was a difference in the quality of the studies as the scores varied from 0.45 to 0.95, where the studies of a better quality have a higher number with a maximum of 1. The scores of the quality evaluations are presented in Table 5.

Table 4. Description of reported data collection details of reviews

Article	Data search described	Inclusion and exclusion criteria stated	Flow chart of study selection process	Quality assessment of studies
[12] Firth 2013	yes	yes	no	no
[13] Goran 2012	no	no	no	no
[14] Harder & Marc 2013	no	no	no	no
[15] Herasevich et al. 2013	no	no	no	no
[16] Hewson-Conroy et al. 2010	yes	yes	no	no
[28] Ko et al. 2011	yes	yes	yes	yes
[18] Kruger & Tremper 2011	no	no	no	no
[19] Shake et al. 2013	no	no	no	no
[20] Sheerwood et al. 2002	no	no	no	no
[22] Taylor 2005	no	no	no	no
[25] Winters & Dorman 2006	no	no	no	no

Table 5. Quality scores of original studies evaluated with a tool by Kmet et al. [11]

Author	Template	Score [interval range, 0-1]
[26] Harris et al. 2007	Quantitative	0,83
[27] Ilan et al. 2011	Quantitative	0,88
[17] Khunlertkit & Carayon 2013	Qualitative	0,95
[29] Nast et al. 2005	Quantitative	0,83
[21] Simpson et al. 2007	Qualitative	0,45
[30] Stahl et al. 2009	Quantitative	0,79
[23] Thomas et al. 2013	Qualitative	0,80
[24] Vardaman et al. 2012	Qualitative	0,80

Different information management efforts have been applied to improve patient safety in the critical care setting for adults. The identified information management efforts may focus on strategic, tactical, operational and clinical levels of decision-making as illustrated in Table 6. Most of the described information management efforts were designed for the clinical level of decision-making, and only a few were designed for each of the other levels of decision-making.

Based on the findings of this review, there is some evidence to support the use of the applied information management efforts to improve patient safety i.e. safety checklists, incident reporting systems, and structured handover. The strongest evidence was found in a systematic review of the use of safety checklists [28] and an integrative review of the use of different checklists [16]. There was also some evidence in three intervention studies to support the use of an adverse event reporting system [26], [27], [29], and furthermore, two single studies to support the use of structured handover [23], [30]. However, all of these studies include a risk of bias, and therefore, the results are not generalizable per se.

Table 6. Information management means to improve patient safety and the different levels of decision-making in critical care

Level of decision-making	Means to improve information management
Strategic	Teamwork model [20] Safety Programs Incident reporting [26], [27], [29] Guidelines for unit design and infrastructure [14] Care quality checklists [21]
Tactical	Incident reporting system [26], [27], [29] Workload index and staffing models [14] Care quality checklists [21] Education to improve nurses' knowledge about medication [12]
Operational	Workload index and staffing models [14] Checklists [16], [19], [21], [28] Daily goal sheet [19], [25]
Clinical	Computer provider order entry systems [12] Bar code medication administration [12] Tele ICU nursing [13], [17] Integrating real-time information displays [18] Electronic health records (EHRs) [14], [18] Designing units to improve patient monitoring [14] Easy access to computers [14] Structured handover e.g. SBAR [14], [23], [24], [30] Patient monitoring systems [14] Clinical electronic decision support systems [15], [18], [22] Checklists and protocols [16], [19], [21], [28,] Daily goal sheet [19], [25]

Difficulties concerning adopted information management efforts were also reported. Firstly, poorly designed EHRs and bad access to information systems may increase clinical charting time, which rises the risk of forgetting to chart important information [14]. Secondly, information overload and false alarms given by patient monitoring systems, may result in omission of important information e.g. a real alarm [14], [18]. These unnecessary alarms were suggested to be a result of the current lack of integration between various systems in use [18]. Thirdly, information and communication technology systems, e.g. Tele-ICU, might lead to medication errors if patient-related information exchanged between the users of the system is insufficient, and furthermore, these systems might be ineffective if the technology itself is not accepted by the users [17].

5   Discussion

The aim of this study was to describe the current research of information management efforts in improving patient safety in critical care. The main findings of the literature review are that 1) research about information management in the critical care setting is still limited from the patient safety perspective, but this research is on the increase. 2) Most of the reported research about information management efforts to improve patient safety identified in this review, focus on the clinical decision-making level. 3) The existing research indicates that quality checklists and structured handovers may improve patient safety, and that easily available incident reporting systems may increase incident reporting in the critical care setting. In addition, 4) the means to improve information management from the patient safety perspective in critical care vary, and both manual and electronic means exist, but there are challenges with the usability aspects of these systems.

This study has several limitations. Firstly, there is a risk of bias in the literature selection and evaluation process as only one researcher was conducting this. However, this process was completed with a systematic approach with defined inclusion, exclusion and evaluation criteria. Secondly, the database search results were quite small, and therefore, a query expansion with a larger set of terms might improve the findings. Thirdly, the quality of all articles was not evaluated with the same validated tool due to the variability of the research designs. No articles were excluded based in the quality evaluations, and therefore, there is a large risk of bias of the findings, even though the literature search was limited to peer review journals. In addition, many of the reviews were reported in such a way that quality evaluation would have been difficult as few of the reviews described the research methods at all. Therefore, as the existing research on this topic from a patient safety perspective still seems to be rather limited, the evidence found about the different information management efforts is not yet very strong, and conclusions should thus be made with caution.

The quality evaluation instrument developed by Kmet et al. [11] has no clearly defined cut-point for studies, which would be based on the quality score. In the guidelines the score for study inclusion and exclusion vary from 0.55 (liberal view) to 0.75 (conservative view). In this review we did not exclude any articles based on the quality evaluations. However, we propose to use the upper limit suggested in the guidelines by Kmet et al. i.e. 0.75, to reduce the risk of bias of results due to poor quality research.

In conclusion, the patient safety perspective of information management in the critical care setting seems to be a fairly unexplored area, but some evidence exists to support the use of structured handover, checklists and easily available incident reporting systems. However, stronger evidence is still needed to support the different means to be implemented in the critical care setting to improve information management and to reduce the risk of harm to patients. Further research is also needed from a patient safety perspective on the impact of the used information systems patient outcomes, workflow and user satisfaction in critical care. Additionally, more research is needed on means to support information management on operational, tactical and strategic levels of decision-making to ensure patient safety throughout the critical care setting and improve care. Finally, the findings did not show any studies discussing an integration of hospital information sources with any external information sources e.g. other health care organisations, state agencies or insurance companies. This kind of research would also be interesting in the future.

References

1. World Health Organization: Patient safety (2014),
   http://www.who.int/patientsafety/about/en/ (April 1, 2014)
2. World Health Organization: WHO patient safety curriculum guide: multi-professional edition (2011), http://whqlibdoc.who.int/publications/
   2011/9789241501958_eng.pdf?ua=1 (April 1, 2014)
3. Bion, J.F., Heffner, J.E.: Challenges in the care of the acutely ill. Lancet 363(9413), 970–977 (2004)
4. Valentin, A., Capuzzo, M., Guidet, B., Moreno, R.P., Dolanski, L., Bauer, P., Metnitz, P.G.: Research Group on Quality Improvement of European Society of Intensive Care Medicine; Sentinel Events Evaluation Study Investigators: Patient safety in intensive care: results from the multinational Sentinel Events Evaluation (SEE) study. Intensive Care Med. 32(10), 1591–1598 (2006)
5. Valentin, A., Ferdinande, P.: Recommendations on basic requirements for intensive care units: structural and organizational aspects. Intensive Care Med. 37(10), 1575–1587 (2011)
6. Haupt, M.T., Bekes, C.E., Brilli, R.J., Carl, L.C., Gray, A.W., Jastremski, M.S., Naylor, D.F., Rudis, M., Spevetz, A., Wedel, S.K., Horst, M.: Guidelines on critical care services and personnel: Recommendations based on a system of categorization of three levels of care, http://www.learnicu.org/pages/guidelines.aspx (April 1, 2014)
7. American Association of Critical-Care Nurses: About Critical Care Nursing, http://www.aacn.org/wd/publishing/content/pressroom/aboutcri ticalcarenursing.pcms?menu=publications (April 1, 2014)
8. Reader, T.W., Flin, R., Cuthbertson, B.H.: Communication skills and error in the intensive care unit. Curr. Opin. Crit. Care 13(6), 732–736 (2007)
9. Pronovost, P.J., Thompson, D.A., Holzmueller, C.G., Lubomski, L.H., Dorman, T., Dickman, F., Fahey, M., Steinwachs, D.M., Engineer, L., Sexton, J.B., Wu, A.W., Morlock, L.L.: Toward learning from patient safety reporting systems. J. Crit. Care 21(4), 305–315 (2006)
10. Murtola, L.M., Lundgrén-Laine, H., Salanterä, S.: Information systems in hospitals: a review article from a nursing management perspective. Int. J. Networking and Virtual Organisations 13(1), 81–100 (2013)

11. Kmet, L.M., Lee, R.C., Cook, L.S.: Standard quality assessment criteria for evaluating primary research papers from a variety of fields. Alberta Heritage Foundation for Medical Research. Edmonton, Canada (2004), http://www.ihe.ca/documents/HTA-FR13.pdf (April 1, 2014)
12. Frith, K.H.: Medication Errors in the Intensive Care Unit: Literature Review Using the SEIPS Model. AACN Advanced Critical Care 24(4), 389–404 (2013)
13. Goran, S.F.: Measuring tele-ICU impact: does it optimize quality outcomes for the critically ill patient? J. Nurs. Manag. 20, 414–428 (2012)
14. Harder, K.A., Marc, D.: Human factors issues in the intensive care unit. AACN Adv. Crit. Care 24(4), 405–414 (2013)
15. Herasevich, V., Kor, D.J., Subramanian, A., Pickering, B.W.: Connecting the dots: rule-based decision support systems in the modern EMR era. J. Clin. Monit. Comput. 27(4), 443–448 (2013)
16. Hewson-Conroy, K.M., Elliott, D., Burrell, A.R.: Quality and safety in intensive care - A means to an end is critical. Aust. Crit. Care 23(3), 109–129 (2010)
17. Khunlertkit, A., Carayon, P.: Contributions of tele-intensive care unit (Tele-ICU) technology to quality of care and patient safety. J. Crit. Care 28(3), 315 (2013)
18. Kruger, G.H., Tremper, K.K.: Advanced integrated real-time clinical displays. Anesthesiol. Clin. 29(3), 487–504 (2011)
19. Shake, J.G., Pronovost, P.J., Whitman, G.J.: Cardiac surgical ICU care: eliminating "preventable" complications. J. Card. Surg. 28(4), 406–413 (2013)
20. Sherwood, G., Thomas, E., Bennett, D.S., Lewis, P.: A teamwork model to promote patient safety in critical care. Crit. Care Nurs. Clin. North Am. 14(4), 333–340 (2002)
21. Simpson, S.Q., Peterson, D.A., O'Brien-Ladner, A.R.: Development and implementation of an ICU quality improvement checklist. AACN Adv. Crit. Care 18(2), 183–189 (2007)
22. Taylor, P.P.: Use of handheld devices in critical care. Crit. Care Nurs. Clin. North Am. 17(1), 45–50, x (2005)
23. Thomas, M.J., Schultz, T.J., Hannaford, N., Runciman, W.B.: Failures in transition: learning from incidents relating to clinical handover in acute care. J. Healthc. Qual. 35(3), 49–56 (2013)
24. Vardaman, J.M., Cornell, P., Gondo, M.B., Amis, J.M., Townsend-Gervis, M., Thetford, C.: Beyond communication: the role of standardized protocols in a changing health care environment. Health Care Manage. Rev. 37(1), 88–97 (2012)
25. Winters, B., Dorman, T.: Patient-safety and quality initiatives in the intensive-care unit. Curr. Opin. Anaesthesiol. 19(2), 140–145 (2006)
26. Harris, C.B., Krauss, M.J., Coopersmith, C.M., Avidan, M., Nast, P.A., Kollef, M.H., Dunagan, W.C., Fraser, V.J.: Patient safety event reporting in critical care: a study of three intensive care units. Crit. Care. Med. 35(4), 1068–1076 (2007)
27. Ilan, R., Squires, M., Panopoulos, C., Day, A.: Increasing patient safety event reporting in 2 intensive care units: a prospective interventional study. J. Crit. Care 26(4), 431, e11–e8 (2011)
28. Ko, H.C., Turner, T.J., Finnigan, M.A.: Systematic review of safety checklists for use by medical care teams in acute hospital settings – limited evidence of effectiveness. BMC Health Serv. Res. 2(11), 211 (2011)
29. Nast, P.A., Avidan, M., Harris, C.B., Krauss, M.J., Jacobsohn, E., Petlin, A., Dunagan, W.C., Fraser, V.J.: Reporting and classification of patient safety events in a cardiothoracic intensive care unit and cardiothoracic postoperative care unit. J. Thorac. Cardiovasc. Surg. 130(4), 1137 (2005)
30. Stahl, K., Palileo, A., Schulman, C.I., Wilson, K., Augenstein, J., Kiffin, C., McKenney, M.: Enhancing patient safety in the trauma/surgical intensive care unit. J. Trauma 67(3), 430–433 (2009)

Information Categories Used to Create Situational Awareness in Emergency Medical Dispatch: A Scenario-Based Study

Teija Norri-Sederholm[1,*], Juhani Seppälä[2], Jouni Kurola[3], Kaija Saranto[1], and Heikki Paakkonen[3]

[1] Department of Health and Social Management, University of Eastern Finland, Finland
[2] Kymenlaakso University of Applied Sciences, Kotka, Finland
[3] Centre for Prehospital Emergency Care, Kuopio University Hospital, Kuopio, Finland
teija.norri-sederholm@uef.fi

Abstract. In emergency medical dispatch it is essential to find out what has happened and what to expect. When this information is collected and processed it creates situational awareness. Dispatchers should have knowledge of relevant, necessary, and missing data to be able to dispatch the right medical response units with right information. The aim of this study was to identify the information categories needed to create situational awareness in emergency medical dispatch. In emergency medical dispatch, the information role and information need are different, depending on the role of dispatch centre personnel. ERC operators use similar types of information, regardless of the incident, whereas for incident monitors the incident affects the use of, and the need for, information.

Keywords: Emergency medical dispatch, situational awareness; dispatch centre; incident monitoring.

1 Introduction

Situational awareness (SA) is about knowing what is going on so that you can work out what to do [1]. This is exactly what Emergency Response Centre (ERC) operators' work is about. They need to find out what has happened and is happening, in order to dispatch the right response units to the scene. SA is also about being aware of what is not the case, what we do not know and may need to find out, and what others are aware and unaware of [2]. During the emergency call, ERC operators carry out a risk assessment, based on the guidelines provided by the respective authorities, to assess the seriousness of the emergency. They collect information from the emergency caller in order to dispatch the right unit(s). They also decide what information is delivered to the response unit(s). [3] These decisions are not made in isolation, but within the context of a dynamically changing situation. Awareness of this situation is therefore crucial. [4]

---

* Corresponding author.

K. Saranto et al. (Eds.): WIS 2014, CCIS 450, pp. 144–158, 2014.

The ERC Administration provides emergency response centre services in Finland. Their duties are to receive emergency calls for the rescue, police and social and health services; handle communications relating to the safety of people, property and the environment; and relay the information they receive to the appropriate assisting authorities or partners. The ERC Administration is an agency under the Ministry of the Interior. [5] ERC operators have training which is planned by the Emergency Services College, Police College, and ERC Administration. The examination (90 credits) can be completed in 1.5 years. [6]

There are two task-based roles in the Emergency Response Centre: ERC operator and incident monitor. An ERC operator's job is to answer emergency calls, assess the seriousness of the emergency, carry out the first phase risk assessment, based on the guidelines provided by the respective authorities, locate the accident scene, estimate the overlapping of missions, conduct a more precise risk assessment, and give guidance and instructions relating to emergency incidents. ERC operators alert all the necessary authorities (rescue, police and social and health services) in urgent missions (classes A and B) to the scene and transfer the non-urgent missions (classes C and D) to incident monitoring. Incident monitoring comprises dispatching the non-urgent missions to response units and making the additional alerts needed. Incident monitors follow and supervise the status information of the response units of the different authorities concerned, the choices ERC operators make relating to the response units, and alert notices. They also answer radio messages, support and assist the dispatched units at the scene and allocate missions with waiting status to ambulance units. [7]

Without information, there is no situational awareness. SA comes from information and its interpretation [8, 9]. In this study, information can be data, information or knowledge. Briefly described (Table 1.), data are raw, and do not have meaning on their own. Information is data that have been given meaning by way of relational connection. This "meaning" can be useful but does not have to be. Knowledge is the appropriate collection of information, with the intent of being useful. [10]

Table 1. Ackoff's definitions of data, information, and knowledge

Category	Definition	Example
Data	Symbols	Accident, ambulance, injury, family, A203
Information	Data that are processed to be useful; providing answers to "who", "what", "where", and "when" questions	Car accident in highway. Two unconscious teenagers in the park. A threat of shooting at shopping centre.
Knowledge	Application of data and information; providing answers to "how" questions	Need to dispatch two ambulances. In this type of case I must follow certain guidelines. This situation might cause…

Information gathering and interpretation differ from one situation to another and also from one actor to another, depending on the task or purpose of the actor in an organization. All these different viewpoints exist in situations where actors are involved. [11] Because the information needed varies, based on the task and the goal, one needs to understand what is important in one's role. SA is derived from various sources of information. Sometimes the cues are overt, but sometimes they can be quite subtle and they might be registered only subconsciously [8]. When receiving information, the ERC operator should also be able to pick up subtle cues. The amount of information regarding the incident can vary. The ERC operator should know what data are relevant, what data are needed, and what data are still missing to be able to dispatch the right response units with the right information.

There is a lot of research related to SA, and different aspects of SA are studied in many areas, for example psychology, education, and cognition. SA is also studied in the Emergency Medical Services (EMS) field, mainly centered on different technologies rather than on the information itself. However, not much research is done in relation to SA and emergency medical dispatch (EMD). Blandford and Wong [4] conducted research from a cognitive perspective and concluded by proposing high-level requirements for information systems. The study was performed in London, where there were four different roles (call-takers, telephone dispatchers, radio operators, and allocators) involved in working with emergency calls. EMD operators who demonstrated an awareness of SA described a mental model that consists of a static set of information (knowledge that does not change or changes infrequently, and that they need to know) and a dynamic set of information, which they needed to keep track of. EMD operators also needed to integrate the pieces of information about the situation which they received from different sources, over a period of time, and by different methods. The researchers also found that in major incidents, where there is usually a large volume of information, complications include ambiguous information and significant time pressure. Decisions depend on the SA of the person making them [12]. SA has a key role in information sharing and especially in predicting what will happen next. SA is about information and inference [2].

The aim of this study was to identify information categories needed to create SA and to compare the differences between the ERC operator and the incident monitor in emergency medical dispatch.

2   Material and Methods

2.1   Design of the Study

Ten ERC operators, who also worked in incident monitoring, from three different Finnish Emergency Response Centres, volunteered to participate in the study. They came from different geographic areas of Finland, and different sizes of centres, for sample diversity. The data were collected using semi-structured interviews in January–March 2012.

Three progressive scenarios based on real-life experiences were used in the study. The scenarios were selected to represent different types of emergency calls focusing on the ambulance service. The first scenario was a winter traffic accident, with eight potential patients, about 30 km from the city centre. The second described a situation on a Saturday night at the beginning of June, at the start of the school summer holiday. Many young adults in different locations in one neighborhood were not feeling well and later became unconscious. The third scenario was a shooting threat outside a shopping centre, ending in one person being wounded. The scenarios involved two to five emergency calls. The interviewees had two roles during the scenario: ERC operator and incident monitor.

The scenarios were designed and pre-tested by prehospital emergency care professionals, and checked in informal pilot interviews, conducted by the corresponding author, with an ERC instructor and a police field commander, who both vouched for the validity of the scenarios.

The scenarios proceeded as emergency calls and practices in ERC do in real life in Finland. The ERC operator answered the emergency call, carried out the risk assessment, and dispatched all the necessary units and authorities directly based on the information received [3]. In some cases they alerted the units during the emergency call and then continued with the call. ERC operators also gave advice to the emergency caller to help them cope until the ambulance unit arrived. There were requests from ambulance services and the police to alert more units, or these units changed the severity of the task. Incident monitoring was also part of all the scenarios. As each scenario proceeded, the ERC operator interviewed switched roles to incident monitoring. The scenario proceeded from the perspective of incident monitoring. In this role, the incident monitor, amongst the other things related to the role, finds the nearest free ambulance unit(s), takes care of communication with the authorities responsible, and needs to be aware of the continuously changing situation relating to incidents and resources in their area, and be prepared for a possible multi-casualty incident [7]. Some scenarios caused a situation where there were not enough ambulances for the mission or no free ambulances in the area.

ERC operators were able to use the same information sources as they use in their daily work, such as the ERC information system, with maps and guidelines, during the interview. After each emergency call, interviewees were asked to describe what type of information they were looking for and why, what information they delivered to the response units, and what were they thinking during the call. The interviews were audio-recorded, and their average duration was approximately 80 minutes.

2.2   Ethics

The University of Eastern Finland Committee on Research Ethics approved the study on 15 December 2011.

2.3   Analysis

Deductive content analysis was used with the data. Content analysis is a research technique where replicable and valid inferences are made from texts in the context of their use [13]. Deductive content analysis can be used when the structure of analysis is operationalized on the basis of previous knowledge and is based on an earlier theory or model. A categorization matrix is used, and the data are coded based on categories [14]. In this study, the information exchange meta-model [11] was used to categorize the interview data, which were transcribed verbatim.

In this article, the information exchange meta-model (Table 2.) is used to find out what type of information is essential in the Emergency Response Centre from a SA point of view. It is a systemic model of the information to be used in planning and decision-making situations.

Table 2. The information exchange meta-model [11]

Values, Competence	Internal Facts	Conclusions	External Facts
Basic Assumptions Hidden assumptions that guide the behaviour of an actor. The fundamental features of a culture.	**Mission, Vision** A subjective and expressed impression of the end state of the actor.	**Decision** A solution based on thinking and assessment.	**Task** Activities or work to be performed, activities originated by upper-level management or by the development of a situation.
Socially True Values Assumptions that are mutually accepted in a certain group to be a basis of thinking and executing activities.	**Means** Activities or methods applied to reach an aim or fulfil a purpose.	**Alternatives to Act** Description of realistically executable acting solutions.	**Foreseen End States** Future situations most certainly reached when activities are finished.
Physically True Values Assumption about structures that can be accepted to be valid, e.g. organisation, division of labour, competencies.	**Resources** Available tangible resources such as people, financial resources, material, machinery and office space.	**Possibilities to Act** Describes possible paths to the goal that the actor can choose and that provide something new to the actor, e.g. strategy alternatives.	**Anticipated Futures** Describes a thing, event or development that can be taught or is expected.
Social Artefacts Structure of a social system, principles of interaction, description of nodes and their mutual positions, and observable behaviour.	**Action Patterns** Describe how an actor can behave, e.g., process descriptions and instructions.	**Restrictions** Things that have to be considered before planning the use of resources and means in the context of anticipated futures.	**Environment** Describes an area or a space that affects an actor, e.g. media activities or market trends, national trends, and global trends.
Physical Artefacts Results of activity, like technical results of a group, written and spoken language, symbols, art.	**Features** Describe the properties of objects such as organisations or equipment, e.g. infrastructure descriptions and properties of equipment.	**Event Model** A description that enables the outlining of the pattern of a situation. For example, reports, documents and analysed conclusions such as quality reports, statistics, pictures and maps.	**Events** Describes time-limited events caused by actors. For example, meetings, and sales reports on stock market prices.

The model contains three main levels of thinking: decision, planning and operating. It describes the human information handling process in the case of SA and situational understanding. It is about the ability to exchange information that is relevant to the situation being dealt with. This ontology of the human information handling structure is used to analyze various information sharing and information exploitation situations. The model framework consists of columns and layers. Each layer of the model represents a specialized task in the overall process of forming situational understanding and using information in the situation follow-up, planning and decision-making process. Layers describe the degree of temporality and abstraction of information. Information in the uppermost row is, relatively, the most abstract and future oriented, and its effects are long-lasting. The lowest level contains information that updates quickly, is concrete, and is observable as immediate events. The leftmost column contains cultural information described by Schein [15, 16]. The second left column contains actors´ internal information. The third left column contains information about expressed conclusions made by the actor. The right column describes information that comes from outside of an actor or is remarkably affected by the world outside the actor itself. [11, 17, 18, 19]

The text was coded one scenario at a time to increase reliability. The codes were the 20 information categories from the information exchange meta-model. The coding itself was done by using Atlas.ti 7 qualitative data software, and text belonging to the code could be either a meaningful whole sentence or a couple of words with a meaningful purpose. ERC operators' and incident monitors' texts were analyzed separately. To ensure the validity of the coding, a check was done by the corresponding author after all the text was coded. An expert from the ERC Administration also checked some information categories.

To enable comparison between categories, the findings are changed to percentages, which are calculated for each scenario. To evaluate the significance of each information category, a mean score is needed. Based on the model, the mean score is five, which comes from 100% divided by 20 (20 categories). According to the model, if the mean score is twice that, i.e.10, the data in this category are highly meaningful.

Firstly, the important categories of information and the differences between the scenarios are described, and secondly, the layerwise and columnwise findings are explained. Lastly, the information profile is presented for ERC operators and incident monitors. The profiles are also compared. The profile describes the kind of information they need and the type of information they should provide for others.

3   Results

The results are presented separately for ERC operators and incident monitors. The total number of findings was 2,720, including 2,189 from ERC operators and 531 from incident monitors (Table 3.).

Table 3. Number of findings

Scenario	ERC operator	Incident monitor	All
Traffic accident	366	206	572
Youth	1121	213	1334
Shooting case	702	112	814
All findings	2189	531	2720

The main categories of information with a highly meaningful value ($\geq$10) in the ERC operators' work were Events (51%) and Means (17%) whereas for incident monitors they were Action Patterns (18%) and Means (18%), as shown in Tables 4 and 5.

Table 4. Relative proportion of data in ERC operator's work and the significance of the data

Layer	Category	Traffic accident	Youth	Shooting case	All findings
Decision-making	Basic assumptions	2	1	0,3	1
	Mission, vision	0	0	0	0
	Decision	8*	8*	8*	8*
	Task	0	0	0,1	0
Means	Socially true values	3	1	3	2
	Means	18**	17**	16**	17**
	Alternatives to act	1	2	2	2
	Foreseen end states	0	0	0	0
Resources	Physically true values	0	0	0	0
	Resources	0,3	1	0	0,4
	Possibilities to act	0	0	0,3	0,1
	Anticipated future	0	0	0	0
Constraint	Social artefact	0,3	0,4	1	1
	Action patterns	7*	4	8*	6*
	Restrictions	1	1	1	1
	Environment	2	1	0,3	1
Event information	Physical artefacts	1	1	1	1
	Features	6*	3	4	4
	Event model	6*	6*	4	5*
	Events	43**	53**	52**	51**

*Indicates meaningful value
** Indicates highly meaningful value

For ERC operators the values for Means were similar in different scenarios. For incident monitors, the youth scenario had a higher value (23%) than average (18%), and the shooting scenario had a lower value (9%). There was also variation in incident monitors' Action Patterns: the traffic accident was 18%, the youth scenario 9%, and the shooting scenario 35%. In incident monitoring, there were also information categories which in some scenarios had a highly meaningful value: Decision in the youth scenario (14%), Task in the shooting case (11%), Socially True Values in the traffic accident scenario (10%), and Event Model in the youth scenario (11%).

Table 5. Relative proportion of data in incident monitor's work and the significance of the data

Layer	Category	Traffic accident	Youth	Shooting case	All findings
Decision-making	Basic assumptions	4	2	2	3
	Mission, vision	0	0	0	0
	Decision	5*	14**	4	8*
	Task	3	1	11**	4
Means	Socially true values	10**	9*	8*	9*
	Means	18**	23**	9*	18**
	Alternatives to act	2	5*	5*	4
	Foreseen end states	0	0	0	0
Resources	Physically true values	0	1	0	0,2
	Resources	1	2	1	1
	Possibilities to act	1	1	0	0,4
	Anticipated future	2	0	0	1
Constraint	Social artefact	8*	2	5*	5*
	Action patterns	18**	9*	35**	18**
	Restrictions	5*	4	5*	5*
	Environment	1	2	0	1
Event information	Physical artefacts	2	6*	6*	5*
	Features	8*	2	1	4
	Event model	5*	11**	4	7*
	Events	8*	8*	6*	8*

*Indicates meaningful value
** Indicates highly meaningful value

As shown in Table 4, the meaningful information categories for ERC operators were Decision (8%), Action Patterns (6%) and Event Model (5%). The Decision category was the only one with a meaningful value in all scenarios. Regardless of the scenario, the value was 8%. The Event Model had a meaningful value (6%) in the traffic accident and the youth scenarios. The following excerpt from the traffic accident scenario is an example of the Event Model category.

> "The emergency caller had not stopped at the scene. She reported that there were several people in two cars on the highway and that none of them had got out of the cars. I assume that these people are injured, because usually people get out of the car. I know that there must be at least two people, the drivers, so I need to dispatch at least two ambulances. Most probably I will need more."

Furthermore, the Features category had a meaningful value in the traffic accident scenario (6%). In incident monitoring, the meaningful information categories were Socially True Values (9%), Decision (8%), Events (8%), Event Model (7%), Restrictions (5%), Social Artefact (5%), and Physical Artefacts (5%). Some scenarios also had a meaningful value: Features (8%) in the traffic accident scenario and Alternatives to Act in the youth and shooting cases (5%).

Remarkable in the results by layers (Table 6) is that in ERC operator data the separate scenarios are quite close to the average of all findings, whereas in incident monitoring data there is meaningful deviation between the scenarios. Also, when comparing the data, it can be seen that incident monitors have higher values in Decision Making (15 v 9), Means (31 v 21) and Constraints (28 v 9), whereas ERC operators have a clearly higher value in Event information (60 v 24). It is notable that the Resources layer is not meaningful in this study. On observing the columnwise data, a feature of interest is found. There is a difference between ERC operators and incident monitors in each column.

Table 6. Comparison of results by model layers and columns

ERC operator

Layers	Traffic accident	Youth	Shooting	All findings
1 Decision-making	10	9	8	9
2 Means	22	20	21	21
3 Resources	0	1	0	1
4 Constraint	11	7	11	9
5 Event information	57	63	60	60
Total (%)	100	100	100	100

Columns				
Conclusions	17	17	14	16
External facts	44	54	52	52
Internal facts	32	25	29	27
Values, Competence	7	4	5	5
Total (%)	100	100	100	100

Incident Monitoring

Layers	Traffic accident	Youth	Shooting	All findings
1 Decision-making	12	17	16	15
2 Means	30	36	21	31
3 Resources	2	3	1	2
4 Constraint	32	17	45	28
5 Event information	24	27	17	24
Total (%)	100	100	100	100

Columns				
Conclusions	18	35	16	24
External facts	14	10	17	13
Internal facts	44	36	46	42
Values, Competence	24	19	21	21
Total (%)	100	100	100	100

An average of the ERC operators' and incident monitors' information interest profiles, with the role and the associated scenario-specific deviations, are presented in Figure 1. While comparing the information interest profiles we find that they are indeed different. The ERC operators seem to act mainly as Situation Followers collecting Event-related information. They also act as Decision Makers with a focus on the Decision and Means information categories.

Role	Categories by layers		ERC operator				Incident monitoring			
			All	Traffic accident	Youth	Shooting	All	Traffic accident	Youth	Shooting
Decision maker	Decision	Basic assumptions								
		Mission, vision								
		Decision	o	o	o	o	x	x	xx	x
		Task								xx
	Means	Socially true values					x	xx	xx	x
		Means	oo	oo	oo	oo	xx	xx	xx	x
Planner		Alternatives to act							xx	x
		Foreseen end states								
	Resources	Physically true values								
		Resources								
		Possibilities to act								
		Anticipated futures								
Analyzer	Constrains	Social artefacts					x		x	x
		Action patterns	o	o	o	o	xx	xx	x	xx
		Restrictions					x	x		x
		Environment								
Situation follower	Event	Physical artefacts					x		x	x
		Features		o				x		
		Event model	o	o	o		x	x	xx	
		Events	oo	oo	oo	oo	x	x	x	x

Fig. 1. Comparison of role-related information interest profiles

Incident monitors act in several roles – Decision Makers, Analyzers and Situation Followers – using more information categories than ERC operators. As Decision Makers, the most important information areas are Means, Decision, and, interestingly, Socially True Values. Also, Alternatives to Act stands out in both the youth and the shooting scenarios. In the Analyzer role, the focus is on Constraints, especially the Action Patterns. In addition, Restrictions, Social Artefacts, and Physical Artefacts need to be considered. As Situation Followers, the incident monitors need Event information, which is also part of the Analyzer role.

4   Discussion

The aim of this study was to identify information categories needed to create SA and to compare the differences between ERC operators and incident monitors in EMD. This was done by using the information exchange meta-model [11]. The results of this study indicate that ERC operators and incident monitors have different information profiles. ERC operators' main roles are as Situation Followers and Decision Makers, whereas incident monitors have, in addition to these, an Analyzer role. This finding demonstrates quite well the nature of their work [7]. An ERC operator's task is mainly to obtain event-related information [20] and, based on that information, they, in a Decision Maker role, decide which units to dispatch. In this process, they have certain Means to receive the information needed before making the decision, and then to deliver the essential information to the units concerned. In incident monitoring, the main task is to have "the big picture" of what is happening in the area, to have an up-to-date plan all the time so that there are enough units available, and to take charge in bigger incidents. This result is supported by Seppälä [7].

Next, the results are discussed from the perspective of both building SA and formulating the information profiles, by starting the discussion from the lowest layers of the Information Exchange Meta Model.

From the SA point of view, the process starts from receiving situational information [11]. ERC operators collected the data needed regarding the incident based on the risk assessment. They received Events information mainly from the emergency caller, and based on that they created the next question. This also explains the very high value for the Events category. Incident monitors typically obtained Events information from the scene, from EMS units and the police. The Event Model for incident monitors included an analysis of the situation in the area, and thinking about the criteria for the prioritization of cases. The ERC operators described in the Event Model what they were thinking before making their decision. Interestingly, the Features category was meaningful in both groups only in the traffic accident scenario. The codes in this category typically involved using the properties of the ERC information system for searching and receiving information, as for example using the map to locate the traffic accident more precisely, finding the nearest free units, receiving information that, based on the address, other emergency calls are made from the same scene, and checking the unit response proposal, based on the mission code. They also used the properties of the ERC information system to deliver the information. With the help of this situational information, and by using their tacit knowledge in event modelling, they build up a picture of the situation.

Staff in the Analyzer role develops an understanding of the possibilities of how the overall situation could develop. In this role, in addition to obtaining Events information, Constraints information was used. ERC operators had only one meaningful category in the Constraints layer, Action Patterns. Therefore, they did not have an Analyzer role. However, their Action Patterns described the ERC operators' work tasks, for example asking the emergency caller to wait for a moment while the ERC operator dispatched the units. They then continued the call, to collect more information and gave instructions to the caller. For incident monitors, Action Patterns was a highly meaningful category. A typical example of Action Patterns was finding and dispatching more units and delivering information to them while the ERC operator was still on the emergency call, collecting information. Receiving or noting information from all the Restrictions is necessary in developing an understanding of how the situation may develop [11]. Restrictions were often related to finding the nearest free ambulance unit when there was a dearth of them in the area. They also involved thinking about distances and the actual time when the unit would be on the scene, the possible use of units from the neighboring town, or free ambulances on the road in the area, on the way back to their own town. Physical Artefacts were official guidelines and instructions, such as risk assessment guidelines, instructions to dispatch the right number and type of the units to the scene, guidelines for communication, and instructions to alert the tactical emergency medical support (TEMS). Social Artefacts related to principles of interaction, such as that the first ambulance unit on the scene gives the first data by information channel, so that all the units on the way to the scene and the ERC hear the given information at the same time. Incident monitors need to have a good understanding of all the different instructions and possible Action Patterns, because they define the basic rules to communicate and use resources. When this knowledge of all Constraints is combined with the Event information, incident monitors can understand both what this all means, and what might happen next, from the perspective of one incident in the overall situation in the area this ERC is responsible for. In order to understand all this, incident monitors need to have received and analyzed a sufficient amount of information. These results are aligned with those from a previous study [4], conducted in emergency medical dispatch.

Finally, in the Decision Maker role, ERC operators and incident monitors should have, and use, a situational understanding [11]. Again, the ERC operators' information profile is more straightforward. They make decisions and have the means to realize them. Decisions related mainly to the mission code, such as B702 (Immediate response – unconsciousness), based on risk assessment or the number of units to be dispatched, whereas Means were actions like dispatching the units to the scene, giving instructions to the emergency caller, sharing information with other authorities, such as the police, and locating the emergency caller or the units on the map. The difference in the profile shows that ERC operators are responsible for one incident at a time, and only up to the moment the emergency call is ended and the response units are dispatched. They are also supposed to make decisions and use different means to achieve their goal as quickly and efficiently as possible. This might also explain why ERC operators do not undertake the Analyzer role and why only two information categories were meaningful in the Decision Maker role.

Incident monitors are responsible for the situation in a whole area [7] and therefore most probably use several information categories as Decision Makers. In this study the Means category was the most meaningful. Typical Means in incident monitoring were delivering information to the dispatched unit and locating units which can be quickly released, if needed. Incident monitors also had other highly meaningful categories. The Decision category included subjects mainly related to deciding which units to dispatch to the scene, in situations where they were in short supply, and where decisions needed to be made to deal with readiness in the area in general. The Task category mainly comprised requests from the police to dispatch TEMS in the shooting scenario, whereas most of the Socially True Values were descriptions of how other authorities communicate with each other. As regards Alternatives to Act, they related mainly to finding the units, asking advice from the prehospital field supervisor or ERC shift supervisor, and communication. When working at this level, they have knowledge about how to deal with different situations and, as mentioned in the literature review [11], the whole spectrum of the tacit dimension is available to the Decision Maker.

Interesting findings can be obtained when looking at the data by layers and columns. In ERC operators' data the values are quite similar, regardless of the scenario. This could be explained by the fact that they do the risk assessment in every emergency call and follow the dispatch instructions. The differences in the Event information layer and the External facts column can be explained by the different number of emergency calls per scenario. When comparing the data between ERC operators and incident monitors we find that the numbers are quite different. This demonstrates the difference in their role, which reflects the need and use of information. However, the Resources layer had very low values compared to other information layers in both groups. The low number in the Resources category is especially interesting. The result may be a consequence of the fact that when the interviewees mentioned resources in particular, it was related their dearth then belonging then to the Restrictions category. Incident monitoring also has differences between the scenarios. This might confirm that in incident monitoring it is not possible to manage all situations with the same type of information. However, with a small sample size, caution must be used, as the findings might not be transferable to every case.

The findings of the present study are quite similar to those from the previous research in prehospital emergency care context, where the participants were prehospital field supervisors [21]. In the previous study the most meaningful categories were Events, Means, Action Patterns, and Decision. These were similar, except the Decision category, which had a meaningful value. However, Decision was the fourth most common category in this study. When comparing the results to those from previous research [9], which was conducted in crisis management situations, with Finnish national administration workers, using the same model, the main information categories were totally different.   They were Alternatives to Act, Foreseen End States, Anticipated Futures, Mission and Vision, Resources, and Tasks. The explanation for this could be the fact that the aim of the study was different. It was about identifying the information requirements of top decision makers during a situation of sudden crisis.

We should also note the information categories where the value is lower than one. Mission and Vision, Foreseen End States, Possibilities to Act, and Physically True Values were lower than one in both groups. ERC operators also had a low value in the Resources or Anticipated Futures, and Environment categories. This might be due to the nature of EMD and the fact that the information exchange model is a generic model, made for all kinds of information exchange situations. When comparing this result with that for paramedic field supervisors, it is similar in relation to Mission and Vision, Anticipated Futures and Foreseen End States [21]. It stands to reason that these factors are, or should be, clear to everyone in prehospital emergency care.

Overall, ERC operators and incident monitors seem to act in several roles from an information point of view. They have different information profiles, with some similarities. The explanations as to which information categories are meaningful are most probably task related, and some may be related to the context, prehospital emergency care. The differences in information profiles should be considered when planning work processes, training and information systems. However, more research is needed to deepen our understanding of what type of data is needed and expected to be delivered in prehospital emergency care within the organizations concerned. Having this knowledge helps to improve SA and to focus on meaningful information flow in communication in prehospital emergency care.

Limitations

The main limitation in this study is that data were not collected from real-life situations. This was not possible without the risk of affecting the quality of the EMD. However, in this study, the focus was on the flow of information, and not on the actions performed in EMD. This study was a part of wider research. The method used to collect the data was tested in the previous study, with paramedic field supervisors, and the progressive scenarios proved to be realistic and functioned quite well as a data collection tool. The nature of the scenarios was very different, to facilitate the identification of differences. The scenarios were created by a multi-disciplinary team, and their validity was checked and tested by the research group and external experts. With regard to the chosen method, as mentioned in the background section above, there is not much research related to SA in emergency medical dispatch, and especially with a focus on the information itself. The model used proved to be suitable for this type of research in the previous study, with prehospital field supervisors, in the context of prehospital emergency care.

One question that should be asked is whether the sample was sufficient and representative. The total number of findings was 2,720, including 2,189 from ERC operators and 531 from incident monitoring. The big difference in the number of findings can be explained by the nature of EMD. The ERC operator collects data from emergency calls, and this gave a total of 1,120 findings. The interviewees came from geographically different parts of Finland and different sizes of dispatch centres. This study was conducted in one country, which uses a type of EMD different from those in most countries [3]. However, regardless of differences in organizations and working methods, the need for information is most probably the same, and SA as a concept is global.

5   Conclusions

This study provided evidence that ERC operators' and incident monitors' information profiles for SA and information needs are different. This study also proved that, regardless of the differences in incidents, the significance of the information category was similar for ERC operators, whereas in incident monitoring the significance varied, depending on the incident. These results were also aligned with those from a previous study, showing that the most meaningful information categories in prehospital emergency care are Events, Means, Action Patterns, and Decision. These results can be used in developing work processes, training and information systems in EMD.

Acknowledgements. We would like to thank the ERC Administration in Finland for their administrative support and expertise in conducting this study.

References

1. Adam, E.C.: Fighter Cockpits of the Future. In: Proceedings of 12th IEEE/AIAA Digital Avionics Systems Conference (DASC), pp. 318–323. IEEE (1993)
2. McGuinness, B.: Quantitative Analysis of Situational Awareness (QUASA): Applying Signal Detection Theory to True/False Probes and Self-Ratings. In: Command and Control Research and Technology Symposium, San Diego, USA (2004)

3. ERC Administration: The first official link in the chain of assistance and safety Provision. Basic facts about the Emergency Response Centre Administration. Emergency Response Centre Administration Finland, Pori (2011)
4. Blandford, A., Wong, W.: Situation Awareness in Emergency Medical Dispatch. International Journal of Human-Computer Studies 61, 421–452 (2004)
5. Ministry of the Interior, Emergency number 112 and emergency response centres, http://www.intermin.fi/en/security/emergency_number_112_and_emergency_response_centres
6. ERC Administration: To be an ERC operator? (In Finnish: Hätäkeskuspäivystäjäksi?), http://www.112.fi/meille_toihin/hatakeskuspaivystajaksi
7. Seppälä, J.: Emergency medical dispatch. In: Silfvast, T., Castrén, M., Kurola, J., Lund, V., Martikainen, M. (eds.) Manual of Prehospital Emergency Care (In Finnish; Hätäkeskustoiminta, in: Ensihoito-opas), Duodecim, Saarijärvi, pp. 343–350 (2013)
8. Endsley, M.: Theoretical underpinnings of situation awareness: a critical review. In: Endslay, M., Garland, D.J. (eds.) Situation Awareness Analysis and Measurement, pp. 3–32. Lawrence Erlbaum Associates, New Jersey (2000)
9. Kuusisto, R.: From Common Operational Picture to Precision Management. In: Managemental Information Flows in Crisis Management Network (In Finnish: Tilannekuvasta täsmäjohtamiseen Johtamisen tietovirrat kriisin hallinan verkostossa), Publications of the Ministry of Transport and Communications 81/2005, Helsinki (2005)
10. Ackoff, R.: From Data to Wisdom. J. Applied Systems Analysis 16, 3–9 (1989)
11. Kuusisto, R.: "SHIFT" Theoretically-Practically Motivated Framework: Information Exchange Viewpoint on Developing Collaboration Support Systems, Finnish Defence University, Department of Tactics and Operations Art, Series 3, No 1/2008. Edita Prima Oy, Helsinki (2008)
12. Busby, S., Witucki-Brown, J.: Theory development for situational awareness in multi-casualty incidents. Journal of Emergency Nursing 37, 444–452 (2011)
13. Krippendorf, K.: Content analysis An introduction to Its Methodology, 3rd edn. SAGE Publications Inc., Los Angeles (2013)
14. Kyngäs, H., Elo, S.: The qualitative content analysis process. Journal of Advanced Nursing 62, 107–115 (2008)
15. Schein, E.H.: Organizational Psychology, 3rd edn. Prentice-Hall, Englewood Cliffs (1980)
16. Schein, E.H.: Organizational Culture and Leadership, 2nd edn. Jossey-Bass, San Francisco (1992)
17. Kuusisto, R., Kuusisto, T.: Information Security Culture as a Social System: Some Notes of Information Availability and Sharing. In: Gupta, M., Sharman, R. (eds.) Social and Human Elements of Information Security: Emerging Trends and Countermeasures, pp. 77–97. IGI Global, Hershey (2009)
18. Kuusisto, R.: User Approach to Knowledge Discovery in Networked Environment. In: Syväjärvi, A., Stenvall, J. (eds.) Data Mining in Public and Private Sectors: Organizational and Government Applications, pp. 358–374. IGI Global, Hershey (2011)
19. Kuusisto, R.: Information Sharing Framework for Agile Command and Control in Complex Inter-domain Collaboration Environment. In: Proceedings of 17th International Command and Control Research and Technology Symposium (2012)
20. Act on the Operation of Emergency Response Centres (692/2010): Finland (2010)
21. Norri-Sederholm, T., Kuusisto, R., Kurola, J., Saranto, K., Paakkonen, H.: A paramedic field supervisor's situational awareness in prehospital emergency care. Prehosp. Disaster Med. 29, 151–159 (2014)

Serious Games and Active Healthy Ageing: A Pre-study

Reetta Raitoharju[1], Mika Luimula[1], Aung Pyae[1], Paula Pitkäkangas[1],
and Jouni Smed[2]

[1] Turku University of Applied Sciences, Turku, Finland
{reetta.raitoharju,mika.luimula,aung.pyae,
paula.pitkakangas}@turkuamk.fi
[2] University of Turku, Turku, Finland
jouni.smed@utu.fi

Abstract. This article describes the results of a pre-study that was conducted in a project called Gamified Solutions in Healthcare. The Gamified Solutions in Healthcare project, funded by Tekes – the Finnish Funding Agency for Innovation, develops new services and effective activity solutions to elderly people through gamification. This research project combines the expertise of many different disciplines and is linked to company-driven projects that develop scalable international serious games solutions for healthcare utilisation. The pre-study consisted of mapping existing games for seniors, conducting a pre-test on console games and interviewing potential users of serious games. The purpose of this article is to report these results and to present a research agenda for future research.

Keywords: Serious games, gamification, active ageing.

1 Introduction

Active ageing is the process of optimising opportunities for health, participation and security in order to enhance quality of life as people age. [1] This term can be applied to both individuals and groups and it emphasises the ability to participate in society while being provided with protection, security and care. Well-being in this matter is understood widely as physical, mental and social well-being. [2] Many everyday services such as banking, insurance and healthcare are becoming more and more digitalised. Younger generations are using information technology to communicate. The digital divide and unequal opportunities of using modern technology can alienate seniors from society. Therefore, including seniors in the development of the information society is very important. One aspect of the information society is the increased gamification of various things such as learning or exercise. Gamification is the process of applying game-design thinking to traditionally non-game applications and functions to make them more fun and – above all – more engaging.

Serious games are games that are used for purposes other than mere entertainment. They can be used in several application areas, such as military, government, educational, corporate, and healthcare. [3] Some research has been conducted on the positive effects of games and they have been found to affect, for instance, analytical

K. Saranto et al. (Eds.): WIS 2014, CCIS 450, pp. 159–167, 2014.
© Springer International Publishing Switzerland 2014

and spatial skills, strategic skills and insights, learning and recollection capabilities, psychomotor skills, visual selective attention [4]. In healthcare, serious games have been used to enhance physical fitness, educate health/self-directed care, distraction therapy, recovery and rehabilitation, training and simulation, diagnosis and treatment of mental illness, cognitive functioning and control; for example see [5, 6].

This paper describes the purpose and research agenda of a project called Gamified Solutions in Healthcare (GSH). GSH project develops new services and effective activity solutions for elderly people through gamification. The purpose is to include elderly people in the development and testing of games that could be used for more than just entertainment purposes (e.g. serious games). Since this field is quite new, we conducted a pre-study in the beginning of the project in order to form our research agenda. The aim of this paper is to describe the results of the pre-study. Our purpose is three-fold: firstly, to map the existing games in the market that could be used as such or could function as an example of features that a game suitable for seniors could have. This search was limited to games that could enhance health and well-being (physical, mental, social). Secondly, we evaluate the features in games that could make them senior-friendly or unfriendly. Thirdly, we examine what kind of barriers or attitudes there could be in the process of introducing games for the elderly.

This paper is structured as follows: we begin with an introduction of the GSH project followed by a summary of serious games especially in healthcare. After that, the methods and results of a pre-study will be summarised and finally, we present the research agenda and discuss the project and field of research.

2   Gamified Solutions in Healthcare

GSH is a joint research project between Turku University of Applied Sciences and the University of Turku. In cooperation with Serious Games Finland Oy, Attendo Finland Oy, City of Turku Welfare Division, and Puuha Group Oy, the project researches and develops new gamified services. The project results are aimed for healthcare utilisation and promote exercise, social inclusiveness and enhanced quality of life. The project is funded by Tekes (the Finnish Funding Agency for Innovation) until the end of 2015.

A basis for this project is a study that was conducted together with Serious Games Finland, Sendai Finland Wellbeing Center, and Sendai National College of Technology. Serious Games Finland was interested to test their serious game called Liitäjä in Japan (see [7] for a detailed report on the results). At the same time, our researchers were cooperating with Puuha Group in their gamified playground project resulting in the first prototype that was presented in the Turku International Book Fair in October 2013 (see Figure 1). Since this prototype is a combination of mechanical engineering and game development it represents a quite unique approach and it opens for the GSH project new research questions to be studied. Moreover, the industrial partners Serious Games Finland and Puuha Group both have interests in the emerging Asian markets.

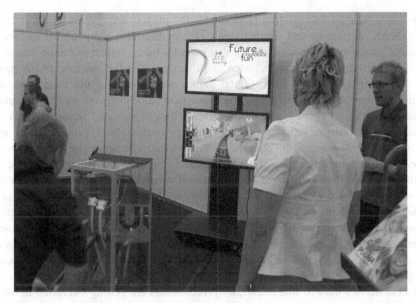

Fig. 1. Puuha's gamified playground instrument presented in the Turku International Book Fair

The solutions studied in GSH include Virtual Service Home Application and Gamified Exercise Environments both for indoors and outdoors. The Virtual Service Home Application connects elderly people still living alone at home with service home activities, enables better communication with family members and offers several gamified and activating concepts virtually. The application has the possibility to monitor and measure the customer's wellbeing. Gamified exercise environments combine digital and mobile technology with traditional playground- and exercise equipment. Outdoor Exercise Environments are targeted for more active users and indoor exercise environments more towards rehabilitative use.

The developed solutions increase an active and independent way of life while measuring the users' activity levels and performance. The project introduces different activities and gamified services through a person's life span from early retirement to service home. By utilising the new gamified concepts, social and healthcare operators can expand their service offering, serve new clientele better and compete on tightening markets. The effectiveness of the developed solutions can be demonstrated through the large number of test users nationally and internationally.

3   Serious Games in Healthcare

Nowadays, digital games are no longer just an activity for the purpose of entertainment. The use of digital games for specific purposes has become more and more popular also in other areas such as education, healthcare, business, and the military. Basically, digital games are designed to make the players experience high levels of motivation and engagement in the game itself [8]. Video games have been known as a form of an engaging platform for the players and gamers because of its entertaining, motivating and fun activities. One of the main motivational factors in computer games is the sense of control that includes users' influence on the course of events and a tight relationship between users' actions and the outcome of the game [9]. According to Prensky [10], digital games are potentially the most engaging pastime in history and it is due to the combination of game elements such as fun, play, problem solving, challenge, rules, and story-telling. Over the years, there is an increasing interest in digital games among professionals, researchers, and practitioners. For example, the concept of edutainment (education and entertainment) is widely accepted in the learning environment. Serious games are also used in specific areas such as military training, physical rehabilitation, and aviation. In the business sector, people tend to use the concept of gamification in their business models and marketing strategies (e.g. Nike and Starbucks gamified their marketing strategies). Among different areas that adopt digital games for specific purposes, digital games for healthcare is one of the promising areas. Many healthcare experts are currently using digital technology in addressing their medical and healthcare needs.

Recent studies showed that healthcare professionals are getting interested in using computer games for stroke rehabilitation [11]. Virtual rehabilitation received great interest from many researchers and healthcare professionals because it is able to provide a natural or real-life environment; individuals have the opportunity to forget about their surroundings and situation and focus directly on a task in the simulated environment [12]. Among commercially available games, Nintendo Wii seems to be one of the most promising technologies to be used as a therapeutic tool in stroke rehabilitation because of its low cost hardware and physical-based input interaction with the game. Wii encourages players to use natural actions to play games and has gained the support of occupational therapists because it is easy to use, entertaining and has a wide variety of games available which can help patients perform therapeutic training [13]. With regard to serious games, it derives game entertainment and fun elements from digital games but its main emphasis may be on serious activities such as training and learning. User experiences from serious gameplay are expected to be used in real-life environments such as defence training, business and marketing, manufacturing, and education among others. According to Stanford University School of Medicine [14], the current needs of healthcare industries are lower healthcare costs and affordable healthcare, better health outcomes and healthier population, and better patient experiences and patient engagement. To address these healthcare needs, serious games have potential. For example the potentials of serious games have been proven in preventative care and behaviour modification (e.g. games for diabetes prevention and behaviour change for sufferers) [14].

In addition to these, researchers are adopting digital games in long-term healthcare (e.g. rehabilitation) as well as chronic diseases (e.g. cancer). According to the non-profit group Cancer Research UK [15], they launched a new game for smartphone users that help the players analyse real cancer data with the goal of helping scientists find potential treatments. In this game called "Play to Cure: Genes in Space" [15], it speeds up the decoding of data to reveal patterns in the genetic faults that cause cancers to grow and spread. While the players perform the gameplay, they are actually looking at the genetic data of real cancer patients and helping to process large amounts of data more quickly than current computers can. Finally, the players' activities in the game are sent to researchers who identify genetics patterns that may lead to cancer. With regard to physical game-based intervention, exergaming is another interesting area that can draw attention from researchers and game designers because it has potential as a remedy to the growing societal healthcare problems of children's obesity and diabetes. The core concept of exergaming relies on the idea of using vigorous body movements and activities as the input for interacting with engaging digital game content that may lead to higher motivation to participate in calorie-burning cardiovascular exercise activities. Such game-based activities with functional body movements can have positive health outcomes for diabetes patients and obese children [16]. According to Ruppert [17], in the past years research findings have shown that adopting virtual environments in the health context can make a significant difference in treating anxiety disorders, drug and alcohol abuse, eating disorders, impulsive disorders, and more. As people are already using these systems for such purposes, this digital game-based technology could play a major role in changing behaviour to prevent obesity as well as in diabetes management training. All in all, it is a fact that digital games and game-based intervention for healthcare are regarded as a promising way of improving the healthcare system, treatment, and clinical outcomes.

4   Pre-study Methods and Results

The purpose of the pre-study was to get a basic understanding of the current stage of games and attitudes towards games among seniors in order to form a more detailed research agenda for the project. The aim of the pre-study was not to get scientific or generalisable information about the topic but rather to help us to formulate the research topics that should be answered during the project. The pre-study consisted of three stages:

Phase 1: Mapping senior-friendly games in the market

Phase 2: Evaluating senior-friendly and unfriendly features in the games

Phase 3: Getting a basic understanding of possible barriers and attitudes when introducing games to the elderly.

In Phase 1, we identified 30 games. Our inclusion criteria were that the game is suitable for senior users and it should improve health and well-being. These 30 identified games were then tested and classified into the following categories: (1) games for physical activity, (2) games for social activity, and (3) games for mental activity. Games for physical activity are mainly console games that used different sensors that recognize movements. Games for social activity are games that one could play with other people such as bingo, chess, and chats. Games for mental activity are games that activate the brain and memory such as memory games, and problem solving games.

In Phase 2, a team of 12 health informatics students tested different console games and their suitability for improving seniors' physical activity. This was done by observing the students' playing. In the console game testing a group of students tested existing console games that were identified to improve physical activity. The purpose was to evaluate the suitability for senior users and the senior-friendly and unfriendly features. Problems that were observed and identified during the test were related to:

- Physical limitations: the games included jumps, fast movements and other elements that were not considered senior-friendly
- Visual elements: the games were full of visual, moving elements
- Usability: the beginning of the games was complicated and took a lot of time, the instructions were in small print and with no language options
- Focus: the focus in many games was more in body building and fitness exercise
- Selection of sports: several games were about roller skating, street dancing and many other sports that are not that familiar or important to seniors

In Phase 3, we conducted three interviews of seniors, who were over 70 years old and were using a health technology service. The themes of the interview were games in general, willingness to play digital games for health and well-being and issues related to the use of information technology in general.

The interviews revealed several interesting issues about gaming among seniors. For instance, attitudes towards games in general may not be as positive as among younger generations. Games were considered to be something for people with nothing better to do. Also the word "exercise" was considered something that younger people or women would do. However, when discussing the topic in more detail, the seniors revealed several games that they have played and could play, for instance chess, coin slots, poker and quizzes. Games that the seniors would play together with others seemed to gain a more positive response than games that you play by yourself. The seniors were also concerned about their information technology skills and some thought they would not have the mental capabilities to learn digital games. Physical limitations were also seen as a problem.

5   Forming a Research Agenda for Serious Games in Active Ageing

As a result of the pre-study, we prepared a research agenda. In the pre-study, we identified some gaps in the current knowledge, which prompt us update the research agenda to fill these gaps and to enhance the usage of serious games among the seniors. Based on the pre-study, project plan and discussions, it became imminent that we should conduct more research about the seniors' attitudes towards gaming and digital games. Especially, we need more focus group interviews as well as some usability testing with console games. This includes also attaining more knowledge about the physical limitations and their influence on gaming. Finally, the research requires systematic analysis about the existing games for seniors, and the attitudes and perceptions of health and social care workers that work with seniors.

The project research can be summarised in four primary topics:
1. gamification mechanisms
2. usability for elderly people
3. effectiveness of game solutions for elderly people (e.g., business and production models)
4. attitudes and acceptance of games by the elderly people

Based on our work, we formed a preliminary schedule for the research shown in Table 1.

Table 1. Research schedule

Time	Research type	Description
January–March 2014	Pre-study	Pre-studies about different topics in order to get familiar with the topic and to formulate the research agenda.
March–June 2014	Attitudes and acceptance	Interviewing the elderly people and care workers about games and gamification, visits and observation in the care units.
April–December 2014	Effectiveness of business and production models	The business potential and production models of games for the elderly are analysed using interviews and financial figures.
June-July 2014	Usability test in Finland and Japan	Investigate usability and user experience with existing games (e.g. Liitäjä, Puuha game) with Finnish and Japanese test subjects.
August-September 2014	Game development	Based on usability tests and previous tests, we design new games and redesign existing games.
August–December 2014	Attitudes and acceptance	Questionnaire and/or interviews about the attitudes and acceptance of the elderly and care workers about games and gamification.
October-November 2014	Usability test	New or redesigned games will be tested with Finnish and Japanese test subjects.
December-January 2015	Feedback analysis and game redesign	Analyzing the feedback and re-designing the game
February-April 2015	Final usability testing in Finland, Japan and Singapore	Evaluating the effectiveness, usability and entertaining of the new developed games, both laboratory and field testing.

6   Discussion

Games and gamification in active healthy aging is a relatively new research topic. Based on our project plan, pre-study and discussions we have drawn some lines on how to proceed in the research. Most of the research will be assisted by students in different laboratories and centre of research. Our aim is to apply methodologies such as CDIO and PBL to successfully implement the research in teaching activities [18, 19, 20, 21]. Cooperation both nationally and internationally is also crucial for the success of this project. Especially, we see important the possibilities to do research in Sendai Finland Wellbeing Center, Japan and Singapore.

Finnish game industry has many globally well-known brands such as Rovio, Supercell, and Remedy. However, Finnish and generally speaking all Western game companies have had some challenges to enter the Asian game markets. At the end of year 2013, Supercell was sold to Japanese investors with 1.2 billion euros. The Finnish way of developing games, needs for new solutions in active healthy ageing, and cooperation with our Asian partners will not only open us better possibilities to build new innovations but also to generate new business opportunities for companies participating in this project. This research field is still quite new, but on the other hand we have seen that researchers all over the world are now activating. Ageing will definitely cause a lot of costs for our societies but will also create new business.

In conclusion, games and gamification offer great possibilities for active healthy ageing. Already existing games can be used with small modifications. As nations are ageing and more and more attention is paid to active healthy ageing, gaming should be considered as a potential tool for enhancing health and well-being. Introducing games and gaming to seniors is also part of avoiding digital divide and to brake negative stereotypes about the seniors.

References

1. Active ageing: A policy framework. World Health Organization, Ageing and Life Cource (2002), http://whqlibdoc.who.int/hq/2002/WHO_NMH_NPH_02.8.pdf?ua=1
2. Peel, N.M., McClure, R.J., Bartlett, H.P.: Behavioral Determinants of Healthy Ageing. American Journal of Preventive Medicine 28(3) (2005)
3. Susi, T., Johannesson, M., Backlund, P.: Serious Games – An Overview. Technical Reports. School of Humatities and Informatics, University of Skövde, Sweden (2007), http://www.diva-portal.org/smash/get/diva2:2416/FULLTEXT01.pdf
4. Mitchell, A., Savill-Smith, C.: The Use of Computer and Video Games for Learning: A Review of the Literature. Learning and Skills Development Agency (2004)
5. Taylor, M.J.D., MacCormick, D., Shawis, T., Impson, R., Griffin, M.: Activity-promoting Gaming Systems in Exercise and Rehabilitation. Journal of Rehabilitaiton Research & Development 48(10), 1171–1186 (2011)
6. Adamo, K.B., Rutherford, J.A., Goldfield, G.S.: Effects of Interacive Video Game Cycling on Overweight and Obese Adolescent Health. Applied Phisiology, Nutrition & Metabolism 35, 805–815 (2010)

7. Nakai, A., Luimula, M., Hongo, S., Vuola, H.: Evaluating a Game Motion-Based Control by Using Kansei Engineering Knowledge. In: Proceedings of the 3rd IEEE Conference on Cognitive Infocommunications, Budapest, Hungary, December 2-5 (2013)
8. Watters, J.C., Oore, S., Shepherd, M., Abouzied, A., Cox, A., Kellar, M., Kharrazi, H., Liu, F., Otley, A.: Extending the Use of Games in Health Care. In: 39th Annual Hawaii International Conference on System Sciences, Kauai, Hawaii, January 4-7 (2006)
9. McCallum, S.: Gamification and serious games for personalized health. In: Phealth 2012: Proceedings of the 9th International Conference on Wearable Micro and Nano Technologies for Personalized Health, IOS Press, Amsterdam (2012)
10. Prensky, M.: Fun, play and games: What makes games engaging. In: Digital Game-Based Learning (2001)
11. Burke, J.W., McNeill, M.D.J., Charles, D.K., Morrow, P.J., Crosbie, J.H., McDonough, S.M.: Designing engaging, playable games for rehabilitation. In: International Conference Series on Disability, Virtual Reality and Associated Technologies, ICDVRAT (2010)
12. Halton, J.: Virtual rehabilitation with video games: A new frontier for occupational therapy. Occupational Therapy Now 9(6), 12–14 (2008)
13. Anderson, F., Annett, M., Bischof, W.F.: Lean on Wii: Physical rehabilitation with virtual reality and wii peripherals. Annual Review of CyberTherapy and Telemedicine 8, 181–184 (2010)
14. Motivation and emotion can be modified in Game Play to improve patient behavior and health, http://www-935.ibm.com/services/us/gbs/gaming/healthcare/ (retrieved March 2014)
15. Anelea, A.: New gaming app seeks to cure cancer (2014), http://digitaljournal.com/tech/technology/new-gaming-app-seeks-to-cure-cancer/article/370906 (accessed: March 30, 2014)
16. Rizzo, A., Lange, B., Suma, E.A., Bolas, M.: Virtual reality and interactive digital game technology: new tools to address childhood obesity and diabetes. J. Diabetes Sci. Technol. 5(2), 256–264 (2011)
17. Ruppert, B.: New Directions in Virtual Environments and Gaming to Address Obesity and Diabetes: Industry Perspective. Journal of Diabetes Science and Technology 5(2), 277–282 (2011)
18. Luimula, M., Roslöf, J., Kontio, J.: Designing Game Development Education - First Experiences of CDIO Implementations. In: Proceedings of the 9th International CDIO Conference, Cambridge, MA, USA, p. 9 (2013)
19. Luimula, M., Roslöf, J., Suominen, T.: Proficiency, Business and Services Expertise in Game Development Education, iNEER Innovations 2013, iNEER, pp. 131–140 (2013)
20. Luimula, M., Skarli, K.: Game Development Projects – From Idea Generation to Startup Activities. In: Proceedings of the International Conference on Engineering Education, Riga, Latvia, June 2-7 (accepted, 2014)
21. Kulmala, R., Luimula, M., Roslöf, J.: Capstone Innovation Project – Pedagogical Model and Methods. In: Proceedings of the 10th International CDIO Conference (CDIO 2014), Barcelona, Spain (accepted, 2014)

A Proxy-Based Security Solution
for Web-Based Online eHealth Services

Sampsa Rauti, Heidi Parisod, Minna Aromaa, Sanna Salanterä,
Sami Hyrynsalmi, Janne Lahtiranta, Jouni Smed, and Ville Leppänen

University of Turku, 20014 Turku, Finland
{sjprau,hemapar,sansala,sthyry,jouni.smed,
ville.leppanen}@utu.fi, minna.aromaa@turku.fi

Abstract. This paper presents an idea of using a proxy-based security solution to protect web-based eHealth applications from client-side attacks.
In today's Internet, eHealth services face many challenges related to information security as the users display and input sensitive information using
web applications. This information may be spied on or modified by a malicious adversary. By obfuscating the executable code of a web application
and by continuously dynamically changing obfuscation, our solution makes
it more difficult for a piece of malware to attack its target. We believe it
would effectively mitigate automated client-side attacks.

Keywords: security in eHealth applications, web-based eHealth services, web application security, man-in-the-browser attacks.

1 Introduction

eHealth refers to healthcare practices supported by electronic processes and communication. eHealth environments provide users with continuosly improving possibilities to promote their own health. In this paper, we concentrate on web-based
health services. Taltioni service used in Finland is such online environment with
various health-related applications [15]. Other examples of health-related online
services include Finnish Omakanta [7] and TheCarrot.com [18].

In this kind of health-related online service, information security is of utmost
importance. Naturally, the users should be able to decide who is granted access
to their health information. For example, in Taltioni, users can share selected
health information with other users or healthcare professionals.

In today's Internet, however, also eHealth services face many information security related challenges [6,20]. Malicious programs, or *malware*, that has infiltrated
into the user's own computer can cause a significant security risk for any online service where the users input and store their personal data. An attack can take place
on the server, the network between the server and the client, or on the client computer. A piece of malware residing in the user's web browser, for example, can steal
or change the information that the user sends to an online service [10]. The same
can also happen in the other direction: the malicious program can tamper with the
information coming from the server to deceive the user.

K. Saranto et al. (Eds.): WIS 2014, CCIS 450, pp. 168–176, 2014.

This paper discusses these client-side security threats in web-based eHealth services. Although Taltioni applications are used as example cases, the security problem is present in all modern web applications that display and store data. To mitigate malicious attacks, we introduce a proxy-based solution to improve the information security.

The paper loosely follows the design science research methodology for information system research [8]. Section 2 presents the problem and motivation – the sensitive nature of the data in eHealth applications. Section 3 further illustrates the problem with examples from practical Taltioni applications. Section 4 presents the client-side security threats present in eHealth applications running in web environment and also outlines some objectives for our solution. Section 5 presents our solution and its evaluation. Section 6 concludes the paper.

2   On eHealth Applications and Possible Threats

According to the World Health Organization, eHealth refers to "the transfer of health resources and health care by electronic means". This definition consists of three main areas: 1) Delivery of health information for consumers or health professionals through the Internet and telecommunications, 2) using IT and e-commerce to improve public health services (e.g. education of health workers), and 3) use of e-commerce and e-business practices in health systems management. [19] On the other hand, the term can be thought to characterize "not only a technical development, but also a state-of-mind, a way of thinking, an attitude, and a commitment for networked, global thinking, to improve healthcare locally, regionally, and worldwide by using information and communication technology." [2]

The definition of eHealth also often covers a broad range of eHealth applications such as electronic health records, health care system portals, online health information websites and health education programs, health communication programs and other applications. These eHealth applications hold potential in increasing both consumer and provider access to relevant health information, enchance quality of care, reduce healthcare errors, increase collaboration and promote health. [5]

Thus, the range of health information transferred through different eHealth applications is very broad in nature. They can contain general health information related to for example health education, but also private information related to consumer's patient records. For example, the HL7 standards are followed in Finland and patient record systems list patient name, date of birth, sex, patient address, phone number, marital status, SSN, religion, citizenship and nationality [4]. The information stored and displayed in these systems can be of very sensitive and private nature [12]. Information related to the patient records is confidential and the access to it is regulated by the law. However, sensitivity of this information also means there can be many motivated attackers. In wrong hands, this sort of information enables many kinds of malicious usage. Several eHealth applications run in web browsers, which makes them especially vulnerable to attacks, as explained in Section 4.

Web-based eHealth services can be targeted by malicious attackers for several reasons:

- *Ransomware.* Individual health records or even whole healthcare information systems can be held captive to extort money [3]. The target can be either a service provider or a private individual.
- *Channel.* The web-based online health service can be turned into a proxy for malware. To use web-based services for healthcare purposes in the first place involves trust, which can be exploited.
- *Harm.* Health devices operated via a web-based service can be accessed and the function of the device, related data, measurement intervals or quality control data may be altered.
- *Fraud.* If the service has information related to compensations, even a small detail such as the user's bank account, it can be altered to serve dubious purposes.
- *Indirect fraud.* The information captured from the service could be used to commit identity theft related frauds.
- *Business.* If the service is used for doctor-patient interaction, the attacker can act as either one. This could be exploited to offer purchase recommendations that can lead the patient to use false online pharmacies.

Modifying the incoming or outgoing data is not as tempting in health applications as it is in the context of online banking, for example, but it is still a possibility that should be taken into account. If using eHealth services online will become more common in future, the client-side security of these services has to be addressed. On the other hand, eHealth services have to be highly secure in order to convince users to adopt them [6].

3   A Short Overview of Taltioni Applications

In Finland, the information on personal health and well-being is stored in the systems of various organizations and health services. It is therefore highly fragmented at the moment. Taltioni aims at building a single service platform and database that contains information on health and well-being for Finns, healthcare providers and producers of well-being services [17]. Taltioni is meant for citizens to create and maintain their well-being related information. The basic idea is that the information in Taltioni is mostly created by citizens but some of it is provided by healthcare professionals as well. The purpose of Taltioni is not to replace Kanta-related databases maintained by healthcare professionals but to complete those databases from citizen side.

Several Taltioni applications are used to display and store different kinds of health-related data [16]:

- Oma Terveys application brings together all kinds of health information – public and private – on the user. The user can display results of laboratory tests, information on vaccinations, times for doctor appointments and prescriptions. The application also gathers data on diseases that need constant attention, for example blood sugar and blood pressure levels. All the user's information from public and private healthcare is meant to be collected to one place.

- Wellmo is an application that helps the user to achieve a healthy lifestyle. It collects all kinds of data related to the user's well-being. More specifically, it stores information on the user's physical exercise, weight, sleep and alcohol use.
- Lääkekortti.fi service helps the user to manage data on medication and vaccinations.
- Kasvuseula.fi is a web service, where the user can keep track of a child's height and weight. The application automatically analyzes this data and predicts the potential growth disorders like overweight, underweight or changes in growth rate.
- iPana Äitiys is a service where a pregnant mother can store information about the progression of her pregnancy and make her own diary entries. The service can also be used to interact with child health centre or hospital, and the mother can also view all the healthcare information related to her pregnancy.

These examples further underline the very sensitive nature of the data in eHealth systems. Many attackers may be interested to spy on it. For example, a user can view his or her medical record online. Messages can also be exchanged between users and healthcare professionals, so the user can also input sensitive information into the system.

All of these previously discussed applications run in a web browser environment. While some of the applications are smart phone applications, they all can also be used with a web browser. This kind of web applications are suspectible to the client-side attacks introduced in the next section. We believe that Taltioni's server and the traffic in network between the server and the client are well protected. In web-based health applications, the client side is exposed to the greatest information security threat.

4   Security Risks on the Client Side

It is usually much easier for an attacker to attack the user's computer than to compromise the server side of an online service. The users' computers, where the security is often insufficient in many ways, are techologically a very weak link in today's information security. Therefore, we will concentrate on the malware residing on the user's computer and see what kind of risks it can cause for eHealth applications running in web browser environment.

Assume a malicious adversary would like to spy on and possibly alter the data the user inputs when using an eHealth application. First, the malicious program used by the adversary infects the unsuspecting user's computer and browser. Whenever a certain web page (application) with a correct URL address is loaded, the malware waits that the user securely logs in and after that it starts to observe the user's actions. When the user submits data, the malware intercepts the transmission, extracts all data and modifies the values according to the adversary's needs. The browser sends the data to the server, including the values modified by the malware.

When the server receives data, it has no way to differentiate between the original values and the modified ones. The server therefore accepts the values and sends its reply to the user's browser. When the browser receives the reply for the modified transaction, the malware again notices this and replaces the modified data in the server's reply with the data that the user originally submitted. The user's browser now displays the reply with the original details. The user thinks that the original transaction was delivered to the server intact. Both the server and the user are oblivious to the fact that their communication has been compromised.

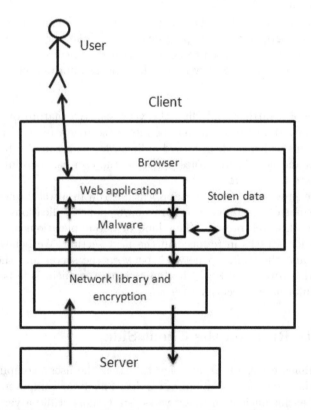

Fig. 1. Spying and modification attacks on the sensitive information

Here, we can differentiate between two different scenarios, *data spying* and *data modification*. In a system where the user stores health-related data, the simplest scenario includes the user's data getting stolen by the malware but not altered in any way. The user may never find out that sensitive information has been disclosed to the adversary.

On the other hand, the information could be modified before it reaches the server. This way the data is possibly shown differently to different people, since the users see the original data they have submitted but other users or healthcare professionals may see the data modified by the malware. This latter scenario is probably less likely than the first one in the context of eHealth applications, but it is still plausible.

Figure 1 illustrates these attacks. The solid lines indicate the flow of data. Malware in the browser attaches itself to the web application in order to modify or spy on the data. This is done when the data is still in plain text form and not yet encrypted. The main difference between the two scenarios is that after a spying attack, the malware sends the data to the attacker. Modification attacks do not need such functionality.

Because of security arrangements in eHealth services like Taltioni, other users of the service cannot see any data on a certain user of the service if the user in question has not specifically allowed them to see it [17]. However, as described above, a piece of malware on the user's machine certainly can see and modify everything flowing between the server and the client.

The security threats described above are definitely not a problem only for Taltioni's services or even eHealth applications in general, but the same threat is present in all web applications where the user inputs data using the application and the information is sent over the network. However, eHealth applications can be considered more critical than many other applications, because health-related data has the potential to be very sensitive.

It is clear that we need new ways to prevent these threats. For example, many banks already use a side channel, like SMS-based verification, in order to make sure the user has really meant to make the money transfer that the bank's server has received information about [13]. Attacks like this are already happening. For example, Zeus is a piece of malware that is able to modify user transactions on the fly [14].

While using a side channel is somewhat acceptable when applied to unexpected money transfers, it is in our view less obvious that users would accept this kind of verification in the context of eHealth services. After all, it has a notable effect on the usability of the service. Also, a side channel causes expenses to the service provider.

We probably need some lighter approach where the user does not need to do anything special to verify actions made in the system. In the next section, we introduce a transparent method to protect the user data. Although it does not guarantee to prevent all tampering, it should considerably mitigate client-side attacks.

5   Our Solution

Malware residing on the user's browser needs to know the web application's structure in order to spy on or modify the data submitted by the user. Our idea is to change the application running on the user's browser so that it will become very difficult for malware to compromise it. In this section, we will not go to technical details of our approach. It has previously been described conceptually in [9] and more detailed discussion about implementation can be found in [11].

Changing the application's executable code while preserving its original functionality is called *obfuscation* [1]. Now, the user will not notice any changes in the functionality of the application, but the code is different on each user's machine. This will make generic, automated malware attacks very difficult, since the malware needs to know what to change about the target application's functionality.

We make attacking the web application even harder by obfuscating it again continuously during its execution. When the structure of the application's code is continuously changed, the malware has very little time to analyze and modify it.

In our solution, we see the obfuscator as a service that acts between the clients and the server side. The obfuscator is independent of the web application that is being protected and also does not depend on the server. As a result, this service can be thought as a proxy component located between the client and the server. The idea of an independent proxy makes our scheme highly generic. The proxy is also totally invisible to the user of the obfuscated application.

The general idea of our obfuscator scheme is the following. The client first requests and displays a proxy page instead of the original one. The proxy page then requests the original application from the server and completely obfuscates the application. This obfuscated application is then returned to the client. Naturally, the client does not know that it is actually communicating with a proxy page. The page keeps obfuscating itself over and over to protect itself from attacks. The frequency of updates can be very high. This functionality is illustrated in Figure 2.

On the client side, the application consists of HTML and JavaScript code that is executed by the browser to run the application on the client machine. The original page created by the server is shown as a diamond in Figure 2. The circles in the figure represent the new obfuscations frequently created by the obfuscator.

The obfuscation can be applied to any part of the JavaScript code. For example, our proof-of-the-concept implementation in [11] scrambled the function signatures in the code. However, the best result is of course achieved by using several different obfuscation techniques in combination. These attacks together essentially transform the original code to completely differently looking code which still implements the same external functionality. This makes the obfuscated code more resilient against attacks.

A more detailed description of different obfuscation techniques is available in [9]. Some obfuscation can also be applied to the HTML code of the web page that is being protected. For clarity, obfuscation is only applied to HTML and JavaScript code but not to the data sent over the network. Normal application-specific cryptography protocols are of course applied to this data.

Our solution works against both scenarios – spying and modification attacks – described earlier. It mitigates the spying attacks by changing the application's

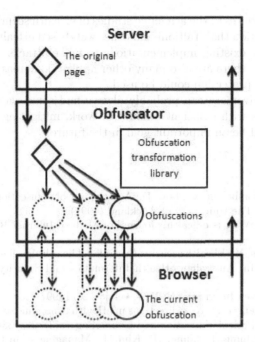

Fig. 2. The obfuscator proxy

structure. The adversary still has ways to capture the data that the user inputs in the application, but a piece of malware is now left with much more data it needs to analyze if it does not know the application's structure. Additionally, it also has to send the captured data to the attacker, and this activity may be detected.

Modification attacks are often even more dependent on the known structure of the application, especially if the data is encrypted by the application before it is sent to the server. Therefore, our approach should effectively mitigate these attacks as well.

Significant performance losses that are noticed by the user are not acceptable as a result of obfuscation. In response to the growing use of JavaScript frameworks and Ajax and competition between web browsers, the performances of JavaScript engines in major browsers have significantly improved in recent years. Therefore, good efficiency and transparency to the user are achievable even when the application is strongly obfuscated and the obfuscation updates are frequent.

6   Discussion

In this paper, we have shown that the sensitive information flowing in web-based eHealth systems can be compromised in client-side attacks performed by malware that has infiltrated into the user's machine. This poses a serious threat to web-based eHealth services and their users.

Our work contributes to the academic studies of eHealth security by proposing a proxy-based solution that Taltioni and other web-based eHealth services could integrate into their existing implementations to make attacks more difficult to perform. Of course, there are also many other application areas where this kind of web application protection could be used.

Although the adversary can probably always find some way to spy or alter online transactions with sufficient amount of work, mitigating automated and generic attacks will be an important goal in the future.

References

1. Collberg, C., Thomborson, C., Low, D.: A taxonomy of obfuscation tranformations. Tech. Rep. 148, The University of Auckland (1997)
2. Eysenbach, G.: What is e-health? Journal of Medical Internet Research 3(2), e20 (2001)
3. Foster, B., Lejins, Y.: Ehealth security Australia: The solution lies with frameworks and standards. In: Australian eHealth Informatics and Security Conference, pp. 21–28 (2013)
4. Health Level Seven International: HL7, version 2.3 (1997)
5. Kreps, G., Neuhauser, L.: New directions in eHealth communication: Opportunities and challenges. Patient Education and Counseling 78(3), 329–336 (2010)
6. Oladimeji, E., Chung, L., Jung, H., Kim, J.: Managing security and privacy in ubiquitous ehealth information interchange. In: Proceedings of the 5th International Conference on Ubiquitous Information Management, pp. 1–10 (2011)
7. Omakanta: Omakanta homepage, http://www.omakanta.fi
8. Peffers, K., Tuunanen, T., Rothenberger, M., Chatterjee, S.: A design science research methodology for information system research. Journal of Management Informration Systems 24(3) (2007)
9. Rauti, S., Leppänen, V.: Resilient Code Protection by JavaScript and HTML Obfuscation for Ajax Applications against Man-in-the-Browser Attacks (under review)
10. Rauti, S., Leppänen, V.: Man-in-the-Browser Attacks in Modern Web Browsers. In: Emerging Trends in ICT Security, pp. 469–480 (2014)
11. Rauti, S., Leppänen, V.: A proxy-like obfuscator for web application protection. International Journal on Information Technologies and Security 6(1) (2014)
12. Rodwin, M.: Patient Data: Property, Privacy & the Public Interest. American Journal of Law and Medicine (36), 586–618 (2010)
13. Safenet: Man-in-the-Browser. Understanding Man-in-the-Browser Attacks and Addressing the Problem. Technical report
14. Dougan, T., Curran, K.: Man-in-the-browser attacks. International Journal of Ambient Computing and Intelligence 4(1), 29–39 (2012)
15. Taltioni: Taltioni homepage, http://www.taltioni.fi/en/individuals/taltioni
16. Taltioni: Taltioniin liitettävät palvelut, http://www.taltioni.fi/fi/kansalaiset/palvelut
17. Taltioni: What is taltioni? http://www.taltioni.fi/en/individuals/taltioni
18. TheCarrot: TheCarrot homepage, http://www.thecarrot.com
19. WHO: E-Health (2014), http://www.who.int/trade/glossary/story021/en/
20. Wilkowska, W., Ziefle, M.: Privacy and data security in E-health: Requirements from the user's perspective. Health Informatics Journal 18(3), 191–201 (2012)

Case Study: Using Assistive Technology to Cope with Unexpected Blindness

Neeraj Sachdeva

University of Turku, Turku, Finland
neesac@utu.fi

Abstract. Some people are born with no vision, whereas some lose their vision later in life. It is important to understand the role of assistive technology in improving the quality of life of these people. Since people who lose vision later in life have altered & diminished perception of the environment around them, their attitude towards assistive technology can be different to those that have been blind since birth. This paper aims to understand perspectives of someone who lost his vision later in life. Using insights drawn from interviews and case study of one blind user, this paper discusses and explains his use of assistive technology to cope with unexpected blindness.

Results indicate that adopting new technology to overcome challenges is not easy. However, through willingness and proper direction, it can be accomplished. Results provide ideas that could improve social rehabilitation for people that have faced unexpected loss in vision.

Keywords: Assistive Technology Adoption, Totally Blind People, Unexpected Loss of Vision.

1 Introduction

Losing vision at a later stage in life can have a strong impact on a person. Someone in this condition has already been able to see for a prolonged period of time (unlike those that have been blind since birth), and their outlook on life could be strikingly different and perceptive to the environment around them. Roberts (2006) has speculated on the lives of blind people in a sighted culture. His comments ring true in most cases and highlight an increasing need for better acclimatization for those that lose vision later in life:

"We are used to conveying and absorbing vast amounts of information visually or in print. Our buildings, offices, homes and appliances are designed with the assumption that everyone has full vision, and our love affair with automobiles has produced urban geographies in most parts of the country that require everyone to drive. Those of us who are sighted routinely assume full sight in others and practice many social behaviors that are sight-based, such as giving directions by pointing, responding to comments with facial expressions." ([1], XIII)

Unexpected loss of vision can be detrimental to personal and professional growth and sustenance, but with positive attitude and a stronger-than-usual will to succeed,

K. Saranto et al. (Eds.): WIS 2014, CCIS 450, pp. 177–185, 2014.

these challenges can be overcome. There have been many documented cases of later-in-life blind people overcoming adversity to succeed, some of which include Joseph Pulitzer, Andrea Bocelli, Claude Monet and Galileo Galilei. While this paper in no way argues that every later-in-life blind person can become an exemplar, it must be noted that there are people who unexpectedly lose vision, yet cope with the challenges thrown at them in this sighted world. Whilst these historic figures hardly used any modern assistive technology for their accomplishments, the availability and relative easy accessibility provides ample opportunities to blind people today.

In health-care, the term "assistive technology" holds a special meaning. Riemer-Reiss and Wacker (2000, Page 44) have said that "assistive technology devices enable individuals with disabilities to participate in society as contributing members". Easy availability and access to these devices ensures that blind people are able to carry out daily tasks with relative ease. Common assistive technologies used by totally blind people include Screen readers [3], Braille printers [4], Personal Digital Assistants (both Braille and Speech operated) as well as Audible Tactile Signs and Warning Surfaces.

The study described here is an exploratory case study of a blind user who had lost his vision later in life. Previous studies have focused on hypothesis and theories to prove certain expected outcomes. Instead, this study is explorative, and is aimed at understanding end-user perception of assistive technology and its role in everyday life. This study deals with usability in a wholesome sense – looking at social and psychological attributes that govern adoption and use of assistive technology.

The rest of this paper unfolds as follows: Section 2. Section 3 discusses the methodology used for this research. Section 4 shows findings from the interviews, categorizing them based on the responses gathered. Section 5, the final section of this paper ends in conclusion and discussion, where emphasis has been maintained on discussing the possibilities of further research to understand this issue. The conclusion focuses on theoretical and practical contributions.

2   Background

2.1   What is Assistive Technology?

Assistive technology provides numerous benefits to people with disability. According to Hersh (2007), assistive technology can be used to overcome the social, infrastructure and other barriers experienced by disabled people that prevent their full and equal participation in all aspects of society. Similarly, Carr, Gibson and Robinson (2001) have pointed out that assistive technology allows people to continue in their normal roles and meet their expectations of life despite their physical impairment and disability. Whilst assistive technology is readily available, its accessibility depends on geographical location, financial capabilities and intrinsic motivation of the end-user. In the case of visually impaired and blind people, while assistive technology is very useful, its implementation and accessibility has been often questioned [7].

With respect to assistive technology adoption and continued use, interesting observations have been documented through the years. Scherer (1996) mentions that people select assistive technology based on how well these technologies satisfy the needs and preferences. Edyburn (2004) posits that developing a unifying theory that clarifies relationships among assistive technology and instructional technology for the sake of learning could lead to better understanding and usage. Assistive technology is useful in multiple scenarios including thinking, remembering, learning [10] and [11] or cognitive rehabilitation [12], to decrease isolation [13], recreation and more. It also provides important socio-psychological benefits such as empowerment [14].

Design Construct. The research setting was designed to accommodate participant requests. The participant was interviewed in a semi-structured interview format in his natural environment – at his work – where he spends a considerable portion of his daily life. Since the case study was explorative, topics such as non-work environment including home and public surroundings also came up. While the intention with these case studies was to understand the role of assistive technology in the participant's life, the interviewer ensured that the questions were not leading to a certain conclusion.

This study is aimed at understanding the perceived and actual impact of assistive technology on the life of someone who had recently lost his vision. Losing vision can have a deep emotional and social impact, repercussions of which are visible in nearly every walk of life. Few studies have looked at the impact of losing vision later in life [15,16,17] but focus has primarily been on negative aspects. Considering this, it becomes necessary to discuss the positive attributes – both personal and social – that affect life after unexpected blindness. Some of these attributes include motivation, strong-will, and community support – anything that could assist individual's unexpected loss of vision.

3   Method

The explorative case study of – with John – took place in three different sessions, each lasting between 40 and 60 minutes. All the interviews were recorded, and the interviewer also took notes during the sessions. The sessions were conducted at John's office, as it was a convenient and non-intrusive location for both interviewee and participant to meet. The setting also allowed possibility of observing John in his natural surroundings. The interviews involved open-ended questions focused on understanding daily life of the participant.

Yin (1981) suggests reporting the case studies in the form of narratives, based on a clear conceptual framework. Stake (1995) also supports narrative-based analysis as it optimizes the opportunity of the reader to gain an experiential understanding of the case. Based on this, a semi-structured questionnaire was designed for this interview. Some questions allowed the interviewer to focus on special issues – such as life at home, traveling between home and work, and general mobility at work.

The participant – John – is an owner of a company in Finland. In an accident 3 years ago, John lost his eyesight completely, and has almost no chance of regaining any vision. Upon leaving hospital after the accident, John decided to rejoin work, to continue what he had built up over the years. His current focus was towards growing the company further while trying to live the kind of lifestyle he had been used to before the accident.

4   Analysis

4.1   Perspectives on Everyday Life

Throughout the interview and observation phase, John's interaction with everyday environment was closely observed and documented. John's willing ness to openly discuss his condition and use of assistive technology was more forthcoming since he felt that this research would help other blind people. Generally, he was positive about the future of assistive technology, and had been involved in beta-testing potential solutions that could help him "see" things, or sense them better.

John had lost his eyesight in a medical accident in 2009. Upon finding about loss of his eyesight, John was saddened but he decided to not let that affect his quality of life, and went back to work immediately. His strong-will is evident from the fact that even though he faced adversity, he decided to continue working. Part of the reason for him going back to work could be that he wanted to focus on his work and move forward rather than feel restricted due to this unexpected loss of vision.

The company – led by John – had moved to new premises in 2008. Since he was used to the surroundings before the accident, it was easier for him to come back to work in the same office and to an extent – the same role. Since the accident, he faced minor issues at the office whereby little changes in furniture hurt him, but overall, he was comfortable with orientation. However, he did stress that it was necessary to have everything in the same place – both at home and at work. This helped him avoid injuries. As a result, the office environment underwent minor modifications such as easier access to his secretary, as well as physical adjustments such as a hand-railing from outside his office that led him close to the toilet, which assisted him in better mobility within the office.

Since his loss of vision, John faced some issues consistently – everyday. For example, he was unable to discern colors, and thus, could not pick out clothes by himself. Moreover, a visually impaired person can find it difficult to commute, especially if the means of transportation are not easily accessible. Public transportation is particularly difficult in these situations [20,21]. Fortunately, John's commute to work was a 10-minute walk, and he was generally accompanied by an assistant or friend(s). Similarly, in case of meetings held within the local area, someone would always accompany John. Moreover, John found that he had trouble walking and talking on phone at the same time, as he had to then concentrate on multiple actions. Dual task and effects have been studied and documented by various studies [26,27].

John mentioned that for any form of travel, detailed planning was required for each and every step. Generally when John would travel to new places, people with him would help him with navigating and understand the new surroundings. However, at one time, he was forgotten at the screening gate at the airport.

4.2   Government Support

Generally, John had a very positive image about assistance provided by the Government. When John was discharged from the hospital, he was sent through a rehabilitation process. Rehabilitation was aimed at acclimatizing him to unexpected loss of vision, and helping him face challenges presented in near future. The rehabilitation unit encouraged use of technology, and put John in touch with Finnish Federation for the Visually Impaired (Näkövammaisten Keskusliitto ry, NKL), which allowed him easy access to people who would provide more details on assistive technology. Access to local unit ensured that John could get timely and location based help for any questions or issues.

The local NKL organization had recommended John to use screen readers on his computer. Upon further research, John found 2 screen readers that could be used – JAWS and NVDA. At €1800, JAWS was costly yet highly recommended and the one most compatible to John's language and usage needs.

However, buying this software with Government support was not as easy as it was originally hoped. John needed permission from KELA and Insurance companies to purchase the software, which delayed the process by 2 months. Additionally, there was confusion regarding who would compensate for John's purchase between the two organizations. John was willing to pay for the software himself, and reimburse later. But lack of assurance from either party made him decide otherwise, and in the end he purchased NVDA to gain quicker access to information. These kinds of delays can be critical in assistive technology adoption and accessibility [2], [22].

The local hospital gave John vouchers to purchase a mobile phone especially suitable for his condition. Communication and data management was always complicated, and John often used his secretary to store and manage data on his computer, as well as his calendar. Previously, he used to use calendars on his computer and mobile, but due to some missed appointments, he decided to seek the help of his wife and secretary. John seemed happy that there were people around him to assist, which by his own admission, also made him "lazy".

Overall, John was happy with the quality of support offered by local organizations. However, from technological perspective, he felt that he could use a complete catalog of devices (hardware and software) that are available in Finland. In fact, if an organization such as NKL could keep such a list, it would be useful for blind (and visually impaired) people, caregivers as well as their prospective employers. However, such a list is not yet available, and due to budgeting constraints, there are no immediate plans to create such a list.

4.3   Dependence on Technology

Since his untimely accident, John had started relying on new techniques to make his daily tasks simpler. One such technique was "touch typing". While John had been accustomed to the one-finger typing system before his accident, he now had to learn touch-typing in order to navigate around the keyboard faster. Touch-typing system has been traditionally recognized as a common part of education for blind people [23].

In terms of computer use and operating system preference, John had noticed that Windows XP and JAWS were incompatible. But since John preferred Windows XP instead of Windows 7 (which instead was compatible with JAWS), he decided to use an alternate solution – NVDA screen reader – a free and open-source solution. He also didn't use Facebook, and his primary reasons to do so were difficult user-interface, and his intention of keeping personal information private.

John also faced difficulties with Digibox (the cable TV system) at home. He was unable to navigate easily, and had to seek assistance to find channels and record programs. In the morning TV-shows where hosts would interview a guest, the guest's name and their position were made available for sighted viewers, but it was not easily accessible to those with visual impairment. Similarly, John didn't like spoken description in movies (at the cinema), as he felt that the description couldn't give a clear idea of the experience. On the other hand, when walking somewhere, John preferred the escort to describe the surroundings to him.

When compared reading for leisure via screen reader compared to listening to audio, John preferred the latter – though this could be a personal preference to gather data – especially since John couldn't clearly explain this preference. Usually, someone else would purchase audio recordings of various books for him. However, he had recently started reading digital version of a weekly magazine, which was delivered via emails.

John used Outlook based emailing system to correspond on work related matters. Whilst the tool was sufficient for daily use, it was not convenient to use for archived and old emails. Interestingly, John mentioned that he only actively uses technical devices when he is checking emails or sending text messages. Other than that, his dependence on technology is limited.

4.4   Perspective on Adoption

John emphasized that since he lost his vision later in life, it is much simpler for him to adopt technology. His past experiences with technology, when he had full vision, allowed him to get a better understanding of the technological setup – something those that have been blind since birth would not have been able to experience. However, if there was a new technology that John had not experienced before – like touchscreen systems – he faced challenges in using it.

Generally, John had trouble browsing internet through screen readers, as most websites don't follow optimal accessibility guidelines, as pointed out by many other studies [24,25]. This often made him frustrated and less reliant on screen reader technology, choosing to depend on other people instead. At the time of interview, John was transitioning to a new laptop – to something that would be durable and last a few years. This transition brought up many challenges such as a new keyboard, different operating system and a new screen reader technology.

Whilst John was used to traveling alone before his accident, he now depended on someone to take him from one place to another, which by his own admission, limited his technology adoption. It is somewhat understandable in some cases, considering local environments such as railway stations are still not completely accessible, though the authorities are consistently working towards rectifying this.

5   Discussion and Conclusion

Assistive technology has been pivotal in improving quality of life through better accessibility of information. This study tried to understand assistive technology availability, accessibility and use from the perspective of a late-in-life blind person. While a comparison in attitudes between a late-in-life blind person, and someone who has been blind since birth is lacking, the series of interviews still provided valuable insights into how assistive technology is perceived by our subject – John. Through hit-and-trial and often by depending on others, John was able to successfully use computers and screen readers (both NVDA and JAWS) post-accident. However, he faced numerous barriers along the way – the delay in making assistive technology accessible being one of them.

Socio-psychological factors can be very important to cope with unexpected disability. John's willingness to face adversity head-on and his intent to adapt highlighted his strong-will and motivation to move forward. However, his circumstances did require stability in his external environment to make his life as comfortable as possible – which was possible, partly due to his influential status. It can be argued that for someone who does not have a highly elevated social status such as this, enough opportunities or resources might not be available. It would be useful to do further studies with other participants to learn more about how they resolve issues that cannot otherwise be resolved unless someone is available to help them.

Social environment plays an influential role in coping with disability, and for most part, the social rehabilitation system helped John adopt assistive technology faster. Yet at the same time, easy availability of other people made him less reliant on assistive technology. Moreover, even though Finland is a sparsely populated country, the availability of local organizations significantly improved John's rehabilitation process. However, even though the Government support was available, in some cases, it was not as easily accessible due to bureaucracy, which for others with disability could prove to be a big challenge.

Most things in life, such as picking out clothes, watching television, transportation, and information gathering are necessary, and in case of blind people, can be – to an extent – simplified with the right assistive technology. Screen readers form an important part of the toolkit as they allow easier information gathering and communication. Even then, due to a lack of consistency in technologies such as Web 2.0, screen readers can falter. Regardless, these technologies are useful to provision a better quality of life, and hence are preferred by people with disabilities – regardless of when they became disabled.

References

1. Roberts, D.L.: The First Year: Age-Related Macular Degeneration: An Essential Guide for the Newly Diagnosed. Da Capo Press (2006)
2. Riemer-Reiss, M.L., Wacker, R.R.: Factors Associated with Assistive Technology Discontinuance Among Individuals with Disabilities. Journal of Rehabilitation 66(3), 44–50 (2000)

3. Leporini, B., Paternò, F.: Increasing usability when interacting through screen readers. Universal Access in the Information Society 3(1), 57–70 (2004), doi:10.1007/s10209-003-0076-4
4. Goldberg, A.M., et al.: A Look at Five Braille Printers. Journal of Visual Impairment and Blindness 81(6) (1987)
5. Hersh, M.A.: Assistive Technology for Visually Impaired and Blind People. Springer (2007)
6. Carr, A.J., Gibson, B., Robinson, P.G.: Is quality of life determined by expectations or experience? BMJ: British Medical Journal 322(7296), 1240–1243 (2001)
7. Abner, G.H., Lahm, E.A.: Implementation of Assistive Technology with Students Who Are Visually Impaired: Teachers' Readiness. Journal of Visual Impairment & Blindness 96(2), 98 (2002)
8. Scherer, M.J.: Outcomes of assistive technology use on quality of life. Disability and Rehabilitation 18(9), 439–448 (1996)
9. Edyburn, D.: Rethinking Assistive Technology. Special Education Technology Practice 5(4), 16–23 (2004)
10. Scherer, K.R.: What are emotions? And how can they be measured? Social Science Information 44(4), 695–729 (2005), doi:10.1177/0539018405058216
11. Edyburn, D.: Assistive Technology and Mild Disabilities. Special Education Technology Practice 8(4), 18–28 (2006)
12. Frank Lopresti, E., Mihailidis, A., Kirsch, N.: Assistive technology for cognitive rehabilitation: State of the art. Neuropsychological Rehabilitation 14(1-2), 5–39 (2004), doi:10.1080/09602010343000101
13. Bradley, N., Poppen, W.: Assistive technology, computers and Internet may decrease sense of isolation for homebound elderly and disabled persons. Technology and Disability 15(1), 19–25 (2003)
14. Hurst, A., Tobias, J.: Empowering Individuals with Do-it-yourself Assistive Technology. In: The Proceedings of the 13th International ACM SIGACCESS Conference on Computers and Accessibility, pp. 11–18. ACM, New York (2011), doi:10.1145/2049536.2049541
15. Krieger, S.: Things No Longer There: A Memoir of Losing Sight and Finding Vision. Terrace Books (2005)
16. Murray, S., McKay, R., Nieuwoudt, J.: Grief and needs of adults with acquired visual impairments. British Journal of Visual Impairment 28(2), 78–89 (2010)
17. Harris, H.J.: How to Survive Losing Vision: Managing and Overcoming Progressive Blindness Because of Retinal Disease. AuthorHouse (2011)
18. Yin, R.K.: The Case Study Crisis: Some Answers. Administrative Science Quarterly 26(1), 58–65 (1981), doi:10.2307/2392599
19. Stake, R.E.: The Art of Case Study Research. Sage (1995)
20. Gallon, C., Fowkes, A., Edwards, M.: Accidents involving visually impaired people using public transport or walking. TRL project report (PR 82) (1995), http://trid.trb.org/view.aspx?id=426204 (retrieved)
21. Hine, J., Mitchell, F.: Better for Everyone? Travel Experiences and Transport Exclusion. Urban Studies 38(2), 319–332 (2001)
22. Murchland, S., Parkyn, H.: Using assistive technology for schoolwork: the experience of children with physical disabilities. Disability & Rehabilitation: Assistive Technology 5(6), 438–447 (2010), doi:10.3109/17483107.2010.481773
23. Edwards, A.D.N.: Soundtrack: An Auditory Interface for Blind Users. Hum.-Comput. Interact. 4(1), 45–66 (1989), doi:10.1207/s15327051hci0401_2

24. Asakawa, C.: What's the Web Like if You Can'T See It? In: Proceedings of the 2005 International Cross-Disciplinary Workshop on Web Accessibility (W4A), pp. 1–8. ACM, New York (2005), doi:10.1145/1061811.1061813
25. Hackett, S., Parmanto, B., Zeng, X.: Accessibility of Internet Websites Through Time. In: Proceedings of the 6th International ACM SIGACCESS Conference on Computers and Accessibility, pp. 32–39. ACM, New York (2004), doi:10.1145/1028630.1028638
26. Hyman, I.E., Boss, S.M., Wise, B.M., McKenzie, K.E., Caggiano, J.M.: Did you see the unicycling clown? Inattentional blindness while walking and talking on a cell phone. Applied Cognitive Psychology 24(5), 597–607 (2010), doi:10.1002/acp.1638
27. Neider, M.B., Gaspar, J.G., McCarley, J.S., Crowell, J.A., Kaczmarski, H., Kramer, A.F.: Walking and talking: Dual-task effects on street crossing behavior in older adults. Psychology and Aging 26(2), 260–268 (2011), doi:10.1037/a0021566

Data Mining in Promoting Aviation Safety Management

Olli Sjöblom

University of Turku, Turku School of Economics, Finland
oljusj@utu.fi

Abstract. Safety is a key strategic management concern for safety-critical industries and management needs new, more efficient tools and methods for more effective management routines. Effective methods are needed to identify and manage risks in both aviation and other safety-critical industries in order to improve safety. Analysing safety related records and learning from "touch and go" situations is one possible way of preventing hazardous conditions from occurring. The eventuality of an incident or an accident may markedly be reduced if the risks connected to it are efficiently diagnosed. With the aid of this outlook, flight safety has witnessed decades of successful improvement. This paper introduces aviation safety data analysis as an important application area for data mining. In this research text mining was utilised to study 1,240 flight safety reports testing three different systems, applying clustering to find similarities between reports, perhaps containing the indications of a lethal trend, without any presumption of their existence. All the different systems produced coherent results, proving that mining could extract information from unstructured data, which might not be possible with conventional methods.

Keywords: Management, Flight Safety, Data Mining, Text Mining, Analysis Method.

1   Introduction

Organisational decision making, especially in safety-critical systems, such as nuclear power and air traffic, is a complicated task. The top priority for the airline industry has always been the improvement of air safety [1]. Worldwide aviation is growing rapidly. Air traffic has generally been forecasted to grow 5 – 6% annually over the next two decades [2], or even over the next 10 – 15 years, the global air travel will probably double [3]. Consequently, the number of accidents will respectively increase if nothing were done to improve it, which development would, clearly, be unacceptable. This has been foreseen already at the shift of the millennium by the European Commission [4] that expressed the need to explore new and efficient ways in order to improve air safety.

The conventional safety tools and methods based on data collection have reached their peak performance because of their inability to create new knowledge. For further improvements new methods and tools, like data mining, are urgently needed [5]. The need for automated means to process data is increasing rapidly, because the amount of generated and stored unstructured data is increasing rapidly [6]. Usually, data accumulates faster than it can be processed [7]. To extract knowledge from the vast

K. Saranto et al. (Eds.): WIS 2014, CCIS 450, pp. 186–193, 2014.

amount of information and data that is now available, organisations search for the methods to making smarter decisions in order to achieve better results, are increasingly utilising the data assets as well as their advances in computational power with software combined with specialised analysts [8].

2   Management in Safety-Related Context

Kettunen et al. [9] emphasise the managerial challenges in the safety-critical industries, which are typically related to finding a balance between diverging demands and expectations, like economy- and safety-related objects without forgetting the priorities-setting and maintaining focus on these components. The key action is a continuous balancing between taking risks and allocating resources for risk management.

The significant development in database and software technologies, i.e. the warehousing of transaction data, has enabled the organisations to build a foundation for knowledge discovery in databases [10]. The unknown lethal factors brought into daylight could be eliminated; at least a significant part of them and a sufficient safety level could be reached with reduced investment allocation. For air traffic, there is theoretically no upper limit to allocate resources to safety in different forms, such as investing into hi-tech equipment and control systems on a redundant scale, investing in personnel training and developing directives and action rules to add safeguards. The relation between safety and cost efficiency could be illustrated explicitly comparing the costs between comprehensive maintenance programs and maintenance-induced accidents, the benefits that outweigh the accident costs [11].The process for allocating extra resources to special projects might become even more troublesome in case there are interdependencies among the projects [12]. Managing risk and safety has been problematic in air transport: very high levels of safety are too costly – high levels of risk are unacceptable. Therefore, safety reports have been collected through decades to investigate and assess risks and to define risk standards, which are consistent with the value systems of the society [13, 14].

3   Flight Safety

Air traffic is full of incidents and deviations that do not contain any hazard as such, but need to be investigated to find out potential lethal trends. These undesirable, but very minor events are valuable investigation subjects for risk and safety specialists to build an understanding about their causes and to detect unsafe trends. Investigation also reveals whether countermeasures are warranted and how to reduce or eliminate potential accidents [15].The appearance of similar recurring cases (a cluster) may indicate a hazardous trend that should be analysed very carefully to find out whether a real danger exists or not. The possibly existing lethal trends are trying to penetrate through the layers of defences, barriers and safeguards (Figure 1) that, fortunately, usually stop them from proceeding. Because serious incidents and even accidents do happen, it can be presumed that after a certain amount of time they pass all the layers but the last one; then they will pass the last layer as well, which leads to accidents. The latest studies on aviation suggest that text mining can be utilised to detect these trends [16], i.e. the chains of events that lead to accidents if intervention does not occur [17].

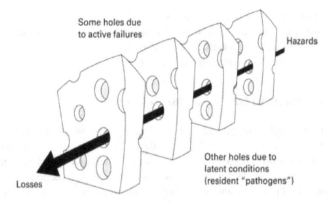

Some holes due
to active failures

Hazards

Other holes due to
latent conditions
(resident "pathogens")

Losses

Successive layers of defences, barriers and safeguards

Fig. 1. The Swiss Cheese model [17, 18]

Searching for similar documents (clustering) is an essential mining function, able to reveal a recurring hazard that might lead to an accident. The clustering results have preliminarily proved its better performance compared with more traditional statistical methods [19]. These, often called "the nuggets of knowledge", are hidden in vast amounts of data and are practically undiscoverable with conventional techniques [20]. Using mining software, knowledge of data is combined by an analyst with advanced machine learning technologies to discover the relationships. Watson [20] also found that with conventional techniques it might take years to find meaningful relationships.

4   The Research Process

Finding trends from narrative data has required significant human involvement. Thus, the analysis process and its possible results rely on the skill, memory and experience of the safety officers [21]. Before data mining systems were developed, there were no tools for analysing textual data with computers. Data mining provides a worthy alternative in the selection of analysis methods in order to illustrate the safety indicators and to reveal undesired trends.

Clustering explores the data set and determines the structure of natural groupings without any preliminary assumptions. It is also directly applicable to Reason's Swiss Cheese model (see Figure 1). The literature in English gives several examples about using clustering in mining flight safety reports. The basic idea of cluster analysis is that all the texts within each cluster have a high similarity in content [22]. Using clustering as method, the main focus is the discovering and identifying of weak signals in the documentation.

The basis of all safety management is the systematic collection and analysis of operational data to identify and quantify potential risks [23]. The research data consisted of the narratives of 1,240 flight safety reports of deviation events from the years 1994-1996 in Finnish, provided by the Finnish Civil Aviation Authority (FCAA). The size of the narratives varied from a few words to a couple of sentences.

A three-year period containing more than 1,000 reports was considered creating a 'critical mass' for producing relevant and reliable mining results. As the material was more than 10 years old, it was guaranteed that the data was already statute-barred and there were no open cases [24].

Three different systems seemed to be appropriate for benchmarking. The author was aware of one prototype (GILTA), one commercial product (TEMIS) with a Finnish module prototype, and one commercial system (PolyVista) with encouraging results mining Spanish, which seemed worth testing in Finnish.

The structure of the research process is presented in Figure 2. The process contains several steps or phases that must be gone through to form knowledge from raw data. To be understandable the information must be presented with reports, graphs or in other suitable forms once found. Both information and knowledge can be refined from collected raw data using conventional tools, but in acquiring further value their limits will be reached. This is clearly seen in the goal of the whole process through which new knowledge can be synthesised from previously held knowledge.

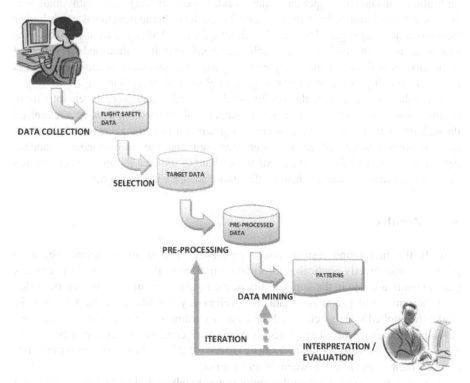

Fig. 2. The structure of the mining process

Mining is an iterative process although it makes no sense to increase the amount of rounds too much. The need for tuning, especially the definition of stop words and synonyms was discovered on the basis of the results of the first mining round. Some pure mistakes, like some common stop words and synonyms forgotten from the list, were noticed. A more significant problem was the appearance of some frequently used "common" words (like 'plane' with its synonyms 'airplane' and 'aircraft') skewing the results. Their role in the data was carefully analysed [25], using a quantitative data analysis application called NVivo to get a deeper analysis.

In case there is a need to change the definitions of the data again, like in this study it appeared to be, the mining process proceeds from the interpretation/evaluation phase back to pre-processing as showed in Figure 2. As there was an obvious need to redefine the stop words and synonyms, the return was necessary. In the picture, a smaller 'loop' also exists, illustrated with a dash line. This path will be used in case there is no need to change the data itself, but for example when a big cluster ought to be re-clustered in order to receive smaller amounts of data to interpret and evaluate.

With structured data, the explanation of a case usually tells the truth to a certain extent, but completed with narrative data it can be close to 100%, at least theoretically. Mining combined with other methods will give significant contributions to the decision processes. Narrative text mining is demanding also because of the multiplicity of languages spoken in the world. Especially languages with small user groups, such as Finnish, have to wait for efficient tools being developed much longer than the major languages. The search technologies are challenged by inflected forms and compounds. In Finnish, for example, the words may have thousands of inflected forms and in addition to that, they can be parts of compounds in almost countless combinations [26]. For search technologies, English is an "easy" language.

The coherent clusters as the results of the second round were taken into more detailed inspection. The progress as the change of distribution can be recognised through the percentage of 'sense making'[1] clusters. Further, the average weight of the most important words of each cluster increased and the correspondent standard deviation diminished significantly. All these changes indicate the movement towards the aimed more homogenous clusters, thus more accurate information.

5   Results

Already the first round results looked promising. The smallest clusters began to produce some directly applicable information indicating that the sizes of the clusters play a significant role in the applicability of the results. This must, however, be scaled with the amount of production data. No preliminary definitions or limitations were made; the applied systems clustered the cases according to their basic determinations. Although the results of all the three systems were coherent, GILTA can be said to have produced the most accurate results clustering 1,240 flight safety reports into 100 clusters, their sizes varied between 58 and 1 report.

PolyVista processed the data determining the number of clusters first to be 6 and then raising it up to 20 in a second step, setting the score 100 for the most content describing word of the cluster and correspondent values to the others. When there were 20 clusters, the smallest of them contained 10 reports and the biggest 232, and in

---

[1] Clusters, from which information can be seen clearly as such.

that case, in eleven of them the scores of the three most important words were more than 50. In the last cluster containing 10 reports, the scores of the 10 most important words were 50 or more, which can be considered a good mining result.

Due to the Finnish module of TEMIS, no pre-processing was necessary. It created 26 clusters leaving out 8 reports as unclassified documents. The size of the clusters varied from 108 to 21 reports. The system was allowed by the operator to create sub clusters in case the size of the cluster exceeds 100 reports and therefore the first cluster was divided into two sub clusters with 58 and 50 documents. After the division, the biggest cluster included 78 reports.

In the target data, about 20 clusters could preliminarily be regarded as containing potentially lethal trends, e.g. a door opening during a flight. Others, like flying into Finnish airspace without air traffic control clearance and illegal smoking on board during the flight as well as gliding-related events can be mentioned. During the second data mining round, refining the definitions after the first one caused a fairly small but remarkable increase in the accuracy of the results. Narratives with a single word were excluded correctly from the clustering as an anomaly by the system. Despite their disparity, the contents of the clusters seemed to be very relevant and were used as material for a more accurate examination by human investigation to find out the existence of the potential hazard in similar recurring events. An additional detail is worth noting - all systems left out almost the same reports.

The testing process proved that data mining might be the only one for uncovering hidden information, supporting the premise that if lethal trends on the whole exist, it reveals important safety information from fast accumulating, vast amounts of data, not accessible with other methods, to be used as an essential factor for strategic safety management. Additionally, because it can find things or traits or tendencies we are not aware of, too, it is an essential tool for being used not only in strategic management but could also be used for allocating resources in safety management.

6   Discussion

Data mining does not give straight answers to the questions, but its role is purely a decision support system although that often provides, indispensable supplementary information for the decision making processes. Thus, the representation of the discovered patterns and the assessing of their value requires that they be consolidated with existing domain knowledge because their value or significance cannot be captured using mining tools. This is why the process requires human participants with vast experience of the subject.

To develop this study further, the other data fields left out in order to simplify the research process, in addition to the narratives only used in this study, might be taken into consideration in the data mining process – in order to gain more accurate results by increasing the coverage of the process.

Despite the fact that data mining has been available as an applicable method already since the 1960s, it is not as widely used as could be expected. Text mining was enabled later than the mining of numerical data being, however, on hand a couple of decades. There are, no doubt several explanations for this. One of the most significant of them, concerning especially text mining, is that these tools are mostly language dependent, a fact which does not favour small language groups like Finnish that also happens to be a substantially complicated language from this point of view, notably requiring resources in order to develop functional tools. Another reason might be that the mining tools have not been as simple to use as the tools the authorities and other actors have been used to. In addition to this, successful data mining does not happen as facilely as the use of, for instance, Excel spreadsheet tools and functions but, as described more minutely before, requires a process including several steps or phases.

Although the accident ratio has diminished since the beginning of the 1960s steadily as well among general aviation as gliders and motor gliders, and there was even a period between 1996 and 2006 without lethal accidents among gliding and motor gliding, the situation is not satisfactory. The lethal accidents have returned to the aviation field having survived ten years totally without and the number of the accidents among ultralight aviation has increased remarkably. This for one's part is the reason why the Finnish Transport Minister ordered in April a wide mapping about the risks among leisure aviation to be made, to be completed at the end of September 2014. This unfavourable development evidently emphasises the significance of the need for sophisticated safety analysis methods and their development.

As mentioned, this study was made with no presumption of the existence of potential lethal trends. In case it is already known what will be looked for, business intelligence (BI) methods could be applicable. Although these systems allow the databases to be queried using numerous keywords to search for known cases of a certain type or their combinations, the results received from them are simpler to interpret compared with those of the mining tools. Additionally, business intelligence can also well be combined with data mining. In case through mining process something worth examining more minutely were found, this data could act as a query basis for BI tools that could pick up more accurate information on the type of cases found. When doing this way, thus applying BI tools in the second phase of the process, additional hazardous factors might be discovered in the data, guiding the safety specialist to those patterns that show where a potential accident could occur.

References

1. Liou, J.J.H., Yen, L., Tzeng, G.-H.: Building an effective safety management system for airlines. Journal of Air Transport Management 14(1), 20–26 (2008)
2. Netjasov, F., Janic, M.: A review of research on risk and safety modelling in civil aviation. Journal of Air Transport Management 14(4), 213–220 (2008)
3. Global Airline Industry Program. Analysis: The Airline Industry. Global Airline Industry Program [WWW-page] (2008), http://web.mit.edu/airlines/analysis/analysis_airline_industry.html [cited 2011 9.5.]
4. European Commission, Proposal for a Directive of the European Parliament and of the Council on occurrence reporting in civil aviation, Commission of the European Communities, Editor 2000, Brussels (2000)
5. Evans, B., Glendon, A.I., Creed, P.A.: Development and initial validation of an Aviation Safety Climate Scale. Journal of Safety Research 38(6), 675–682 (2007)

6. Delen, D., Crossland, M.D.: Seeding the survey and analysis of research literature with text mining. Expert Systems with Applications: An International Journal 34(3), 1707–1720 (2008)
7. Wang, X., Huang, S., Cao, L., Shi, D., Shu, P.: LSSVM with Fuzzy Pre-processing Model Based Aero Engine Data Mining Technology. In: Alhajj, R., Gao, H., Li, X., Li, J., Zaïane, O.R. (eds.) ADMA 2007. LNCS (LNAI), vol. 4632, pp. 100–109. Springer, Heidelberg (2007)
8. Cleary, D.: Predictive Analytics in the Public Sector: Using Data Mining to Assist Better Target Selection for Audit. Electronic Journal of e-Government 9(2) (2011)
9. Kettunen, J., Reiman, T., Wahlström, B.: Safety management challenges and tensions in the European nuclear power industry. Scandinavian Journal of Management 23(4), 424–444 (2007)
10. Blake, M.B., et al.: A Component-Based Data Management and Knowledge Discovery Framework for Aviation Studies. International Journal of Technology and Web Engineering 1(1) (2006)
11. Castro, R.: A Holistic Approach to Aviation Safety. In: Flight Safety Digest, pp. 1–12 (1988)
12. Kirkwood, C.W.: Strategic Decision Making. Wadsworth Publishing Company, Belmont (1997)
13. Janic, M.: An assessment of risk and safety in civil aviation. Journal of Air Transport Management 6(1), 43–50 (2000)
14. Sage, A.P., White, E.B.: Methodologies for Risk and Hazard Assessment: A Survey and Status Report. IEEE Transaction on Systems, Man, and Cybernetics SMC-10(8), 425–446 (1980)
15. Kirwan, B.: Incident reduction and risk migration. Safety Science 49(1), 11–20 (2011)
16. Sjöblom, O.: Data Mining in Aviation Safety. In: 5th International Workshop on Security. Information Processing Society of Japan, Kobe (2010)
17. Reason, J.T.: Human error: models and management. British Medical Journal 320(7237), 768–770 (2000)
18. Reason, J.T.: Managing the Risks of Organizational Accidents, 252p. Ashgate Publishing Limited, Aldershot (1997)
19. Saracoglu, R., Tütünkü, K., Allahverdi, N.: A new approach on search for similar documents with multiple categories using fuzzy clustering. Expert Systems with Applications: An International Journal 34(4), 2545–2554 (2008)
20. Watson, R.T.: Data Management: Databases and Organizations, 2nd edn. John Wiley & Sons (1999)
21. Nazeri, Z.: Application of Aviation Safety Data Mining Workbench at American Airlines. Proof-of-Concept Demonstration of Data and Text Mining, Center for Advanced Aviation Systems Development, MITRE Corporation Inc., McLean, Virginia, US (2003)
22. Rosell, M.: Text Clustering Exploration. Swedish Text Representation and Clustering Results Unraveled. School of Computer Science and Communication, p. 71. Kungliga Tekniska Högskolan, Stockholm (2009)
23. GAIN Working Group B, Role of Analytical Tools in Airline Flight Safety Management Systems, W.G.B.A.M.a. Tools, Global Aviation Information Network (2004)
24. Sjöblom, O., Suomi, R.: Data Mining in Aviation Safety Data Analysis. In: Rahman, H. (ed.) Social and Political Implications of Data Mining: Knowledge Management in E-Government, p. 349. Information Science Reference, Hershey (2009)
25. Lindén, K.: Word Sense Discovery and Disambiguation. In: General Linguistics, p. 191. University of Helsinki, Helsinki (2005)
26. Karlsson, F.: Yleinen kielitiede. Yliopistopaino, Helsinki (1994)

Safe Community Designation as Quality Assurance in Local Security Planning

Brita Somerkoski and Pirjo Lillsunde

National Institute for Health and Welfare, Helsinki, Finland
{brita.somerkoski,pirjo.lillsunde}@thl.fi

Abstract. This study is written to encourage the Finnish municipalities to apply the Safe Community designation and to improve the implementation of national programmes on a local level. The existing sustainable safety work in Finnish communities was utilized for writing the guidelines. The infrastructure for fulfilling the requirements for Safe Community designation was appropriate in the Finnish municipalities because of the national programmes and the local safety plans. The third Internal Security Programme "A Safer tomorrow" (2012) and the fifth National Target and Action Programme for the Prevention of Home and Leisure injuries 2014–2020 both focus on how to solve the everyday problems of safety and security as well as prevention of injuries. The objectives and measures outlined in these programmes are encouraged to be taken into account in local security plans. The majority of Finns (95%) live in a municipality that has a local security plan. These plans include leadership in sustainable multi-sector safety collaboration, targets and measures that improve safety and reduce injuries of vulnerable groups, both genders at all ages in any environment. Local plans also include preparedness for disasters. Although the national safety and security planning infrastructure already exists in Finland, the benefit of the Safe Community designation is that the implementation of the measures are audited and controlled in the certification process. The national strategy and the local security and safety planning can be combined with the Safe Community designation requirements. Obtaining a designation as a Safe Community can be seen also as quality assurance of the safety management system in Finland.

Keywords: safety, security, quality assurance, Safe Community designation, local security planning.

1 Accidents, Injuries, Alcohol and Social Exclusion as a Major Risks for Internal Safety

Finland is considered as a relatively safe country, especially by international comparison. The key elements are well-being of citizens, strong social cohesion, a sense of community or economic stability.[1-2] On the other hand injuries and accidents are a major public health and safety problem since annually about 2,800 Finns die accidentally.[3] Statistically, home and leisure accidents are seen to be the

K. Saranto et al. (Eds.): WIS 2014, CCIS 450, pp. 194–202, 2014.
© Springer International Publishing Switzerland 2014

greatest risk to human health and life. Also alcohol consumption plays an essential role; for instance one third of the fatal accidents occur under the influence of alcohol. In addition the number of fire deaths in relation to the total population is high in Finland compared to the corresponding figure in the other Western countries. [4] Other key challenges in the Finnish society are social exclusion, everyday security challenges, business security and threat of violence and other crime. [5]

Later on in this study we will introduce the fifth Finnish Target program for the Prevention of Home and Leisure Accident Injuries 2014–2020. When preparing the new target programme, same kind of risk factors were found: high level of alcohol consumption and binge drinking; increased alcohol consumption by older persons; increasing health inequalities; resources available for preventive work; increased workloads and rushing at work; higher number of older persons; scaling down of institutional care and living in one's own home for as long as possible; growing number of people who live alone; more technology in homes; engaging in Do-It-Yourself activities; growing number of people who lack everyday skills; rising trend of risk-taking and thrill-seeking; taking less exercise; increasing multiculturalism; increasing tourism and independent travel in particular; different level of safety awareness of foreign tourists in Finland; working less and having more free time. The purpose of the strategic safety and security programs is to enhance the safety culture on both national and local level. As a result of the effective prevention work the number of traffic and occupational accident injuries has decreased in the long term. Also there are some signs of the improved security level in society for instance the reduced number of accident injuries to children and also fires in residential houses. [6]

Preventing injuries can be described as working with "non-events" The domains are also the economic benefit and evidence-based quality in practice. Community-wide interventions have been studied by Popay and Young (1993). The researchers found out that there are two dominant dimensions: firstly the health planning approach which emphasizes behavior change and safety education and secondly the community participation approach, which points out changing the environment. [7]

Welander, Svanström and Ekman state that the idea behind Safe Community to prevent injuries in all areas, considering all ages, environments and situations, reaching the most vulnerable groups and involving not just the governmental but also the non-governmental community sections. This statement is based on the WHO manifesto for safe communities and WHO Health for All strategy [and is a key element of the International Safe Community movement [8, see also 23-24].

Here we can say that the concept of prevention as it relates to health has shifted from *protection* to *intervention* or *prevention* with a broad safety context. [9]

2   The Aims and Conceptual Remarks

The aim of this study was to create guidelines in order to encourage the Finnish municipalities to apply the Safe Community designation and to improve the implementation of national programmes on local level.

The concept of safety has been classified from many points of view. It is said that to attain an optimum level of safety, it requires individuals, communities and governments involvement. Safety can be described as a climate of social cohesion, peace and equity. There should be methods for preventing injuries and accidents, the respects of the value. Also in some studies safety is classified as objective assessed by environmental parameters and secondly subjective, feeling of safety. Some researchers have also started to talk about safety identity. [10, see also 11]. Researchers point out that safety is a state in which hazards and conditions leading to physical injury, psychological or material harm are controlled to preserve the well-being of individuals. On the other hand it is not possibly to define safety in absolute terms, since it is a dynamic state and can also be described from subjective or objective point of view. [11]

According to WHO, safety is a condition where factors that are a threat to a society are managed in such a way that the citizens have the feeling of well-being and prosperity. Safety can also be seen as a condition where one is at the highest possible state of being free from danger. In English, the concept 'safety' has two separate meanings. Safety implies a human-aspect, freedom from accident or injury, while security implies deliberateness or intent, as well as protection from dangers. The word safety is frequently used in connection with accidents and the word security is used refer to protection against undesirable threats. In Finnish, the concept 'turvallisuus' covers both meanings. [12]

The concept of resilience is closely linked to safety. Resilience is the conscious and proactive ability to adapt and function in circumstances of disruption and to recover and to develop afterwards. It can be seen as the ability to cope with unforeseen threats and disruptions. Resilience is also the ability to recover from adversities and learn from them. [13]

Safety promotion consists of measures aimed at maintaining and achieving the ideal conditions by means of fostering interaction and co-operation. Everyone should strive to achieve shared safety objectives. Also legislation requires actions that promote safety.

The feeling of safety is made up of a number of factors, such as health, the functionality of social safety nets and a living environment that is considered safe. The service offering has been fragmented across many different operators, for example, authorities, organizations and the private sector. Promotion of the feeling of safety is not the most important priority of any actor, however. The feeling of insecurity involves the vulnerability of an individual. Vulnerability is seen to be linked to various factors, such as gender, age, ethnicity and victim experiences. Vulnerability affects ability to cope and act in various situations. Insecurity, extra vigilance and psychological stress can manifest as continuous anxiety, fear and even as a panic disorder. [14-20]

3   Preventive Acts on National Level

The objective of the Internal Security Government Programme is to make Finland the safest country in Europe – one in which people feel that they live in a fair and equal society regardless of how they identify themselves.

The key content of the Internal Security Programme consists of prevention of security problems that are the most important from the perspective of everyday life. For instance the program states that the main domestic challenges are the prevention of social exclusion and social polarization. The Internal Security Government Programme is inter sectoral and was prepared on the basis of the comprehensive concept of security. The programme consists of the following subject areas: improving everyday safety and security in the home; improving the safety of young people; combating safety and security threats caused by alcohol and other substances; preventing violent extremism; further developing support services for crime victims; improving the safety of the elderly and improving business security. The programme includes 64 measures to improve safety and security. Each measure designates a responsible party and includes a timetable for implementation. The programme was prepared in broad-based cooperation with the authorities, both governmental and non-governmental organizations and the business sector. [21]

Ministry of Social Affairs and Health launched last year The Target Programme for Prevention of Home and Leisure Accident Injuries 2014–2020. In this programme key aspects of preventing home and leisure accidents are stressing the citizens' personal responsibility and increasing awareness, building safe housing and living environments and supervising product safety. Also in this program it is stated that the shared efforts of all professionals and the voluntary sector will be needed to increase the awareness and inclusion of citizens. Especially personal safety identity is emphasized: the basic point of view is that we can only be personally responsible for our safety when we have the required knowledge and skills. Various organizations must also assume responsibility for the safety. The packages of measures and actions in the program are: improving the safety culture and strengthening safety work; preventing accident injuries caused by the use of medicines, alcohol and drugs; promoting equality and improving the safety of vulnerable groups in particular, improving the safety of the environment and products and preventing injuries caused by falling and tumbling. [21-23]

Based on the ongoing programs it seems very clear what the basic risk factors are considering the safety and security issues in Finnish communities. Instead more practical measures should be introduced to reduce the amount of home and leisure accident injuries and fatals. The international Safe Communities movement can be seen as such an act: a quality assurance for local level safety and security measures. In this study the Finnish communities are encouraged to join to the Safe Community network to gain the quality assurance for the local safety promotion measures.

4   Preventive Acts on Local Level

Like the Internal Security Program, the Local Safety planning is based on the comprehensive concept of security, according to which everyday crimes and disturbances are prevented in cooperation with local communities in Finland. Local security plans cover not only protection against crime but also other, broad dimensions of safety, such as fire safety, traffic safety, security under emergency conditions, and accidents. Local security planning aims to prevent and stop accidents, crime and disturbances, and to reinforce people's sense of security. One of the aims is to better inform residents of how their security will be improved. Municipalities can make a security plan on their own or in partnership with several other municipalities with a cross-sectorial approach. It is possible to draw up a regional level security plan as well. Local security planning is led by a management group: municipal leaders will work together with police and rescue services. [21-24]

To support the local security planning The Association of Finnish Local and Regional Authorities launched few years ago an Electronic welfare report. This database is a tool that provides information on the different dimensions of welfare: quality of life, mental well-being, work ability and functional capacity, participation and influence, security, education and work, equity and justice, housing and the environment, livelihood and services for residents. Local authorities may use this information in their operational and financial planning. A table is drawn up which shows the objectives, measures, the parties responsible, resources and evaluation indicators for the different administrative branches in terms of promoting resident welfare. [25] Electronic welfare report lays the foundation for local strategy work and for operational and financial planning. So far over 70 % of Finnish local authorities have credentials to the electronic welfare report tool. The advantage of this database is that the welfare perspective is included in local strategic management and on the other hand all administrative branches take more responsibility for the welfare of residents.

5   Safe Community Designation as Quality Assurance in Local Security Planning

The World Health Organization (WHO) Manifesto for Safe Communities states that "all human beings have an equal right to health and safety. The emphasis of the Safe Communities approach is on collaboration, partnership and community capacity building to reduce the incidence of injury and promote injury reducing behaviours. The WHO premise "All human beings have an equal right to health and safety" is a fundamental aspect of the WHO Health for All strategy. [26-27]

A basic guideline for Safe Communities movement is" Community interventions to reduce accidents and injuries occur alongside a number of other initiatives with the same goal. These are important because they add a new dimension to the fight against injury in both developed and developing countries. They will not replace other initiatives but will complement them, creating a new way of tackling the pattern of accidents and injuries and dealing with problems which have proved insoluble using traditional top-down approaches by utilizing the strengths of the people to bring about necessary changes in awareness, behavior and environment." [27]

Health and safety promotion often involve complex activities and multiple approaches. The measures taken should be sustainable and also policy-makers as well as citizens should be able to participate in the activity. To evaluate effectiveness of prevention strategies means, that the community should identificate the effective strategies to reduce morbidity and mortality. [28-29]

An evaluation study in Sweden points out that the fundamental features of community based injury prevention is its shift away from focusing on individual responsibility towards more communitywide approach so that everyone in a community is involved in safety promotion. [30]

To be a member of the International Safe Community Network a community makes an application. As a part of the designation process the community is then audited by a certifier accredited by WHO Collaborating Centre on Community Safety Promotion. The certifier reviews the work in the community and the following seven indicators must be fulfilled. These are :"An infrastructure based on partnership and collaborations, governed by a cross-sector group that is responsible for safety promotion in their community; long-term, sustainable programs covering genders and all ages, environments, and programs that promote safety for vulnerable groups; programs that are based on the available evidence; programs that document the frequency and causes of injuries; evaluation measures to assess their programs, processes and the effects of change; on-going participation in national and international Safe Communities networks. The quality assurance is done by the certifier, who makes a site visit. [31]

6   Discussion

The majority of Finns (95%) live in a municipality that has a local security plan. The plans include leadership in sustainable multi-sector safety collaboration, targets and measures that improve safety and reduce injuries of vulnerable groups, both genders at all ages in any environment. Local plans also include preparedness for disasters. Throughout Finland the local security plans are prepared using national guidelines.

Safe Community is an international movement of the World Health Organization (WHO) that designates that a community has met international requirements for safety and security. With this paper we propose that these Finnish municipalities that have local security plans, could also qualify for the designation as a Safe Community. The third Internal Security Programme "A Safer tomorrow" (2012) and the fifth National Target and Action Programme for the Prevention of Home and Leisure Accident Injuries 2014-2020 both focus on how to solve the everyday problems of safety and security as well as prevention of injuries. The objectives and measures outlined in these programmes are encouraged to be taken into account in local security plans. The infrastructure for fulfilling the requirements for Safe Community designation is appropriate in the Finnish municipalities because of the national programmes and the local safety plans. The national strategy and the local security and safety planning can be combined with the Safe Community designation requirements. It is possible to utilize the existing sustainable safety work in Finnish communities when fulfilling the Safe Community designation guidelines (fig 1.).

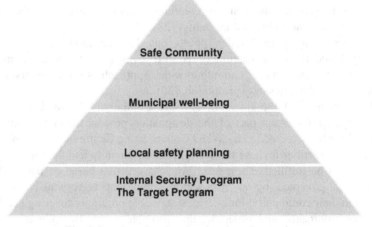

Fig. 1. Local, regional and national work on safety

The guidelines [32] give answers on how to fulfill the designation requirements in national settings. Although the national safety and security planning infrastructure already exists in Finland, the benefit of the Safe Community designation is that the implementation of the measures are audited and controlled in the certification process. The Safe Community designation can be seen as quality assurance of the safety management system.

Safety planning is an integral part of normal work when it is promoted by legislation as well as the actions of the authorities, municipal administrative sectors, communities, businesses, organisations, associations and citizens. Local work on safety and accident prevention involves several sectors and organizations. The improvement of safety is thus a common cause. Safety problems can be solved by several simultaneous actions that have similar goals. The development of the safety culture will happen when practical measures are taken in Finnish communities.

References

1. http://www.intermin.fi/download/37324_STOeng_64s_web_eng.pdf ?e7e9b7241c05d188 (May 3, 2014)
2. http://www.intermin.fi/download/37324_STOeng_64s_web_eng.pdf (May 3, 2014)
3. http://www.intermin.fi/en/security/fire_safety_and_accident_ prevention (May 3, 2014)

4. http://www.intermin.fi/en/security/fire_safety_and_accident_prevention (May 3, 2014)
5. http://www.intermin.fi/download/37324_STOeng_64s_web_eng.pdf ?e7e9b7241c05d188 (May 3, 2014)
6. Target program for the Prevention of Home and Leisure Accident Injuries 2014–2020
7. Welander, G., Svanström, L., Ekman, R.: Safety promotion –an Introduction, 2nd Revised edn. Kristianstads Boktryckeri, Kristianstad (2004)
8. Welander, G., Svanström, L., Ekman, R.: Safety promotion –an Introduction, 2nd Revised edn. Kristianstads Boktryckeri, Kristianstad (2004)
9. Andersson, R., Menckel, E.: On the prevention of accidents and injuries. A comparative analysis of conceptual frameworks. Accident Analysis and Prevention 27(6), 757–768 (1995)
10. Maurice, P., Lavoi, M., Charron, R., Chapdelaine, A., Bonneau, H., Svanström, L., Laflamme, L., Anderson, R., Romer, C.: Safety and Safety Promotion: Conceptual and Operational Aspects (1998)
11. Somerkoski, B.: Turvallisuus yläkoululaisen kokemana. Teoksessa J. Mäkinen (toim.) Asevelvollisuuden tulevaisuus. Maanpuolustuskorkeakoulu. Johtamisen ja sotilaspedagogiikan laitos. Julkaisusarja 2/2013. Artikkelikokoelmat (9). 133–143 (2013)
12. Welander, G., Svanström, L., Ekman, R.: Safety promotion –an Introduction, 2nd Revised edn. Kristianstads Boktryckeri, Kristianstad (2004)
13. Hanén, T.: Turvallisuusjohtaminen ja rajavartiolaitos: yksittäisten onnettomuuksien tutkinnasta strategisten häiriöiden hallintaan. Maanpuolustuskorkeakoulu. Johtamisen laitos, julkaisusarja 1, tutkimuksia (30), 20–25 (2005)
14. http://www.julkari.fi/bitstream/handle/10024/102923/eskola.pdf ?sequence=1 (April 15, 2014)
15. Kokonaisturvallisuuden ja varautumisen sanasto, draft (in publicationprocess October 30, 2013)
16. Somerkoski, B., Lillsunde, P., Impinen, A.: A safer municipality–The Safe Community operating model as a support for local safety planning. Yliopistopaino. Juvenes Print (2014)
17. Suominen, P., Hyvärinen, S.: Palovaroitin, parisuhde vai pamppu? Selvitys vammaisten ihmisten ja mielenterveyskuntoutujien turvallisuuden kokemiseen vaikuttavista tekijöistä. ASPA-julkaisuja 02/2013. Eräsalon Kirjapaino, Tampere (2013)
18. Waitinen, M.: Turvallinen koulu? Helsinkiläisten peruskoulujen turvallisuuskulttuurista ja siihen vaikuttavista tekijöistä. Väitöstutkimus. Helsingin yliopiston tutkimuksia 334. Unigrafia, Helsinki (2011)
19. Zohar, D.: Thirty years of safety climate research: reflections and future directions. Accident Analysis and Prevention 42, 1517–1522 (2010)
20. Ruuhilehto, K., Vilppola, K.: Turvallisuuskulttuuri ja turvallisuuden edistäminen yrityksessä. TUKES-julkaisu 1/2000. Turvatekniikan keskus, Helsinki (2000)
21. http://www.intermin.fi/en/security/internal_security_programme (May 13, 2014)
22. Lillsunde, P., Langel, K., Blencowe T., Kivioja, A., Karjalainen, K., Lehtonen, L.: Psykoaktiiviset aineet ja onnettomuusriski tieliikenteessä. Duodecim 128, 53–62 (2012), DRUID Deliverable D 2.3.5, http://www.druid-project.eu (updated November 28, 2011)
23. Koti- ja vapaa-ajan tapa-turmien ehkäisyn kansallinen tavoiteohjelma vuosille 2014–2020 [webdocument]. Sosiaali- ja terveysministeriö julkaisuja 2013:16, http://www.stm.fi/julkaisut

24. http://www.intermin.fi/internalsecurity/local_security_plann
    ing (May 13, 2014)
25. http://www.hyvinvointikertomus.fi
26. Spinks, A., Turner, C., Nixon, J., McClure, R.J.: The WHO Safe Communities model for
    the prevention of injury in whole population (review). The Cochraine Collaboration. John
    Wiley & Sons (2009)
27. World Health Organisation, WHO. Manifesto for Safe Communities. Safety – A Universal
    Concern and Responsibility for all. Adopted in Srockholm, September 20th 1989, at the
    first World Conference on Accident and Injury Prevention. Geneva (1989), http://
    www.ki.se/csp/pdf/Manifesto.pdf
28. Moller, J., Sanstrom, L., Havanonda, S., Romer, C.: Guidelines for Safe Communities
    WHO Collaborating Centre on Community Safety promotion. Karolinska Institutet,
    Department of Social Medicine, Kronan Health Center, Sundbyberg, Sweden (1989)
29. Welander, G., Svanström, L., Ekman, R.: Safety promotion –an Introduction. 2nd Revised
    edn., pp. 125–130. Kristianstads Boktryckeri, Kristianstad (2004)
30. Lindqvist, K., Timpka, L., Risto, O.: Evaluation of a child safety program based on the
    WHO Safe Community model. Injury Prevention (8), 23–26 (2002)
31. http://www.ki.se/ (May 5, 2014)
32. Somerkoski, B., Lillsunde, P., Impinen, A.: A safer municipality–The Safe Community
    operating model as a support for local safety planning. Yliopistopaino. Juvenes Print
    (2014)

Patients Using Open-Source Disease Control Software Developed by Other Patients

Jose Teixeira

University of Turku, Turku, Finland
jose.teixeira@utu.fi

Abstract. Healthcare information systems are traditionally developed within the R&D labs of medical instrumentation providers, software houses, technology consultancy firms, medical faculties and hospitals. Professionals with either medical or IT backgrounds are the perpetual analysts and developers of most health-care information systems on the market. However, we tackle an exceptional variance where patients are themselves creators of their own health-care information systems.

This user-innovation phenomenon was already addressed in academia but mostly by looking at the systems per se or their development. In this paper, we turn to the users by exploring the consumer behaviors of patients using such patient-innovated systems, i.e. we explore the consumer behaviors of patients using open-source disease control software developed by other patients.

In a Netnographic approach we screened the product pages and relevant Internet forums around three open-source projects providing disease control software: GNU Gluco Control, MySHI (My Self Health Information) and PumpDown-load. A rich set of qualitative data was collected from Internet sites and analyzed with the Grounded Theory method. We developed a theory that unveil two key motivations for the use of disease control software: the patients desire for a more active role in managing their diseases, and the patients annoyance with defective by design vendor lock-in mechanisms from the most common products.

Our contributions increase the understanding on the symbolism, meaning, and consumption patterns of this niche consumer group by screening publicly avail-able data on the Internet, with potential implications to the body of theoretical knowledge in healthcare information systems, chronic care management and practitioners within the industry of disease control.

Keywords: Keyworks: E-Health, Chronic Care, Patient Empowerment, Open-source, User innovation.

1   Introduction

Healthcare information systems are traditionally developed within the R&D labs of medical instrumentation providers, software houses, technology consultancy firms, medical faculties and hospitals. Professionals with either medical or IT backgrounds are the perpetual analysts and developers of most health-care information systems on the market. However, we are aware of a new phenomenon where patients are themselves creators of their own health-care information systems.

K. Saranto et al. (Eds.): WIS 2014, CCIS 450, pp. 203–210, 2014.
© Springer International Publishing Switzerland 2014

This user-innovation phenomenon was already addressed by academia [1], [2] but mostly by looking at the systems per se or their development. In this paper, we turn to the users by exploring the consumer behaviors of patients using such patient-innovated systems, i.e. we explore the consumer behaviors of patients using open-source disease control software developed by other patients.

Taking a Netnographic approach, a novel approach with roots in cultural anthropology, we screened the product pages and relevant Internet forums around three open-source projects providing disease control software: GNU Gluco Control, MySHI (My Self Health Information) and PumpDownload. A rich set of qualitative data was collected from Internet sites, capturing the   users backgrounds, lifestyles, medical conditions and their reasons behind the usage of alternative open-source disease control software.

The Grounded Theory method was employed to analyze the data and the method theory-building functions used to propose a theory emphasizing two key motivations for the use of disease control software: the patients desire for a more active role in managing their diseases, and the patients annoyance with defective by design vendor lock-in mechanisms within the traditional and marked dominant disease-control products.

Our contributions increase the understanding on the symbolism, meaning, and consumption patterns of this niche consumer group by screening publicly available data on the Internet, with implication to the body of theoretical knowledge in healthcare information systems, chronic care management and practitioners within the industry of disease control.

In the following section we introduce our methodological approach unveiling the details of how we collected the data from the Internet and analyzed it in accordance to established guidelines on Netnography and Grounded theory. Presented our findings, we discuss its implications for scholars and practitioners and conclude with future oriented remarks.

2   Method

2.1   Data-Collection

The research questions are how do patients use open-source disease control soft-ware developed by other patients and why. Given the novelty of the phenomenon being study, and given the nature of the research questions, adopted Netnography. Netnography, also know as ethnography on the Internet, is new qualitative research method that adapts ethnographic research techniques to the study of cultures and communities emerging through computer-mediated communication [3], [4].With roots on the Marketing discipline, Netnography is now recognized as a methodological innovation with crescent legitimacy across disciplines, including Information Systems [5].

The Interned was our medium, and for addressing the research questions we screened and retrieved product pages and relevant Internet forums around three open-source projects providing disease control software. The retrieved data was natural occurring and neither provoked or influenced by the researchers. The researcher tried to learn as much as possible about the products, forums, groups and the individuals we seek to understand without interacting directly with them.

From earlier research [1], [2], we have identified GNU Gluco Control, MySHI (My Self Health Information) and PumpDownload as open-source disease control software developed by patient to patient. In a first phase, and given the software products, we screened their associated Internet pages maintained by the software developers. In a second phase, we searched for complementary electronic bulletin boards, newsgroups, usegroups, usenet groups, webpages, online forums, blogs, indexed e-mail mailing lists, etc where consumers/patients meet to discuss their use of such software products. We limited our research to Internet pages written in the English and Spanish language.

The following Table 1, lists the retrieved Internet sites that we subjected to our analysis. The first three sites are product web-pages maintained by software developers that in our case are also chronic patients.   The remaining sites are patient virtual communities, i.e. Internet sites that gather together chronic patients with a particular chronic condition such as diabetes. Patients use such virtual communities to seek and provide medical advise, look for peer support, review new products and services, discuss treatment approaches, advertise products and services, etc.

Table 1. Retrieved Internet sites

Internet page	Description	Link
GNU Gluco Control	Product webpage	http://ggc.sourceforge.net
My Self Health Information	Product webpage	http://sourceforge.net/projects/myshi
Pump Download	Product webpage	http://pumpdownload.sourceforge.net
Tudiabetes	Patients virtual community (International)	http://www.tudiabetes.org
Juvenation	Patients virtual community (International)	http://juvenation.org
Diabetesdaily	Patients virtual community (USA)	http://www.diabetesdaily.com
Diabetessupport	Patients virtual community (UK)	http://www.diabetessupport.co.uk
Shotuporputup	Patients virtual community (UK)	http://www.shootuporputup.co.uk
Midiabetes	Patients virtual community (Chile)	http://midiabetes.cl
Wordgnat blog	Patients virtual community (Canada)	http://worldgnat.wordpress.com

The authors neither provoked the research data neither influenced the research sites. In other words, the authors did not participate in the forums, but just read them. Moreover, the author did not use any of the chat-room features available in some of the virtual communities. Those facts have positive implication to the validity of this research as pointed out by [6]. The selection of the research sites,   captured in Table 1, took in consideration the nature of the research question and the segment, topic and group   being studied, i.e. chronic patients using open-source software developed by other chronic patients. All towards purposing sampling [1], [2] and in consideration with the established research sites evaluation principles as proposed in [3].

2.2   Data-Analysis

As "netnographers", the authors benefit from the nearly automatic transcription of downloaded Internet sites using a simple Internet web-browser. Give the very special nature of the research topic, the authors did not suffer from information overload that many "netbgraphers" experience. As we addressed an emergent and novel phenomena, the size of the data was manageable for the data analysis, without need for sampling or filtering.

Before applying more sophisticated qualitative data-analysis techniques,   the authors performed a first pass or "grand tour" interpretation of the collected textual data. Going back and forward with the data allowed the researchers to be more "familiar" with the data. Some initial categorizations were performed for organizing information regarding how patients use this kind software and why patients use it. Most of the collected patients/consumers collected textual data revels how they use those systems, but patients/consumers also reveal the motives and pre-conditions of their use of such software. On the esprit of grounded theorizing [6] the initial categorizations were open and did not seek a fit towards the established theoretical body of the knowledge[7], [8].

Given the manageable size of the semi-automatically collected data, we screened all the data as long as new insights on important topical areas were popping up [3], [7]. Regarding the nature of the screened Internet forums,   the natural occurring sentences had sufficient descriptive richness depth for revealing the behaviors of patients/consumers using open-source software open-source disease control software developed by other patients. Many reflective textual field-notes were taken by the researchers white reading back and forward the retrieved textual data.   Those field-notes were not subjected to coding for the theory-building phase, but they are a recommendable procedure [3] that increased our understanding of the data.

By adopting netnography over the traditional ethnography we lost track of the valuable personal emotions that could be revealed by taking a more face-to-face on-site research approach. But on other hand, we could expand our data-collection much faster by semi-automatic manners. Data-collection and data-analysis were not made in a   sequential   manner,   a   very   common   execution   strategy   in   the   traditional ethnographic studies. In this study, data-collecting was expanded   several times during the data-analysis, as data linked us to new Internet sites that worthed being collected and analyzed.   Given the manageable number of Internet sites, their content and messages, we did not use any qualitative software packages such as NVivo and Atlas.ti . Coding, linking, content analysis and theory building were performed with pen, paper, pencil and paper basket, the last as deposit of several coding and theory-building efforts that led to not so interesting findings.

In consistency with established guidelines on how to conduct behavioral consumer research [3], [9], [10] we searched for a rich, penetrating metaphoric and symbolic interpretation over meticulous classification. In other words, we were more interested in understanding the how and why of this particular phenomenon that on "putting on boxes" the studied consumers. Our approach relying on netnography [3]–[5] is better suited to the classical approach of studying the act [6] in which the ultimate unit of analysis is not the person, but the behavior or the act. In this last point our "netnographic" approach diverges from the established ethnographic approaches [2], [7]–[9] as the research data occur through computer- mediation, are publicly available, generated in written text form, and the identities of the informers being studied are much more difficult to discern [4].

Given the nature of Internet forums, some textual data was marked as "to not consider". By common sense manners we did no consider for our coding analysis textual sentences revealing extremism, intense hate expressions, intense non-related publicity and apparently off-topic useless talk. We wanted to focus our analysis towards the central topic of the use of open-source disease control software developed by other patients. The employed the Glasserian Grounded Theory [10]–[12] as the core method of data-analysis and technique for theoretical building. We pursued ontological and epistemological consistency with established works in Information Systems Research [13]. The employed the Glasserian aproach to Grounded Theory is already established in Information Systems Research as evidenced in [13]–[16].

Within an qualitative interpretative paradigm and with open and non-strict initial research questions , we enter within the "Glaserian" coding phases employing open-coding, theoretical-coding and theoretical memos. We could identify two kind of main actors within the semi-automatically retrieved textual data: the developers of such software and chronic-patients that are potential-users of such software. In this special case, the software developers are themselves also potential-users of such software. However we could notice that most potential-users do not have the technological and engineering skills required to develop software.

2.3   Theory Building

After coding line by line, sentence by sentence and paragraph by paragraph , in time-consuming multiple interactions, until reaching theoretical saturation. We finally proposed the following categories and selective codes that drove the inductive and deductive theory building process of grounded theorizing as outlined in Table 2.

Table 2. Theorizing selective codes and categories

Selective codes	Category
Call for the use of own mobile devices Call for involvement on the choice of medical device Call for access to own patient data Call for the control of own patient data Call for self-care Call for proximity care Call for multi-geographical care	More active role on the management of their own chronic disease.
Loss of patient data upon device change. Lack of chronic-care data standards Encrypted patient data. Dissatisfaction with the lack of export features. Dissatisfaction with lack of device-change functionalities.	Perceived defective by design vendor lock-in mechanisms within the established medical products.

After multiple iterations where we sorted and grouped open-codes into selective codes, the author then proceeded to theoretical coding, where the relationships between selective codes were considered. From the emerging categories we propose the following two theoretical proposition for increasing our understanding on how and why patients use open-source disease control software developed by other patients:

Theoretical proposition 1 – Chronic patients use open-source disease control software developed by other patients for having a more active role on the management of their own chronic disease.

Theoretical proposition 2 – Chronic patients use open-source disease control software developed by other patients due their perceived defective by design vendor lock-in mechanisms within the established medical products.

3   Findings and Implications

After the detailed data-analysis process relying on the grounded theory method, we identified two key motivations for the use of disease control software: the patients desire for a more active role in managing their diseases, and the patients annoyance with defective by design vendor lock-in mechanisms within the traditional and marked dominant¬ disease-control products.

This study ads on previous research on the same phenomena [17], [18]. If [17] raised the awareness on this new empirical trend where patients turn themselves in the creators of medical software and [18] aggregated users-feedback on such products; we addressed the behavioral motivation on the use of such systems. The potential implications to the theoretical body of knowledge in information systems, medicine, chronic care, patient behaviors, consumer behaviors, virtual communities, health-care policy and wellbeing is to be addressed in future research after an systematic multi-disciplinary literature review on IT and chronic-care.

Our contributions increase the understanding on the symbolism, meaning, and consumption patterns of this niche consumer group by screening publicly available data on the Internet, with potential implications to the body of theoretical knowledge in healthcare information systems, chronic care management and practitioners within the industry of disease control.

4   Conclusion and Future Oriented Remarks

We took an ethnographic approach for understanding the behaviors and motiva-tions of patients using open-source disease control software developed by other pa-tients. Data was collected from three product websites and seven related virtual com-munities (i.e. Internet sites) that gather together chronic patients with a particular chronic condition such as diabetes. After intensive data-analysis, we propose two motives for explaining how and why patients use open-source disease control software developed by other patients: First, the patients desire for a more active role in managing their diseases, and second, the patient perceived defective by design vendor lock-in mechanisms within the market products.

For future, we aim at testing and validating our two proposed behavioral explana-tions by using complementarity research methods that could enable the triangulation of research results. Interviews or survey instruments could be employed directly with the patient/consumers. However, there are a set of ethical and methodological dilem-mas that must be careful mitigated before studying chronic patients with more evasive methods, i.e. the self-awareness of chronic patients that realize that they are being studied due their medical condition can affect the collected data either in the for of interviews or surveys.

This qualitative grounded theory study did not review a-priori a lot of the estab-lished knowledge in information systems, medicine, chronic care, patient behaviors, consumer behaviors, virtual communities, health-care policy, wellbeing, etc. In the spirit of grounded theory [13], [19], [20] this is not necessary a disadvantage at the time of the data-analysis; the established knowledge did not affected the categoriza-tion or coding of the retrieved textual research data. Extracted two theoretical propositions regarding the patients desire for a more active role in managing their chronic diseases and the patients perception of defective by design vendor lock-in mechanisms within established medical products, the authors will further review multi-disciplinary literature on the subject towards the discovery of theoretical implications that should be reported.

References

1. Guba, E.G., Lincoln, Y.S.: Competing paradigms in qualitative research. Handbook of Qualitative Research 2, 163–194 (1994)
2. Silverman, D.: Doing qualitative research. SAGE Publications Limited (2009)
3. Belk, R., Kozinets, R.V., Fischer, E.: Qualitative consumer and Marketing research. Sage (2012)
4. Kozinets, R.V.: The field behind the screen: using netnography for marketing research in online communities. Journal of Marketing Research, 61–72 (2002)
5. Kozinets, R.V.: Netnography: Doing ethnographic research online. Sage Publications Limited (2009)
6. Mead, G.H.: The philosophy of the act (1938)
7. Myers, M.: Investigating information systems with ethnographic research. Communications of the AIS 2(4), 1 (1999)
8. Myers, M.D., Avison, D.: Qualitative Research in Information Systems: A reader. SAGE Publications, Incorporated (2002)
9. Eriksson, P., Kovalainen, A.: Qualitative methods in business re-search. SAGE Publications Limited (2008)
10. Glaser, B.G.: Theoretical sensitivity: Advances in the method-ology of grounded theory, vol. 2. Sociology Press, Mill Valley (1978)
11. Glaser, B.G.: Emergence vs forcing: Basics of grounded theory analysis. Sociology Press (1992)
12. Glaser, B.G.: Doing grounded theory: Issues and discussions. Sociology Press (1998)
13. Urquhart, C., Fernández, W.: Using grounded theory meth-od in information systems: the researcher as blank slate and other myths. Journal of Information Technology (2013)
14. Hekkala, R., Urquhart, C.: Everyday power struggles: living in an IOIS project. European Journal of Information Systems 22(1), 76–94 (2013)
15. Myers, M.D., Newman, M.: The qualitative interview in IS research: Examining the craft. Information and Organization 17(1), 2–26 (2007)
16. Orlikowski, W.J.: Case tools as organizational change: investigating incremental and radical changes in systems development. MIS Quarterly 17(3) (1993)
17. Teixeira, J., Suomi, R.: Chronic Patients as Developers of Innovative Healthcare Information Systems. In: Proceedings of the 4th European Conference on Information Management and Evaluation: Universidade Nova de Lisboa, Lisbon, Portugal, September 9-10, p. 381 (2010)
18. Teixeira, J., Suomi, R.: Open Source Disease Control Soft-ware Development: The Role of Patients. In: Proceedings of the 5th European Conference on Information Management and Evaluation, UniversitàDell'Insubria, Como, Italy, September 8-9, p. 467 (2011)
19. Glasser, B., Strauss, A.: The discovery ofgrounded theory. Weidenfeld& Nicolson, London (1967)
20. Urquhart, C.: Grounded theory for qualitative research: A practical guide. Sage (2013)

Local Pilots, Virtual Tools - Experiments of Health Promotive and Inclusive Services in Different Settings in the Western Uusimaa Region

Hanna Tuohimaa, Elina Rajalahti, Anne Makkonen, Liisa Ranta,
Ulla Lemström, and Aila Peippo

Laurea University of Applied Sciences, Lohja, Finland
{hanna.tuohimaa,elina.rajalahti,anne2.makkonen,liisa.ranta,
ulla.lemstrom,aila.peippo}@laurea.fi

Abstract. In this paper we want to present five concepts for wellbeing related services and activities that have been piloted in the Western Uusimaa region as examples of ways of bringing health and wellbeing to different settings and different user groups. The pilots have been conducted for children in the kindergarten and secondary school, for adults in the health centre and for the unemployed in a variety of every day settings. We also want to present how local experiments can be put into wider use by virtual means and present the concept of the virtual wellbeing backpack family. The paper is based on work done in Laurea University of Applied Sciences (Laurea UAS) in a subproject of a cross regional project Pumppu funded by the European Regional Fund during 2011-2014.

1 Introduction

Sustainable living environments meet the needs of the present without compromising the ability of future generations to meet their own needs, as the Brundtland's Comission stated in their report [1]. The needs of the present and the needs of the future require different things of the living environment, with environmental sustainability more concerned with the needs of the future while social, political and economic sustainability more concerned with the needs of the present [2]. To fulfill the Brundtland's Comission's definition of sustainable development, all the perspectives are needed.

In this article, we are discussing the social sustainaibility prespective of sustainable living environments especially from the perspective of the ability of the living environment to foster health and enhance healthy living. Health is defined by the World Health Organization as "a state of complete physical, mental and social well-being and not merely the absence of disease or infirmity" [3] and health promotion as "the process of enabling people to increase control over their health and its determinants, and thereby improve their health" [4]. We share this understanding of health as a holistic concept taking into consideration both physical aspects as well as mental and social aspects. Following Antonovsky's salutogenic model [5] we see

K. Saranto et al. (Eds.): WIS 2014, CCIS 450, pp. 211–218, 2014.

health as a continuum where both improvement and deterioration are always possible. We acknowledge that health promotion is not merely disease prevention and that we need to see people as they are, complex living beings with certain risks as well as assets in their life making it either a bit easier or more difficult to feel well and be happy. Although we also acknowledge the role of governments in tackling poverty, unemployment and other social determinants of health, in this paper we want to focus on the role of services in supporting wellbeing and enabling movement towards health.

The paper is based on work done in Laurea University of Applied Sciences (Laurea UAS) in a subproject of a cross regional project Pumppu funded by the European Regional Fund during 2011-2014 (A31860). The project partners developed wellbeing services in a citizen centric manner with service providers from both the public, private and the third sector in four regions in southern Finland. All the subprojects had their different focuses (person centred planning, service structure development, technology usage and service vouchers). In our subproject our focus has been on developing services and activities for health promotion and for enhancing inclusion in society in the Western Uusimaa region. The uniting theme in all the subprojects was citizen centrism and seamlessness of care and shared workshops and benchmarking visits were organized on these themes.

In the subproject of Laurea UAS, our main interest has been in finding ways to motivate and empower the individual in his/her life for actively pursuing health related goals through developing better services and supportive activities and enhancing the health literacy skills. In our vision health promotive services are seamlessly connected and easy to access with personal health goals as the starting point and information and support available throughout the personally tailored service path. Health literacy is seen not as merely basic literacy skills but also as an interactive process of participating in changing circumstances and the critical ability to evaluate information and gain greater control of one's life [6].

The settings approach of health promotion focuses on transforming the places or social contexts in which people engage in their daily activities into supportive, health promotive environments [7]. In the project, we wanted to take health issues to the everyday settings of the residents in the area, to kindergartens and schools for example. We wanted to enhance the collaboration of different service providers and other actors in the region in matters related to wellbeing. At the same time we also wanted to define the role of the UAS as a health promoter in the region. Laurea UAS works according to the Learning by Developing pedagogic model [8] where students work in projects in close collaboration with local partners conducting real life research, development and innovation (R&D&I) tasks. The tasks offer students authentic working life experiences and bring about learning opportunities for all the parties involved. At the same time the region and its residents benefit of the end results, in this case of the new services.

In the project, we have taken a wide definition of wellbeing services. Our main goal has been to find ways to support wellbeing and promote health in the salutogenic sense [5], with a holistic approach to health and wellbeing. The human being is seen as an empowered, functioning individual, involved in diverse social relationships. We have not been interested in services in the sense of having a service provider delivering services for the paying customer in the market. Instead, we have been interested in developing all kinds of activities that may have a positive effect on the individual taking part in them.

As we live in an information society where information technology is widely in use both in the organizations offering services as well as by the residents using the services, we also wanted to consider using technology as a tool for health promotion. Although the service pilots presented here are based on face-to-face interaction, also the possibilities of technology have been examined.

2   Pilots for Health Promotion and Social Inclusion in Different Settings

In this paper we want to present wellbeing service concepts that have been piloted in the region during the project as examples of ways of bringing health and wellbeing to different settings and different user groups to promote healthier living environments and enhance the wellbeing of the residents in the region. An overview of the pilots is presented in Table 1. We also want to present how local experiments can be put into wider use by virtual means and present the concept of the virtual wellbeing backpack family.

The Early support for mental health concept was designed to offer easy access discussion support for the pupils (aged 13 to 16) in secondary school. The concept was piloted in one school for two 10 week phases with two nurse students having an open practice during the breaks where the pupils could come and talk about every day issues. The nurse students also visited classes during lessons. The hypothesis was that low threshold services would make it easier for the pupils to discuss about matters close to heart and make it easier to seek help. The pilot was evaluated in two phases, first with a questionnaire to eight graders (aged 14 to 15 n=118) in the middle of the first pilot phase [9] and then with focus group interviews to the staff and the nurse students after the second pilot phase [10]. As the feedback was gathered after five weeks of piloting, only one in five of the eight graders had visited the open practice, mostly talking about life in general. 53% of the students thought that it would be important to have the open practice in the school also in the future. Two thirds considered it good to have an adult to talk with. Only seven pupils had something negative to say, e.g. that not everybody wants to talk about his/her life. In the interviews for the staff the open practice was considered as an important unofficial place for discussion in addition to the official counseling services. In the short time perspective of the pilot phase it is not possible to evaluate the effects of the pilot on a longer time scale but the feedback acknowledges the benefits of having easy access services available.

In the *Learning sessions* pilot the goal was to increase the health literacy skills of teenagers through the use of participative methods in the secondary school setting.

Table 1. Short description of the pilots

Pilot	Target group	Setting	Focus	Feedback method	Results
The Early support for mental health	13 to 16 year old pupils	Secondary school	Low threshold services for mental wellbeing	Questionnaire: 118 pupils Interview: 3 staff members and 3 nursing students	53% saw the need to continue the pilot The pilot was seen as an important proactive, low threshold service in addition to the official counceling services
Learning sessions	15 year old pupils	Secondary school	Health literacy skills and understanding of national diseases	Questionnaire: 71 pupils	89% gained new knowledge 68% started thinking about their health 33% planned to change their lifestyle
Good for the Child	3 to 6 year old children	Kindergarten	Health literacy skills and understanding of healthy nutrition and sleep for the children as well as the parents	Questionnaire: 17 parents	100% saw health promotion as appropriate in the kindergarten setting 47% saw an effect of the nutrition theme at home
Pop up counseling point	The unemployed	Different everyday settings: shopping centres, events, health centres	Low threshold services and counseling on available services for those that are difficult to reach	Questionnaire: 23 visitors at the counseling point	91% got good counseling 59% agreed or mostly agreed that the web page responded well to their specific needs
Self care stations	The adult population in two municipalities	Health centres	Support for self care	Questionnaire: 21 users of the self care station	95% saw the station as important in their self care 71% got answers to specific questions on their mind

The nursing students planned and implemented training sessions in four secondary schools for 15-year-old pupils. The sessions included subjects related to Finnish national diseases (such as coronary heart disease, diabetes and cancer) and first-aid. The hypothesis was that pupils would benefit from interactional sessions and the learning methods would make health related subjects easy to understand. For example, one group drew the human figure on the floor of the gym hall. They marked four points on this figure; head, heart, limbs and guts. In each point nursing students discussed with the pupils, what it means to the specific part of the body if you are smoking, drinking alcohol, eating unhealthy food or not exercising. Pupils also had crossword-puzzles, where they could find the right answers at each point. After the sessions feedback was gathered of the pupils (n=71). The results showed that the pupils benefited from the training sessions, gaining a deeper understanding about the diseases (89 percent) and first-aid skills (92 percent). 33 percent of the pupils claimed that they would change their lifestyle for the better. Of the rest many pointed out in the open comments that they already lead a healthy life and did not see a need to make any changes. As the results of the pilot were promising about the participative methods in teaching health related subjects, the idea was further developed into the gamification of the subject matter. As a result, a small health promotive internet based game has been constructed in the project.

The *Good for the Child* –concept was designed for the kindergarten to bring health related subjects to the everyday activities of children of 3 to 6 years old and their families. The hypothesis was that through the children it would be possible to also reach the parents and influence the health behavior of the whole family. In the first pilot phase two students gathered materials and tested activities related to healthy nutrition and sleep. Besides activities for the children also activities for the parents and the whole family were designed. The activities included e.g. tasting foods, painting about dreams and sewing plush toys out of old pyjamas. For the parents, discussion evenings were organized. Feedback was gathered from the parents (n=17) by a questionnaire. In the feedback fifteen parents considered the pilot as a very good or a rather good experience and all saw health promotive activities as suitable for kindergartens. The most discussed activity at home was the sewing of the plush toys.

In the feedback, two thirds of the children had talked about health related issues at home with regard to nutrition but less than one third with regard to sleep. 47% of the parents thought that the activities related to nutrition had had some kind of an effect at home, only one in five saw effects of the activities related to sleep. For example, the children had learned to eat lettuce and the families had paid more attention to healthy food. Although the effects on sleep were more uncommon, some children had become more aware of the benefits of going to bed early at night. The results showed that even a small scale piloting phase can have an effect at home, however the results depend on the subject matter. For instance, although the sewing of the plush toy was discussed at home, it did not always result in discussing sleep related matters.

In The Good for the Child –pilot the students gathered all the material and instructions that they had used in the pilot phase in a briefcase to be used later on by other students in other kindergartens. The instructions were also left at the kindergartens for further use. In the following pilot phases, new materials were developed for other themes such as exercise. As we wanted to share the material with as many kindergartens as possible, we decided to make a virtual backpack of the materials. In fact, the idea escalated into a whole family of virtual backpacks for different purposes and case groups available online for all interested parties.

One of the concepts that had been developed earlier in the project was further developed prior to piloting to include a virtual backpack from the start. The idea was to take a counseling desk to places where unemployed people would be, to put up a *Pop up counseling point* for contacting the unemployed. The hypothesis was that it would be easier to reach the unemployed if contacting them in places that they visit rather than trying to get them to come to some service point. Through the virtual backpack, the counselor would have all the information that she/he needs on a tablet, instead of separate leaflets. At the same time the material would be available online for the unemployed themselves, too, as well as other service providers. The material included e.g. information about the rights of the unemployed, paths towards employment, wellbeing related information and tips for low budget activities in the region.

The Pop up counseling point was piloted in several settings in the region: at the shopping centre, hospital, health centre and at a career event for the youth. Feedback was gathered from the people who were contacted at the counseling point (n=23). 47% of the ones giving feedback were currently not in the labour force (they were e.g. unemployed or on unemployment pension), 30% had a job and 22% chose the alternative "other" (not specified further). In the feedback, 91% agreed or mostly agreed that they got good counseling at the counseling point. 59% agreed or mostly agreed with the statement that the web page used for counseling responded well to their specific needs and 57% with the statement that the web page offered new information for taking care of their health. This feedback shows that low threshold guidance services are appreciated although the subject matters still need some tuning.

Although in the project, we wanted to take health related issues to different every day settings, we did not want to undermine the role of the health center in promoting health, either. In fact, a local public health care provider was one of our key partners in the project. One of the pilots in the project was developing the *Self care stations* for two local health centres. At the Self care stations, the residents have the opportunity to e.g. measure their blood pressure levels and calculate their body mass index independently, yet having help available if necessary. There are also a variety of leaflets and other materials available, both related to health as well as related to the services and activities available in the region. The hypothesis was that the equipment and information available at the Self care stations would support self care and encourage personal activity in health related matters. The residents and the health centre staff have had the opportunity to participate in the development of the Self care stations to better respond to their needs.

User feedback of the Self care stations was gathered after the opening of the stations through a questionnaire and a return box at both of the Self care stations (21 respondents). Most of the users used the Self care station to measure their blood pressure levels. The users generally thought that the station had enough materials and leaflets. Some suggestions for further development were made e.g. in relation to also measuring the sugar levels or having better equipment for measuring the height.

The results showed that 95% of the Self care station users giving feedback saw the station as important in their self care. 71% got answers to specific questions on their mind. The Self care stations clearly benefitted the users.

Also materials related to self care have been put in a virtual wellbeing backpack. The materials have already been utilized in the next Self care station piloting in the spring of 2014 in another health centre. When having a computer at the Self care station, the materials of the virtual backpack can be viewed by the clients at the station. The backpack can also be utilized by service providers interested in developing their own Self care stations. The same way as the other backpacks this backpack could be further developed later on, after the project, by new student groups to include new materials and viewpoints. The backpack can include both general material as well as region specific instructions.

3   Conclusion

The pilots presented here offer examples of new ways of grasping health and wellbeing related issues in different settings and for different case groups. The feedback results show that even a small scale pilot can have a positive effect on the individual or the whole family. Potential for long term development work to analyze long term effects clearly exist. Through consecutive piloting rounds the materials and tools can be tuned to offer the best outcomes.

The pilot phases have been conducted by nursing students as part of their studies, in collaboration with the staff in the schools and kindergartens and other actors in the region. Through the virtual backpack family the materials can be made available for all interested parties and the concepts developed further for different locations. The experiments may also lead to new innovations, as with the health promotive game that was developed for the youth after the Learning sessions pilot.

Some of the pilots can be continued as such by the service providers in the region. For instance, the activity sessions for the kindergartens can be carried on by the staff as part of the daily activities. However, the pilots also showed the role that the nursing students can have as health promoters in the region. The nursing studies include training periods in kindergartens, schools and other facilities besides the health centres and hospitals. With the developed materials every training period can be seen as an opportunity for health promotion. With the project based Learning by Developing pedagogic model other study units can also be harnessed to developing and piloting new kinds of services, crossing sector lines and seeking new forms of collaboration with partners in the region.

References

1. United Nations: Report of the World Commission on Environment and Development. Our Common Future (1987)
2. Satterthwaite, D.: Sustainable Cities or Cities that Contribute to Sustainable Development? Urban Studies 34(10), 1667–1691 (1997)

3. WHO: Preamble to the Constitution of the World Health Organization as adopted by the International Health Conference, New York, 19-22 June, 1946; signed on 22 July 1946 by the representatives of 61 States (Official Records of the World Health Organization, no. 2, p. 100) and entered into force on 7 April 1948 (1948)
4. WHO: Ottawa Charter for Health Promotion. WHO, Geneva (1986)
5. Antonovsky, A.: The SalutogenicModel as a Theory to Guide Health Promotion. Health Promotion International 11(1), 11–18 (1996)
6. Nutbeam, D.: Health Literacy as a Public Health Goal: a Challenge for Contemporary Health Education and Communication Strategies into the 21st Century. Health Promotion International 15(3), 259–267
7. WHO: Health Promotion Glossary. WHO, Geneva (1998)
8. Raij, K.: Learning by Developing. Laurea Publications A-58. Laurea University of Applied Sciences (2007)
9. Tarilo, C.: Kyselylomake sairaanhoitajaopiskelijoiden vastaanottotoiminnasta 8-luokkalaisille. Kyselylomakkeiden sisällönanalyysi. Workingpaper (2013) (unpublished)
10. Mattila, P.: Sairaanhoitajan ennakoiva toiminta yläkoulussa. Thesis. Laurea University of Applied Sciences, Vantaa (2014)

The websites of the project:

- www.laurea.fi/pumppu (The Laurea UAS subproject webpage in Finnish)
- www.laurea.fi/en/cofi/projects/Pages/Pumppu.aspx (The Laurea UAS subproject webpage in English)
- www.laurea.fi/hyvinvointireppu (The Laurea UAS subproject Wellbeing backpack pages in Finnish)
- pumppu-hanke.blogspot.fi/ (the webpage of the whole Pumppu project in Finnish)

The Influence of Tourists' Safety Perception during Vacation Destination-Decision Process: An Integration of Elaboration Likelihood Model and Theory of Planned Behavior

Ping Wang

Turku school of economics, University of Turku
ping.wang@utu.fi

Abstract. Safety has long been an important consideration in tourism industry due to the nature of intangible and experiential of tourism. Despite the fact that tourists' destination decision-making has attracted lots of concentration, it is noteworthy that few of them touched the relationship between safety perception and destination decision in the perspective of influence process. In order to better understand the influence process of safety perception on travel destination decision-making is still scant, an integrated model based on the two well-tested model, elaboration likelihood model (ELM) and theory of planned behavior (TPB), is proposed in the paper. Cultural dimension of uncertainty avoidance, which related directly to safety issues, are extended to the model. Altogether seven hypotheses are given based on the conceptual framework. Conclusions on the contribution of this paper, and limitations and future research are also discussed.

Keywords: perceived safety, destination decision, ELM, TPB, uncertainty avoidance.

1   Introduction

Safety has long been an important consideration in tourism industry due to the nature of intangible and experiential of tourism. As more vulnerable to unexpected incidents when moving away from home, tourist's safety perception plays a vital role in destination decision process. A survey conducted among Chinese outbound tourists in 2013 revealed that 61.8% tourists regard safety to be one of the most important factors influencing their destination choice. Specifically, safety remains among the top three factors (ranked only the second to attraction) which travelers care the most when making destination choice in recent three years (with 70.4%   in 2012 and 68.1% in 2011of respondents)[1].

With the pervasion of information and communication technology (ICT) and advent of Web 2.0, tourism emerged to be a very promising industry. Tourist's decision-making power has been strengthened enor-mously thanks to the availability

---

[1] Data source: http://go.huanqiu.com/zhuantiyongwen/2013-03/3739055_6.html

K. Saranto et al. (Eds.): WIS 2014, CCIS 450, pp. 219–229, 2014.

of rich information about destination through various online information sources. It's more realizable for potential tourist individuals to make their vacation plan based on various online information sources, and online travel services [1]. As a result, the traditional power positions among travel destinations, travel intermediaries, and tourist have been shifted [2].

Safety concerns are vital for vacation travel decision and a promising travel experience [3]. Despite the fact that tourists' destination decision-making has attracted lots of concentration [4, 5], it is noteworthy that few of them touched the relationship between safety perception and destination decision [6]. What's more, our understanding on the following questions is still scant: what's the influence process of safety perception on tourist's attitude and behavior, especially in the age of information explosion? What types of information influence tourists' safety perception the most? Will the influence tend to be persistent or temporal? What's the different safety perception regarding to tourists from different cultural background?

This study is theoretically grounded on the combination of elaboration likelihood model (ELM) and theory of planned behavior (TPB). Those two theories are applied to build hypotheses concerning how tourists' decision making are affected by safety perception towards potential vacation destination through various information sources. Specifically, influence of safety perception towards vacation destination on is analyzed theoretically, and hypotheses are given to discover the influence of safety perception on tourist behaviors.

2   Literature Review

2.1   Safety Perception in Tourism

Tourism is a safety dependent industry [7].The safety perception of a destination is one of the most important factors influencing tourist's vacation destination choice, especially when travel internationally. The concerns of safety in the context of tourism are associated with different types of risks. As indicated in prior consumer researches, any choice involves risk elements when the outcomes are accompanied with uncertain decisions [8]. According to Haddock (1993), there are two types of risks identified: absolute risk that is real, and perceived risk which is subjective [9]. Absolute risk is assessed by commercial providers, and it can be minimized through implementing safety procedures; while perceived risk is assessed by individual consumers in specific context [9, 10]. This study focuses on perceived risk as associated with perceived safety, because (1) it is consumers' subjective impression concerned with safety when they are making purchase decision [11, 12]; (2) subjective risk (perceived) can be easily measured compared with the objective one, which is believed to be exist in theory [13].

A large and growing body of literature has investigated risk types related to tourism [14-16]. Floyd and Pennington (2004) identified eight types of risk posed to pleasure tourism and clustered respondents into two groups based on their risk perception [3]. The eight types of risks include financial (risk of losing money), health (risk of becoming sick), physical (risk of possibly and accident), crime (risk of being a crime victim), terrorism (risk of being involved with a terrorist act), social (risk of friends/family/associates disapproving of vacation), psychological (risk of having disappointing experience), and natural disasters (risk of natural disasters, hurricane, weather, forest fire). Reisinger and Mavondo [10] concluded five major risks associated with tourism based on a series of former research, they are terrorism, war and political instability, health, crime, cultural and language difficulties. They also point out that all the risks are of growing importance in global tourism. As associated with tourism, they identified 13 types of risks: crime, cultural, equipment, financial, health, performance, physical, political, psychological, satisfaction, social, terrorism and time. Tasci and Boylu [17] conduced six types of general risk in tourism: functional, financial, time, physical, psychological, and social risk. They also indicated that one or more risks, perceived or real, will be taken into consideration when making a decision under uncertainty.

2.2   Tourist's Decision-making

Leisure travel decision-making has attracted lots of concentration through various perspectives in prior researches. The main streams are classified into two perspectives in present paper: the travel process decision model perspective, and tourists' profile perspective.

Travel process orientation perspective demonstrates that decisions of purchasing tourism services occur in stages [18-21]. Concretely, information gathering stage, alternatives assessing and eliminating stage, alternative choosing stage, and finally travel undertaking stage [22]. In addition, constraints from both external and internal, for instance socio-demography, prior travel experience, etc. [23] , will make differences during these stages, and resulting in different decision-making. Theoretically, researches of this group tend to construct decision-making model based on several social science theory, asserting that tourism marketing and research should be based on consumer perceptions and preferences, and tourists' actual destination choice is predicted by their intention and attitude[24, 25].One of the first models out of this which has drew much attention is the general model of traveler leisure destination awareness and choice presented by Woodside and Lysonski in 1989 [24].

Researches from visitor profile perspective insist that vacation decision-making is an ongoing process that cannot be characterized by several sequential stages, and there'll be no end for the decision making [26, 27]. They made classification of different types of vacationers based on tourists' lifestyle, or variation in decision-making styles. Vacationers of different types will behavior differently according to their characteristics during their decision-making process, while different types of decision-making may also be influenced by opportunities, emotions, etc.

In the current study, a decision-making process model is constructed based on the travel process model, cultural background among different types of tourists are also taken into account due to its possible influence in international travel experience [15]. Specifically, five main stages identified during a whole out-bound travel experience according to the travel process, as shown in the Figure 1. Potential outbound travelers searching travel information through various channels: both online sources and offline sources, professional sources and unprofessional sources. Then, in decision progress, they decide where to go, how to go, including destination decision, travel style decision and booking style decision. After all these decisions, they will purchase all or parts of the whole outbound travel related product or services in advance. During their travel experience, they could perceive a real image about destination. At last, various after travel behavior occurs, like sharing travel experience online, recommend the destination to their familiars or not, revisit the attraction or not.

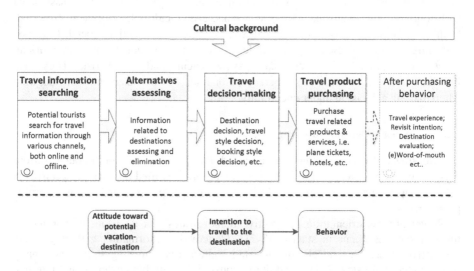

Fig. 1. An Overview of Travel Process

3   Theoretical Framework

This current research is based on well tested theories asserting that human behavior is determined by behavior intention. Determinant of the individuals' behavior intention are their attitude toward performing the behavior, while attitude can be influenced through both central route and peripheral cues [28-31].

3.1   Theory of Planned Behavior

Theory of planned behavior (TPB) is one of the most researched theory, which enjoys high reputation in the field of psychology, to invest the relationship between motivation and behavior extended from the theory of reasoned action (TRA) [28]. In this model, behavior is the final dependent determined by behavior intention. Factors of social and psychological are considered in consumers' decision-making process, they are variables of subjective norm, and attitude toward the behavior in the model (see Fig. 3). The most basic doctrines in this model hold that, intentions to perform different kinds of behaviors can be predicted from attitudes towards the behavior, subjective norms, and perceived behavioral control with a relatively high accuracy. In addition, attitudes, subjective norms, and perceived behavioral control are shown to be related to sets of relevant beliefs about the behavior [28].

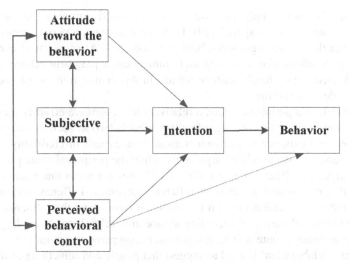

Fig. 2. Theory of planed behavior Ajzen [28]

Theory of planned behavior is proved to be a validate model in the context of destination-decision making. Several previous studies applied theory of planned behavior in the field of tourism to explore the relationship between tourists' attitude and behavior intention, in order to predict tourists' actual behavior [25, 32, 33].

The limitation of theory of planned behavior for understanding the influence of tourists' safety perception on their destination decision-making behavior is that, while it illustrate the relationships of attitude, behavior intention, and behavior, it does not consider how the way information sources perceived by tourists works in the most initial attitude formation stage. Potential tourists in nowadays information era are exposed to super large amount of information sources , even can be described with overlapping information, with the pervasion of information and communication technologies. Information searching is the first stage during a potential tourist's travel decision (see Fig. 1). A perception of safety about the unknown destination is formed after that. A dilemma will occur in choosing between safety and new, unique and novel experience that will be provided [17]. The problem is how the influence process for an attitude formation after the acquirement of information about safety problems at or near the chosen destination. To supplement TPB in this way, we draw on the Elaboration likelihood model.

3.2   Elaboration Likelihood Model

Elaboration likelihood model (ELM) is a dual-process persuasive theory widely used in social and consumer psychology [29, 34]. It views attitude change in two distinct routes: central route and peripheral cue.

Central route views attitude change as a result from "a person's diligent consideration of information she/he feels is central to the true merits of a particular attitudinal position", while peripheral route to attitude change refers to "a person may accept an advocacy simply because it was presented during a pleasant lunch or because the source is an expert." [29]. In the central route, a person scrutinizes more carefully on the related arguments, both pros and cons. After a critical consideration, together with information assessing and elimination, a judgment related to behavior will be formed. As a result, attitude formed in this central route would be persistent after an in-depth scrutinize.

In contrast, in a peripheral route, a relatively less cognitive effort is needed, where a person simply relies on cues regarding the target behavior, such as prior users, prior related personal experience, and endorsement from experts or credibility. The central route processes message-related arguments, while the peripheral route processes cues [35]. As argued by Bhattacherjee (2006), ELM does not mean that people influenced through different routes resulted in different outcomes. Different individuals may come to the same decision through two different routes, and the influence process of the same individual may vary according to time and technology. Accordingly, attitude formed in peripheral route will be less persistent compared to central route.

The term 'elaboration' is used to suggest that people add something of their own to the specific information provided in the communication [34, 35]. It is suggested that people with high elaboration likelihood state are more likely to engage in careful scrutinization, and tend to be more persuaded by argument quality then by peripheral cues. Contrarily, those in low elaboration likelihood will be in lower motivation to think carefully, and then tend to be motivated by peripheral cues. As shown in Fig. 3:

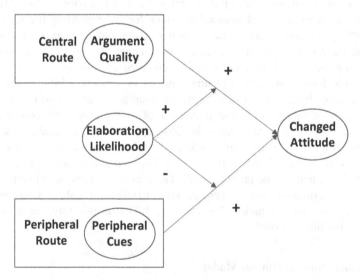

Fig. 3. Elaboration likelihood model Petty, Cacioppo [29]

Two variables emerging from this model is the central route of augment quality and peripheral route of cues. Motivation and ability discussed in the ELM are intention and behavioral control in TPB respectively [28]. Specifically, in TPB, Ajzen (1991) assumes that a person's likelihood of behavioral achievement can be dictated to some extent by the resources available to a person, which is the variable of perceived behavioral control. Therefore, the elaboration likelihood is explained with different level of perceived behavioral control. If people believe they have little control over performing the potential behavior because lack of requisite resources, they likelihood will be low, and vice versa [36].

Therefore, the combined model of TPB and ELM for the current research is shown as follows, Fig 4:

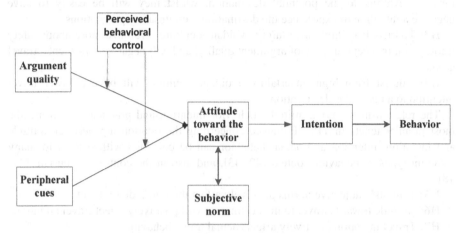

Fig. 4. The Combination of TPB and ELM

4   Conceptual Model and Hypotheses

As mentioned above, the integrated model is constructed based on TPB and ELM, which will be the basis of our conceptual model. Elaboration likelihood model demonstrates a dual-route, multi-process model in which persuasive message works. The cause for two different routes is individual's involvement level, i.e. people of high involvement tent to central route of argument quality, which has been empirically tested in prior research [37, 38]. Perceived behavioral control as related to potential destination expresses tourists' confidence to their ability to perform the behavior [36], which is individual's ability as discussed in the ELM. Thus, Hypothesis 1 and Hypothesis 2 are made as follows:

H1: Tourist with higher perceived behavioral control will concentrate more on the argument quality of available safety information about potential destination.

H2: tourist with lower perceived behavioral control will refer to peripheral cues of safety information about destination.

Cultural dimension of uncertainty avoidance relates to the level of stress in a society in face of an unknown future [39]. Despite that more information on destination available now through various information channels, the nature intangible and experiential of tourism greatly increase uncertainty, especially those without prior experience to the same destination. As a result, tourists from high uncertainty avoidance cultures will perceive higher safety incidents, and a negative attitude to visit the destination will form. Uncertainty avoidance has been successfully tested in the context of tourism [15, 40]. For instance, the effect of uncertainty avoidance on international tourists' behavior in information searching , planning and purchasing to categorize tourists [15], tourists' behavior towards disasters [40], international visitors' culinary choices [41]. Drawing from this empirical conclusion, we propose that people from high uncertainty avoidance culture will be more likely to be persuaded by safety related information in a central route and have a negative attitude toward travelling to the potential destination, whilst they will be easily to have negative a intention to experience the destination with unsafety perceptions.

H3: Tourists from high uncertainty avoidance culture scrutinize more about safety information in a central route of argument quality, and will negatively influence travel attitude.

H4: Tourist from high uncertainty avoidance culture will have a lower travel intention to a particular desti-nation.

The relationships among attitude, behavior intention and practical action are the most premier tenets in TPB. Evidence concerning the relationship between attitude and intention, intention and actual behavior can be collected with respect to many different types of behavior context [42, 43], and also in the context of tourism [44-48].

H5: Tourists' subjective norms positively affect their attitude to travel.

H6: Attitude towards travel to the destination will positively affect travel attention.

H7: Travel intention positively affects actual travel behavior.

The final conceptual framework for this paper and hypotheses are presented in the Figure 5 bellow.

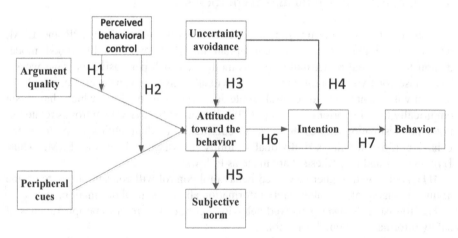

Fig. 5. Conceptual model and hypotheses

5   Conclusion

The premier object for the current research is to discover the influence routes of information sources on behavior in the context of tourism. In particular, the influence routines of safety perception related information on tourists' attitude towards travel to potential destinations.

This research provides a synthesized theoretical framework based on two well-known models, which completes each other in a naturally manner. Each model includes the areas of undeveloped for each other. This model is aimed to explore the influence process of one of the most vital element, safety perception, on vacation travelers' behavior. Safety perception comes from different types of risks are identified in prior researches [3], and are empirically proved to be strong predictors of international tourists' choice [49]. Whereas, how these safety perceptions influence tourists' behavior remains uncovered. Our research contributes a predictive model of behavioral in the context of safety perception in tourism.

This research makes sense in tourism industry for implications on better understanding the role of safety perception in tourist destination decision. As to tourism stakeholders, they can gain further insight in tourist segmentation, and how to inform tourist of different cultural dimensions, different perceived behavioral control about safety issues. More effective marketing strategy for marketers and better destination manage policy could be constructed on the basis of testing the hypotheses proposed in the paper.

6   Limitations and Future Research

The integration of the two well-tested theory of TPB and ELM enables researches in both IS field and tourism to have a full schematic of the relationship of online information sources to final decision making. While the paper proposed a theoretical conception model and hypotheses, but the empirical validation of the hypotheses need to be tested in future research.

References

1. Pan, B., Fesenmaier, D.R.: Online Information Search. Annals of Tourism Research 33(3), 809–832 (2006)
2. Berne, C., Garcia-Gonzalez, M., Mugica, J.: How ICT shifts the power balance of tourism distribution channels. Tourism Management 33(1), 205–214 (2012)
3. Floyd, M.F., Pennington-Gray, L.: Profiling risk perceptions of tourists. Annals of Tourism Research 31(4), 1051–1054 (2004)
4. Gardiner, S., King, C., Grace, D.: Travel Decision Making: An Empirical Examination of Generational Values, Attitudes, and Intentions. Journal of Travel Research 52(3), 310–324 (2013)
5. Mutinda, R., Mayaka, M.: Application of destination choice model: Factors influencing domestic tourists destination choice among residents of Nairobi, Kenya. Tourism Management 33(6), 1593–1597 (2012)
6. Wong, J.-Y., Yeh, C.: Tourist hesitation in destination decision making. Annals of Tourism Research 36(1), 6–23 (2009)
7. Tarlow, P.E., Santana, G.: Providing safety for tourists: A study of a selected sample of tourist destinations in the United States and Brazil. Journal of Travel Research 40(4), 424–431 (2002)

8. Hsu, T.H., Lin, L.Z.: Using fuzzy set theoretic techniques to analyze travel risk: An empirical study. Tourism Management 27(5), 968–981 (2006)
9. Haddock, C., Wisheart, P., Council, N.Z.M.S.: Managing risks in outdoor activities. New Zealand Mountain Safety Council (1993)
10. Reisinger, Y., Mavondo, F.: Cultural Differences in Travel Risk Perception. Journal of Travel & Tourism Marketing 20(1), 13–31 (2006)
11. Bauer, R.A.: Consumer behavior as risk taking. Dynamic Marketing for a Changing World, 398 (1960)
12. Stone, R.N., Winter, F.: Risk in buyer behavior contexts: a clarification. College of Commerce and Business Administration, University of Illinois at Urbana-Champaign (1985)
13. Mitchell, V.-W.: Consumer perceived risk: conceptualisations and models. European Journal of Marketing 33(1/2), 163–195 (1999)
14. Sonmez, S.F., Graefe, A.R.: Influence of terrorism risk on foreign tourism decisions. Annals of Tourism Research 25(1), 112–144 (1998)
15. Money, R.B., Crotts, J.C.: The effect of uncertainty avoidance on information search, planning, and purchases of international travel vacations. Tourism Management 24(2), 191–202 (2003)
16. George, R.: Visitor perceptions of crime-safety and attitudes towards risk: The case of Table Mountain National Park, Cape Town. Tourism Management 31(6), 806–815 (2010)
17. Tasci, A.D.A., Boylu, Y.: Cultural Comparison of Tourists' Safety Perception in Relation to Trip Satisfaction. International Journal of Tourism Research 12(2), 179–192 (2010)
18. Smallman, C., Moore, K.: Process Studies of Tourists' Decision-Making. Annals of Tourism Research 37(2), 397–422 (2010)
19. Smallman, C., et al.: Case Studies of International Tourists' In-Destination Decision-Making Processes in New Zealand. In: Hyde, K.F., Ryan, C., Woodside, A.G. (eds.) Field Guide to Case Study Research in Tourism, Hospitality and Leisure, pp. 297–315 (2012)
20. Walls, A.R., Okumus, F., Wang, Y.: Cognition and Affect Interplay: A Framework for the Tourist Vacation Decision-Making Process. Journal of Travel & Tourism Marketing 28(5), 567–582 (2011)
21. Sirakaya, E., Woodside, A.G.: Building and testing theories of decision making by travellers. Tourism Management 26(6), 815–832 (2005)
22. Mansfeld, Y.: From Motivation to Actual Travel. Annals of Tourism Research 19(3), 399–419 (1992)
23. Sharifpour, M., et al.: Investigating the Role of Prior Knowledge in Tourist Decision Making: A Structural Equation Model of Risk Perceptions and Information Search. Journal of Travel Research 53(3), 307–322 (2014)
24. Woodside, A.G., Lysonski, S.: A general model of traveler destination choice. Journal of Travel Research 27(4), 8–14 (1989)
25. Hsu, C.H.C., Huang, S.: An Extension of the Theory of Planned Behavior Model for Tourists. Journal of Hospitality & Tourism Research 36(3), 390–417 (2012)
26. Serrato, M.A., et al.: Visitor profile, satisfaction levels and clustering of tourists for decision making in Michoacan, Mexico. International Transactions in Operational Research 17(1), 119–143 (2010)
27. Decrop, A., Snelders, D.: A grounded typology of vacation decision-making. Tourism Management 26(2), 121–132 (2005)
28. Ajzen, I.: The theory of planned behavior. Organizational Behavior and Human Decision Processes 50(2), 179–211 (1991)
29. Petty, R.E., Cacioppo, J.T., Schumann, D.: Central and peripheral routes to advertising effectiveness: The moderating role of involvement. Journal of Consumer Research 10(2), 135 (1983)

30. Sparks, B., Pan, G.W.: Chinese Outbound tourists: Understanding their attitudes, constraints and use of information sources. Tourism Management 30(4), 483–494 (2009)
31. SanfordSource, A.B.A.C.: Influence Processes for Information Technology Acceptance: An Elaboration Likelihood Model. MIS Quarterly 30(4), 805–825 (2006)
32. Chien, G.C.L., Yen, I.Y., Hoang, P.-Q.: Combination of Theory of Planned Behavior and Motivation: An Exploratory Study of Potential Beach-based Resorts in Vietnam. Asia Pacific Journal of Tourism Research 17(5), 489–508 (2012)
33. Jalilvand, M.R., Samiei, N.: The impact of electronic word of mouth on a tourism destination choice Testing the theory of planned behavior (TPB). Internet Research 22(5), 591–612 (2012)
34. Petty, R.E., Wegener, D.T.: The elaboration likelihood model: Current status and controversies (1999)
35. Bhattacherjee, A., Sanford, C.: Influence processes for information technology acceptance: An elaboration likelihood model. Mis Quarterly 30(4), 805–825 (2006)
36. Madden, T.J., Ellen, P.S., Ajzen, I.: A Comparison of the Theory of Planned Behavior and the Theory of Reasoned Action. Personality and Social Psychology Bulletin 18(1), 3–9 (1992)
37. Ho, S.Y., Bodoff, D.: The effects of web presonalization on user attitude and behavior: an integration of the elaboration likelihood model and consumer search theory. MIS Quarterly 38(2), 497–520 (2014)
38. Tang, L., Jang, S., Morrison, A.: Dual-route communication of destination websites. Tourism Management 33(1), 38–49 (2012)
39. Hofstede, G.: Hofstede Culture Dimensions - an Independent Validation Using Rokeach Value Survey. Journal of Cross-Cultural Psychology 15(4), 417–433 (1984)
40. Min, J.C.H.: Tourism behavior toward disasters: A cross-cultural comparison. Social Behavior and Personality 35(8), 1031–1032 (2007)
41. Tse, P., Crotts, J.C.: Antecedents of novelty seeking: international visitors' propensity to experiment across Hong Kong's culinary traditions. Tourism Management 26(6), 965–968 (2005)
42. You, D.R., Chen, Y.W., Wang, E.P.: The perceived risk in online shopping and consumer-related factors. International Journal of Psychology 39(5-6), 316 (2004)
43. Chennamaneni, A., Teng, J.T.C., Raja, M.K.: A unified model of knowledge sharing behaviours: theoretical development and empirical test. Behaviour & Information Technology 31(11), 1097–1115 (2012)
44. Wang, J., Ritchie, B.W.: Attitudes and perceptions of crisis planning among accommodation managers: Results from an Australian study. Safety Science 52, 81–91 (2013)
45. Wang, J., Ritchie, B.W.: Understanding accommodation managers' crisis planning intention: An application of the theory of planned behaviour. Tourism Management 33(5), 1057–1067 (2012)
46. Song, H., et al.: Behavioral intention of visitors to an Oriental medicine festival: An extended model of goal directed behavior. Tourism Management 42, 101–113 (2014)
47. Quintal, V.A., Lee, J.A., Soutar, G.N.: Risk, uncertainty and the theory of planned behavior: A tourism example. Tourism Management 31(6), 797–805 (2010)
48. Lam, T., Hsu, C.H.C.: Predicting behavioral intention of choosing a travel destination. Tourism Management 27(4), 589–599 (2006)
49. Sönmez, S.F., Graefe, A.R.: Influence of terrorism risk on foreign tourism decisions. Annals of Tourism Research 25(1), 112–144 (1998)

Patient Safety and Patient Privacy When Patient Reading Their Medical Records

Rose-Mharie Åhlfeldt[1] and Isto Huvala[2]

[1] School of Informatics, University of Skövde
Box 208, SE 541 08 Skövde
rose-mharie.ahlfeldt@his.se
[2] Department of ALM, Uppsala University
Box 625, SE 571 26 Uppsala
isto.huvila@alm.uu.se

Abstract. When patients get access to their personal health information new security demands arise. This paper presents results from a study aiming to improve the understanding of how the patients' different perceptions of their own personal health and health information preferences can be linked to anticipated positive and negative security concerns. The analysis and discussion focuses on investigating how the security issues and patients' perception on the benefits and threats of accessing their medical records relate to each other. The results show that a more holistic systemic perspective to information security is needed to support the effective use of medical records in the healthcare in information and data driven society in order to improve both patient safety and patient privacy.

Keywords: information society, information security, patient safety, patient privacy, well-being.

1 Introduction

In healthcare, patient information is a critical factor. The right information at the right time is necessary for providing the best and safest possible care for patients. Patient information must also be protected from unauthorized access in order to protect patient privacy. The healthcare sector faces a great challenge concerning how patient information security can be managed in healthcare in order to achieve both patient safety and patient privacy for the citizens [1,2,3,4]. In the contemporary information society, patients are also interested in taking part of their patient information and are involved in their care. Residents, patients and relatives can participate actively in the care on their own terms and achieve public and personal health information, treatment and care [5]. Better access to own patient information and becoming more involved in care, raises also questions of the impact of these developments on patient safety and patient privacy [4].

Even if information security research has clearly demonstrated that security, safety and privacy are complex intertwined phenomena, the earlier literature has had a tendency to discuss privacy as a separate issue and not as a part of the concept of infor-

K. Saranto et al. (Eds.): WIS 2014, CCIS 450, pp. 230–239, 2014.

mation security [6]. "Information security and privacy" is an often-mentioned term in the research literature. One particular reason for this is that information security is often conceptualised solely from the perspective of organizational goals while the notion of privacy tends to place more emphasis on individuals and, from an organizational point of view, on "customers" instead of the organization [7]. Information security controls are primarily based on the aims and objectives of the organization. However, even if the notion of security is closer to the organisational agenda, in most of the legal contexts, privacy is a statutory obligation organizations need to address as well. There is a risk that privacy is regarded more as a complementary than an inclusive part of the security arrangements and policies. Furthermore, a specific aspect of this problem in healthcare is that it is not unusual that patient privacy issues may be weighed against patient safety. In these cases it can be difficult to find a balance between the two [2], [4]. To bridge the gap between organizational objectives and privacy concerns and to obtain a high level of information security, it is necessary to incorporate the overlying goal of healthcare – good quality of care – and privacy aspects as integral parts of a holistic information security work in the organization [4].

Another gap in the earlier research is that safety and privacy related studies on information security are mainly dealing with the technical aspects of the issues[6]. Other aspects of information security work related to, for instance, management and the administration, have been largely omitted in the earlier work. In the context of healthcare, when patients get access to their patient information digitally, for example, by accessing their own medical records, health records or other types of public e-health services, the need for a holistic perspective of the information security work (including safety and privacy as well as technical and administrative aspects) increases [4].

The aim of this study is to improve the understanding of how the patients' different perceptions of their own personal health and health information preferences can be linked to anticipated positive and negative security concerns. The study is based on a survey of patients (N=254) who had ordered a paper copy of their medical record from a Swedish county council according to the legislation that allows all citizens to access information on themselves held by public bodies. The analysis and discussion focuses on investigating how the security issues and patients' perception on the benefits and threats of accessing their medical records relate to each other. The analytical framework is derived from the model of information security characteristics [1]: confidentiality, integrity, availability (CIA) and accountability. The findings are discussed in relation to the concepts patient safety and patient privacy.

2   Background

2.1   Information Security in Healthcare: Safety and Privacy

According to the European Health Strategy [1], the aim of healthcare is to provide citizens with good health while respecting the dignity and equal worth of every individual. Hence, the care providers should provide patients with opportunities for the best

---

[1], European Commission (2007). *Together for Health: A strategic Approach for the EU 2008 - 2013.* Brussels: Retrieved from http://ec.europa.eu/health-eu/doc/whitepaper_en.pdf.

care and ensure that care decisions are based on the right information at the right time. They should make every effort to obtain as high level of *patient safety* as possible. Lack of information should not lead to incorrect treatments or unnecessary interventions, such as unneeded visits to the doctor only because patient information from a one healthcare provider is unavailable with another organisation. On the other hand, sensitive patient information must be protected from being distributed to unauthorized persons, that is, one should strive to maintain *patient privacy*. [5].

In order to empower the patient, it is necessary to give patient access to their personal health information. Patients are no longer passive receivers of healthcare services. Instead they will become active players in the management of their own health [8].

2.2   Patient Safety

The Swedish Patient Safety Act[2] defines patient safety as a safeguard against medical injury. Medical injury is defined as affliction, malaise, physical or mental injury, illness or death caused by healthcare and not an inevitable consequence of the patient's condition. The definition is similar to that of WHO Europe [9]: prevention of errors and adverse effects to patients associated with healthcare. It is obvious that patient safety is closely related to patient information. In order to be able to suggest solutions for improving patient safety and increasing the quality of care, it is necessary to secure the management of patient information. In the Swedish context, under the principle that all citizens should be provided access to the information on themselves held by public bodies, a part of this process is to provide patients with a means to get an oversight of their personal medical information. Besides the democracy-related benefits of this oversight, when patients get access to their own information, they get an opportunity to become more knowledgeable of their health and more involved in their own care. The increased informedness has a capability to lead to improved health outcomes and, in long term, also improve patient safety [8].

2.3   Patient Privacy

In contrast to patient safety, there is no similar consensus of the definition of patient privacy. The notion of privacy is highly complex and tends to involve different perspectives and dimensions. As a consequence, there is no single universal definition of *privacy* [10]. In general, privacy has been defined as the right to be free from secret surveillance and to determine whether, when, how, and to whom, one's personal or organizational information is to be revealed [11]. The Swedish Patient Data Act[3] states, "the healthcare record must be designed with respect to the patient's integrity".

---

[2] SFS 2010:659 *The Patient Safety Act*. Available from
http://www.notisum.se/rnp/sls/fakta/a0100659.htm
[3] SFS 2010:659 *The Patient Data Act*. Available from
http://www.riksdagen.se/sv/Dokument-Lagar/Lagar/
Svenskforfattningssamling/Patientdatalag-2008355_sfs-2008-355/
?bet=2008:355

According to the regulation SOSFS 2008:14[4], this is self-evident. Patient information is sensitive and must be protected from unauthorized access for the respect of patients and to achieve trustworthiness in healthcare. When patients get access to their personal health information, new privacy issues may arise. Patient information is not only transferred and communicated inside the healthcare systems. New risks, including both technical and administrational security threats, arise when patient information is transferred outside health organisations [12].

2.4   The Information Security Model

The conclusion of the discussion so far is that patient safety and patient privacy are closely related to patient information and consequently, also to information security. Using the information security model of Åhlfeldt [2], [13], the different information security related requirements of patient information can be mapped to four major aspects (characteristics) of information security (Fig. 1). In order to achieve patient safety, the right patient information (integrity) at the right time (availability) is needed. Similarly, in order to achieve patient privacy, only the right person (confidentiality and accountability) should have access to patient information. The premises of the model and the relation of patient safety and patient privacy, and information security are discussed in more detail in [2] (c.f. Fig 1).

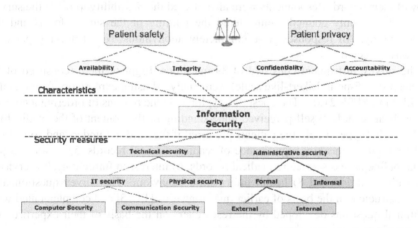

Fig. 1. Information Security Model related to patient safety and patient privacy [2]

However, even if the premise of information security is to achieve high levels of availability, integrity, confidentiality and accountability, it should be noted that these connections are not absolute. There are cases when confidentiality and accountability need to be emphasised in order to achieve patient safety, and vice versa. What is nec-

---

[4] SOSFS 2008:14 Socialstyrelsens föreskrifter om informationshantering och journalföring i hälso- och sjukvården. Available from http://www.socialstyrelsen.se/sosfs/2008-14. (In Swedish).

essary is to find a balance between patient safety and patient privacy. A sufficient level of information security is a sum of all of its main characteristics.

In addition to explicating the relation of information security and patient safety and privacy, the information security model emphasizes the importance of both technical and administrative security measures in achieving a comprehensive level of information security. The lower part of the model presents information security measures organized in a hierarchical order [2]. Since the notion of "information security" is an amalgam of several types of security measures, the model is useful as a basis for achieving a conceptual understanding of its constituent elements.

3   Material and Methods

In order to investigate the safety and privacy aspects of accessing medical records and using e-health services, patient attitudes were investigated using a combined postal and web survey sent to 1000 patients living in a Swedish county that had ordered a paper copy of their medical record in June-August 2012. The aim of the survey was to investigate patient attitudes to reading their medical records to form a baseline before the implementation of a new online access system as a complement of an earlier paper-based model. Response rate was 35,4% (N=354). An invitation to participate in the study and a survey form was mailed to the respondents in the same envelope as a copy of their record. Respondents were also offered the possibility to fill in the survey online. The county council administered the mailing of the survey forms and the online survey. All responses were completely anonymous. No identifying personal data was collected.

The survey instrument consisted of 39 questions. Eight of them (consisted of 53 statements on 5-point Likert-like scale) were analysed using exploratory factor analysis (EFA) in SPSS 21.0.   The questions explored 1) the reasons of ordering a copy of the medical record, 2) self-perceived understanding of the content of the medical record, 3) what type of help the patients preferred if they did not understand something in the record, 4) meaning/significance of reading medical records, 5) views of a potential online access service to medical records, 6) interest in future e-health services, 7) health condition and 8) health information behaviour. The survey questionnaire was constructed on the basis of earlier questionnaires [14,15] and complemented with additional questions developed by the researchers on the basis of their expertise and the specific research questions of this study.

4   Results

Seven factors emerged in the exploratory factor analysis   (Table 1). The factors were interpreted as attitudes related to health services and medical records. The ranking order of the factors provides additional information about their relative strength (one being the strongest). A detailed description of the whole analysis and results are published in [16]. The means for the directly security related questions "I am generally worried of the security of the service"(mean   3.06, sd   1.451) and "I am worried that the medical records are not managed securely enough in the healthcare information systems if they can be read online" (mean 3.18, sd 1.422) were not especially high.

Table 1. Results of the factor analysis (EFA)

Factor	Description
P1	Hypothetically positive to e-health services generally
P2	Positive to reading medical records due to implications
P3	Positive to all Internet use including medical records online
P4	Distrustful and wants to be in control of health treatment
P5	Worried about health
P6	Wants communication with healthcare professionals
P7	Does not understand their medical record

The first factor is noted, P1, "Hypothetically positive to e-health services generally", since the variables associated with P1 all relate to supportive e-health services. The second principal factor, P2, is associated with variables, which are associated to being "Positive to reading medical records due to implications". This is due to the variables indicating a desire to access medical record as a means to improve communication with healthcare, receive better care, better understand their health situation and to be better at taking care of oneself.

The principal factor P3 is interpreted as representing "Positive to all Internet use including medical records online". The variables associated with P3 indicate proneness to use social media to get help if there are problems in understanding something in the medical record, a positive attitude to reading their medical record online and then not worry about security issues, and a positive attitude to communicating with medical staff via email, searching for health information on internet including using social forums.

The label for factor P4 is "Distrustful and wants to be in control of health treatment". The variables associated with P4 indicate likelihood of having ordered the medical record to get an overview of their health condition, check details in their medical record and the received treatment, and to follow up what was said during a healthcare visit. It is also related to distrust of the healthcare providers and willingness to be able to check who has accessed the medical records.

The variables associated with the factor P5 indicate persons who are not in good health and have worries about their condition. P5 is thus labelled "Worried about health". The factor P6 is associated with variables representing a preference to ask healthcare professionals either online, via phone, or at their next visit if they do not understand something in their medical record. The label chosen for P6 is "Wants communication with healthcare professionals". The last factor, P7, "Does not understand their medical record" is associated with variables that indicate difficulties in understanding both the medical record in general and the part they are specifically interested in.

Besides the apparent repercussions in healthcare, information management and systems design contexts, we argue that all the seven identified attitudes have specific implications from the security and privacy perspective. In Table 2, the factors have been mapped into the four information security characteristics (Fig. 1) using a plus (+1) to mark a significant factor from the point of view represented by the factor or minus (-) if the aspect is explicitly trivialised by the standpoint represented by the factor.

Table 2. Factors P1-7 mapped to the four information security characteristics (+ significant aspect for factor; - (empathetically) unsignificant aspect)

	Availability	Integrity	Confidentiality	Accountability
P1	+			
P2	+	+		
P3	+	-	-	-
P4	+	+	+	+
P5	+			
P6				
P7				

Availability is the characteristic that can be related to the largest number of factors. An analysis of the vantage points represented by the factors indicate that access to information has a significant (+) relation to very different types of health related needs and wants. The attitude represented by P1 and P3 are in support of the general availability of eHealth services and online information exchange. P2 can expected to be benefitting of availability of information due its capability to facilitate communication with and participation in healthcare with an aim of receiving more adequate care. Availability of information can help patients to better understand their health and ultimately take better care of their health. Patients' desire for improved communication with healthcare is also consistent with their desire to use various eHealth services for this purpose. In P4, it is possible to see frustration among patients that they did not feel that have received enough information and therefore does not have control over their healthcare. A similar experience of the lack of availability is also indicated by the standpoint represented by the factor P5, patients that are worried about their health. As a whole, it seems that the availability of information may be considered as a crucial element for the experience of a good quality of care that is relevant even if the patients' would have very different attitudes to eHealth services the their current care providers.

Integrity indicates the significance of right and correct information. In case of the attitude P2, it is important to be able to assess that a particular piece of information is correct and the patient has an opportunity to access information using various communication channels and to follow up what was said during a healthcare visit. Moreover, there is frustration among the patients on not getting an overview of their health condition not being able to check details in their medical record and accessing information about their treatment. Hence, the integrity aspect is of crucial importance regarding the patient's confidence in healthcare especially with the factor P4. On the other hand, for P3 that represents a largely carefree attitude of the eventual risks, the patients' uncritically positive attitude to be able to get access to various eHealth services may lead to unwarranted trust on unreliable information. Information can be retrieved from a variety of sources with different levels of quality without any guarantees that the accuracy of information could be ensured. This type of an attitude is a challenge for eHealth service providers and puts pressure on, for instance, the coordination and standardization of patient information.

Confidentiality aspects is not the primary concern of the patients. The generally very positive attitude (represented by P3) to all types of Internet-mediated use of healthcare services may be seen as an indication of a belief that healthcare provides secure eHealth services. Otherwise these services would not exist. However, when more information is disseminated about the patients via the Internet, the likelihood of unauthorized access to patient information increases. In contrast, patients' frustration of not being in control of their treatment (P4) can lead to a naive attitude of overemphasising confidentiality and simultaneously disparaging the benefits of letting relevant professionals access, for instance, the contents of the medical record. In general, however, looking at the results of the factor analysis, the availability and integrity of information seem to be more important for the patients than the risk of having their information revealed by others.

Accountability seems to be similarly to the confidentiality, a relatively minor concern for the patients. Accountability of information tends also to be more a technical question. This aspect becomes crucial for the patient first when an incident has taken place and the question of accountability gets practical relevance. For a person with a generally positive attitude towards online services (P3), accountability is plausibly similarly to confidentiality, a non-question that is taken for granted. On the other hand, when the patient wants to have a better control over their healthcare (P4), traceability and accountability is an apparent issue with an immediate relevance.

5   Discussion and Conclusions

When the results of the factor analysis are mapped to the dimensions of information security, it becomes apparent that there is a clear bias in the patients' privacy and safety concerns and priorities. In general, the patients' attitudes may be characterised as relatively naive. There are three factors that are largely unrelated to privacy and safety, and even in the factors that incorporate information security related reasoning, in contrast to access, safety is not a central aspect in how people conceptualise medical records and how they are accessed. It seems plausible to suggest that security is more or less taken as granted even if it is apparent that the picture may be more complex that it seems. The present analysis of the collected quantitative data does not provide us means to elaborate the relation of the attitudinal constellations revealed by the factor analysis and, for instance, how the different individuals in practice act in their daily life and cope with their eventual concerns on information security.

Similarly, the present factor analysis based approach does not give us possibilities to measure actual levels of concerns and awareness in the population. It merely provides a glimpse into the different types of priorities patients have concerning their health information.

A closer analysis of the intersection of the security characteristics and the factors presented in the paper does provide, however, some clues how the security thinking might be broadened in the future in the different clusters of attitudes represented by the factors P1-P7. Partly, it would be important to counter the occurrence of highly naive attitudes, but also to take into account the diversity of concerns, wants and needs of different aspects of information security. Even if a trustful and distrustful patient benefits of the general improvement of information security, it may be necessary to be more explicit about the precise mechanisms of confidentiality and accountability for distrustful persons and provide them guidance how to manage their personal settings than for a trusting person who would probably be satisfied with more general settings. Similarly, an online-oriented person (P3) could be assumed to expect a more general availability of information, whereas an implications oriented individual might be assumed to be content with a more limited availability. Restricting the availability of information according to the practical needs and demands of individual patients helps to prevent unnecessary transferring of confidential information on the net (cf. [12]).

Our conclusion is that a more holistic systemic perspective to information security [17,18] is needed to support the effective use of medical records in the healthcare in information and data driven society. Availability and integrity, and confidentiality and accountability are all necessary elements of an eHealth service as demonstrated before [2], [13] and their significance is related both to the general quality of the services, but also to the specific needs and wants of particular groups of their users. Safety and privacy are neither mechanistic aspects of technical systems, but issues that pertain to the entire healthcare process [6], [4]. A more systematic approach does not only improve the safety and privacy of patients, but would also enhance the general understanding and possibilities to unleash the real potential of patient access to medical records in improving the care and well-being of patients.

References

1. Kaelber, D.C., Bates, D.W.: Health information exchange and patient safety. Journal of Biomedical Informatics 40(6), S40–S45 (2007)
2. Åhlfeldt, R.-M., Söderström, E.: Patient Safety and Patient Privacy in Information Security from the Patient's View: A case study. Journal of Information System Security (JIS-Sec) 6(4), 71–85 (2010) ISSN:1551-0123
3. Haas, S., Wohlgemuth, S., Echizen, I., Sonehara, N., Muller, G.: Aspects of privacy for electronic health records. Int. J. Med. Inform. 80, e26–e31 (2011)
4. Baker, D.B.: Privacy and security in public health: Maintaining the delicate balance between personal privacy and population safety. In: 22nd Annual Computer Security Applications Conference, ACSAC 2006, pp. 3–22. IEEE (2006)

5. Ministry of Health and Social Affairs, National eHealth – the strategy for accessible and secure information in health and social care: Ministry of Health and Social Affairs (2011)
6. Appari, A., Johnson, M.E.: Information security and privacy in healthcare: current state of research. International Journal of Internet and Enterprise Management 6, 279–314 (2010)
7. Acquisti, A.: Privacy and security of personal information Economics of Information Security, pp. 179–186. Springer (2004)
8. Ünver, Ö., Atzori, W.: Questionnaire for Patient Empowerment Measurement Version 1.0, pp. 1–74 (2013)
9. WHO Europe. Patient Safety (2014), http://www.euro.who.int/en/health-topics/Health-systems/patient-safety (accessed Mars 2014)
10. Leino-Kilpi, H., Välimäki, M., Dassen, T., Gasull, M., Lemonidou, C., Scott, A., Arndt, M.: Privacy: a review of the literature. International Journal of Nursing Studies 38(6), 663–671 (2001)
11. Business Dictionary, Definition Privacy (2014), http://www.businessdectionary.com/definition/privacy.html (accessed Mars 2014)
12. Baker, D.B., Masys, D.R.: PCASSO: a design for secure communication of personal health information via the internet. Int. J. Med. Inform. 54(2), 97–104 (1999)
13. Åhlfeldt, R.-M., Spagnoletti, P., Sindre, G.: Improving the Information Security Model by using TFI. In: Venter, H., Eloff, M., Labuschagne, L., Eloff, J., von Solms, R. (eds.) SEC 2007. IFIP, vol. 232, pp. 73–84. Springer, Boston (2007)
14. Ekendahl, M.: En modell för att hantera journaluppgifter på internet för patienter. Tech. rep., INERA, Stockholm (2011)
15. Fowles, J.B., Kind, A.C., Craft, C., Kind, E.A., Mandel, J.L., Adlis, S.: Patients' interest in reading their medical record: relation with clinical and sociodemographic characteristics and patients' approach to health care. Arch. Intern. Med. 164(7), 793–800 (2004)
16. Huvila, I., Cajander, Å., Daniels, M., Åhlfeldt, R.-M.: Reading Medical Records Serve Different Needs for Patients: Patients' Perceptions of their Medical Records from Different Subject Positions. Journal of the Association for Information Science and Technology (in print, 2014)
17. Leveson, N.: Engineering a safer world: systems thinking applied to safety. MIT Press (2011, 2012)
18. Young, W., Leveson, N.G.: An Integrated Approach to Safety and Security Based on Systems Theory. Commun. ACM 57(2), 31–35 (2014)

Author Index

Åhlfeldt, Rose-Mharie   230
Ahlmén-Laiho, Ulla   1
Aromaa, Minna   168
Asteljoki, Sari   68

Dahlberg, Tomi   16

Ek, Stefan   46
Eriksson-Backa, Kristina   46

Haapasalo-Pesu, Kirsi-Maria   30
Haatainen, Kaisa   78
Hansen, Bruno   36
Heimonen, Juho   57
Henriksen, Finn Lund   36
Holmberg, Kim   46
Huvila, Isto   230
Hyrkkänen, Ursula   88
Hyrynsalmi, Sami   168

Ilola, Tiina   30

Jalonen, Harri   100
Järvi, Ulla   1

Kainu, Ville M.A.   94
Kalliokoski, Kari   57
Kauhanen, Lotta   57
Kimppa, Kai K.   94
Kinos, Sirppa   68
Kivekäs, Eija   78
Kokki, Hannu   78
Kontio, Elina   88
Koskinen, Jani S.S.   94
Kurola, Jouni   144

Laaksonen, Camilla   100
Lahtinen, Riitta   109
Lahtiranta, Janne   168
Larsen, Mogens Lytken   36
Lemström, Ulla   211
Leppänen, Ville   168
Leskinen, Tuija   57
Lillsunde, Pirjo   194

Luimula, Mika   159
Lundgrén-Laine, Heljä   131

Makkonen, Anne   211
Mubarak, Farooq   120
Murtola, Laura-Maria   57, 131

Norri-Sederholm, Teija   144

Ojala, Stina   109

Paakkonen, Heikki   144
Paavola, Jarkko   100
Palmer, Russ   109
Parisod, Heidi   168
Peippo, Aila   211
Pitkäkangas, Paula   159
Pyae, Aung   159

Raitoharju, Reetta   159
Raivo, Elina   57
Rajalahti, Elina   211
Ranta, Liisa   211
Rauti, Sampsa   168

Saarenpää, Teppo   88
Sachdeva, Neeraj   177
Salakoski, Tapio   57
Salanterä, Sanna   57, 131, 168
Saranto, Kaija   78, 144
Schakow, Henrik   36
Schorling, Per   36
Seppälä, Juhani   144
Sjöblom, Olli   186
Smed, Jouni   159, 168
Somerkoski, Brita   194
Suominen, Sakari   1
Suvivuo, Pia   68

Teixeira, Jose   203
Tuohimaa, Hanna   211
Tuominen, Risto   1

Wang, Ping   219